FOUNDATIONS OF EDUCATION

An EMS Approach

FOUNDATIONS OF EDUCATION

An EMS Approach

National Association of EMS Educators

Editor

Debra Cason, RN, MS, EMT-P
Associate Professor and Program Director
University of Texas Southwestern Medical Center
Emergency Medicine Education
Dallas, Texas

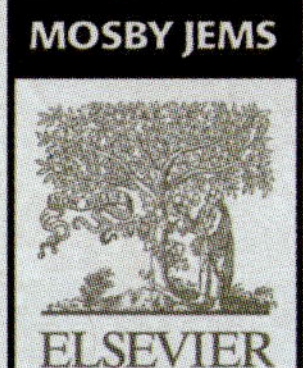

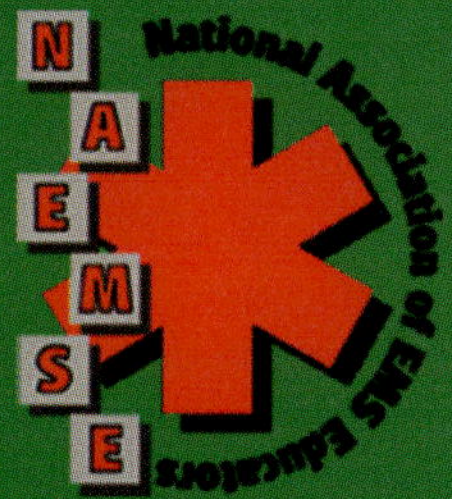

MOSBY JEMS
ELSEVIER

11830 Westline Industrial Drive
St. Louis, Missouri 63146

FOUNDATIONS OF EDUCATION: AN EMS APPROACH

ISBN 13 978-0-323-02867-7
ISBN 10 0-323-02867-5

Notice

Neither the Publisher nor the editors assume any responsibility for any loss or injury and/or damage to persons or property arising out of or related to any use of the material contained in this book. It is the responsibility of the treating practitioner, relying on independent expertise and knowledge of the patient, to determine the best treatment and method of application for the patient.

The Publisher

ISBN 13 978-0-323-02867-7
ISBN 10 0-323-02867-5

Executive Editor: Linda Honeycutt
Senior Developmental Editor: Laura Bayless
Publishing Services Manager: Pat Joiner
Senior Project Manager: Karen M. Rehwinkel
Designer: Kathi Gosche

Printed in the United States of America

Last digit is the print number: 9 8 7 6 5 4 3 2 1

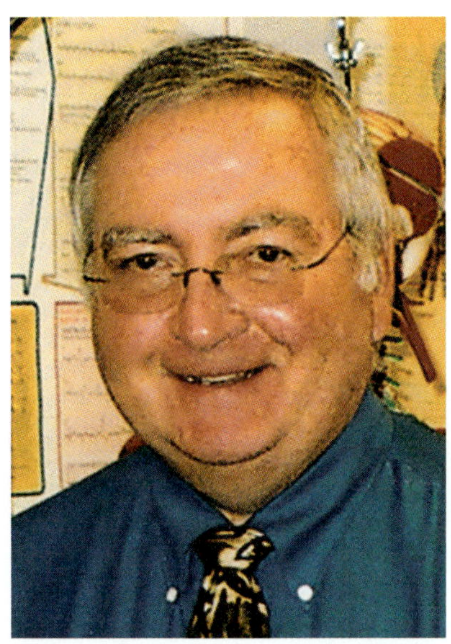

This book is dedicated to the memory of Daniel L. Storer, MD. Dan was an emergency physician who believed deeply in the value of EMS and dedicated much of his time, energy, and passion to helping EMS educators develop quality educational programs. He spent over 27 years as an EMS teacher and medical director, and devoted over 18 years working on behalf of the Committee on Accreditation for EMS Professions. His kind and encouraging manner touched many EMS educators at national meetings, site visits, and when he consulted with programs all across the United States. Throughout his career as an EMS educator he instilled in all of his students a commitment to excellence and a deep respect for human dignity. Dan always displayed a calm, wise, and thoughtful manner and a generous nature. His efforts will have a profound and lasting effect on the future of emergency medicine. He was a role model, mentor, and friend to many, and his guidance will be sorely missed.

NAEMSE & DC

To Kenny, Christopher, and Kate,

whose love sustains me and gives special purpose to my life!

DC

Acknowledgments

The National Association of EMS Educators and Editor Debra Cason wish to acknowledge the tireless efforts of the talented contributors who wrote and re-wrote—theirs was truly a labor or love.

CONTRIBUTORS

Angel Clark Burba, MS, EMT-P
Associate Professor and Program Director
Howard Community College
Columbia, Maryland
Principles of Adult Learning (3), Domains of Learning (7), Goals and Objectives (8), Introduction to Teaching Strategies (12), Remediation (22)

Debra Cason, RN, MS, EMT-P
Associate Professor and Program Director
University of Texas Southwestern Medical Center
Emergency Medicine Education
Dallas, Texas

Alice "Twink" Dalton, RN, MS, NREMT-P
Clinical Educator
Pridemark Paramedic Services
Boulder, Colorado
Teaching in All Domains (13)

Heather Davis, MS, NREMT-P
Education Program Director
Los Angeles County Fire Department
Commerce, California
Attributes of Effective Educators (1), EMS Educator Roles (2), Appendix A: Resources for the EMS Educator

Bill Garcia
Paramedic
Cantonsville, Maryland
Tools for Field and Clinical Learning (18)

George W. Hatch, Jr., EdD, EMT-P
Chairman, Emergency Medical Service Department
Houston Community College System
Houston, Texas
Introduction to Teaching Strategies (12), Teaching in All Domains (13), Tools for Small Group Learning (15)

Arthur Hsieh, MA, NREMT-P
Program Director
Hospital Consortium Education Network
San Mateo, California
Principles of Adult Learning (3), Diversity (5)

Sandy Hunter, MA, NREMT-P
Associate Professor
Paramedic Program
Dizney 225
Eastern Kentucky University
Richmond, Kentucky
Diversity (5)

Gary L. Ireland, MA
Iowa EMS Bureau Chief, Retired
Executive Director, Iowa EMS Association
West Des Moines, Iowa
Administrative Issues (23)

Christopher J. Le Baudour, MS Ed, NREMT
Reach Air Medical Services
Santa Rosa, California
Introduction to Teaching Strategies (12), Tools for Individual Learning (14)

Ranaye J. Marsh, PhD
Idaho State University
Pocatello, Idaho
Legal Issues for the Educator (10)

Mickey Moore, AAS, EMT-P
Central Georgia Technical College
Macon, Georgia
Audiovisual Basics (11), Appendix A: Resources for the EMS Educator

Christopher Nollette, EdD, NREMTP, LP
Director, Emergency Medical Services
Moreno Valley Campus
Riverside Community College
Moreno Valley, California
Attributes of Effective Educators (1), Introduction to Teaching Strategies (12), Teaching in All Domains (13), Tools for Small Group Learning (15), Tools for Large Group Learning (16)

Madeleine O'Donnell, BNg, BEd, MEdS
Teringie, Australia
Tools for Small Group Learning (15), Tools for Large Group Learning (16), Tools for Distance Learning (17)

David Page, MS, NREMT-P
Faculty, Emergency Health Services Department
Inver Hills Community College
St. Paul, Minnesota
The Learning Environment (6), Introduction to Teaching Strategies (12), Tools for Individual Learning (14), Tools for Small Group Learning (15), Tools for Field and Clinical Learning (18)

William Raynovich, MPH, BS, NREMT-P
Assistant Professor
Director, EMS Education
Creighton University
Omaha, Nebraska
Attributes of Effective Educators (1), EMS Educator Roles (2), Principles of Adult Learning (3), Teaching in All Domains (13)

Judith A. Ruple, PhD, RN, NREMT-P
Associate Professor
College of Health & Human Services
The University of Toledo
Toledo, Ohio
Attributes of Effective Educators (1), The Learning Environment (6), Administrative Issues (23)

Jane Smith, MA, NREMT-P
EMS Chief
San Francisco Fire Department
San Francisco, California
Diversity (5)

Cy Stockhoff
Albuquerque, New Mexico
Attributes of Effective Educators (1), EMS Educator Roles (2), Principles of Adult Learning (3)

Mark Terry, BA, NREMT-P
Battalion Chief—Training
Johnson County MedAct
Lee's Summit, Missouri
The Learning Environment (6), Principles of Evaluation of Student Performance (19), Using Written Evaluation Tools (20), Other Evaluation Tools (21)

Bruce Walz, PhD, NREMT-P
Chair, Department of Emergency Health Services
University of Maryland, Baltimore County
Baltimore, Maryland
Principles of Adult Learning (3), Learning Styles (4), Lesson Plans (9), Introduction to Teaching Strategies (12), Teaching in All Domains (13), Tools for Small Group Learning (15), Administrative Issues (23)

Additionally, we were fortunate to have contributors who wrote for our NAEMSE Magazine, *Domain 3*. These contributors are gratefully acknowledged.

Melissa Alexander, MS, NREMT-P
EMS Academy Director
University of New Mexico
Albuquerque, New Mexico

Elizabeth Criss, RN, MEd, CEN
Clinical Educator
Emergency Services
University Medical Center
Tucson, Arizona

Kevin L. Parrish, RN, CCEMT-P, EMT-P
Instructor, Center for Emergency Medicine of Western Pennsylvania
Pittsburgh, Pennsylvania

Dean G. Vokey, BEd, ACP
Atlantic Training Solutions
York, PE Canada

Richard T. Walker, MBA, RRT
Executive Director
CoAEMSP
Bedford, Texas

Other individuals contributed in significant ways to the development and production of this book: Past President Art Hsieh, President Linda Abrahamson, NAEMSE Board of Directors, Heather Davis, and Executive Director Joann Freel conceived, funded, and supported this project. Without their vision and commitment, this project would not have taken off. Co-Directors of the *NHTSA DOT Guidelines for EMS Education* Judy Ruple and Angel Burba, along with the Task Force, are to be credited for creating the foundational materials for this text. Their wise and careful work provided important content and structure.

Our editors from Elsevier, first Claire Merrick and Kelly Trakalo, and then Linda Honeycutt and Laura Bayless, provided much-needed guidance and insight into various aspects of the project that have made it better. Kelly has been a true colleague and friend, and we thank her for her insight and wisdom in the conceptual and incubator stages of this project. Kelly is a consummate professional and maintained her commitment to the project during and after her role as developmental editor.

Cover artist Ruth Araceli was very patient with our abstract ideas and created an outstanding cover. Many thanks to the photographers on this project who used their expertise in the area of education to create photos that tell the story: Kenny Navarro, Angel Burba, Dawn Pecora, Mickey Moore, and Art Hsieh for their contributions. And thanks to Lynne Dees, who provided art suggestions that enhance the material.

Several individuals warrant personal thanks. First is Joann Freel, NAEMSE executive director, who has functioned in many roles during this project. Along with President Linda Abrahamson, Joann has been our cheerleader during many ups and downs, missed deadlines, and more changes. She has managed the many chapter versions, contributor and reviewer issues, and reviewed every word of every chapter. Her tireless efforts and her friendship are greatly appreciated. Nancy Peterson, our NAEMSE developmental editor and consultant, has been an invaluable resource from the very beginning. Her editorial experience, organized mind, ability to listen and synthesize thoughts and feelings, and her understanding of the process has been a critical part of this book in many ways. She has also been a dear friend. [THANK YOU SO MUCH!] Additionally, there have been several key individuals who always responded to cries for help, no matter how quickly we needed the information or feedback: Angel Burba, Bruce Walz, Dave Page, and Kelly Trakalo are amazing sources of knowledge and insight and were extremely helpful personally and professionally. Mark Terry was also an incredible source of writing and insight into the content.

Sincerely,
NAEMSE & DC

Reviewers

We also wish to acknowledge the many insightful reviewers. Their wise feedback was taken to heart and resulted in substantive changes to the scope of the text and other improvements. Their suggestions and input were invaluable to the project.

Linda Abrahamson, BA, RN, EMT-P
NAEMSE President
EMS Education Coordinator/Adjunct Faculty
Silver Cross Hospital/Joliet Junior College
Joliet, Illinois

William Bake, MPH, EMT-P
Training Officer and Community Outreach Coordinator
Eastern Area Prehospital Services
Pittsburgh, Pennsylvania

Ann Bellows, RN, NREMT-P, EdD
Training Coordinator/Southwest Med Evac
Las Cruces, New Mexico

Angel Clark Burba, MS, NREMT-P
Associate Professor and Program Director
Howard Community College
Columbia, Maryland

Will Chapleau, EMT-P, RN, TNS
Chief
Chicago Heights Fire Department
Chicago Heights, Illinois

Arthur Cooper, MD, FACS, FAAP, FCCM
New York, New York

Alice "Twink" Dalton, RN, MS, NREMT-P, MS
Clinical Educator
Pridemark Paramedic Services
Boulder, Colorado

Heather Davis, MS, NREMT-P
Education Program Director
Los Angeles County Fire Department
Commerce, California

Lynne Dees, MFA, LP, NREMT-P, AAS, BFA
Assistant Professor
University of Texas Southwestern Medical Center
Dallas, Texas

Philip D. Dickison, RN, NREMT-P
Columbus, Ohio

James N. Eastham, Jr., ScD
President and CEO
EMSED.COM, LLC
Shrewsbury, Pennsylvania

Marcie Fisher, MA, EMT-P
Program Director
Florida Community College
Orange Park, Florida

Robert W. Folden, EdD, EMT-B
Clinical Assistant Professor
Texas A&M University—Commerce
Greenville, Texas

Joann Freel, BS, CMP
Executive Director
National Association of EMS Educators
Pittsburgh, Pennsylvania

Joseph A. Grafft, MS
President-Elect NAEMSE
EMS Manager–Minnesota State Colleges & Universities
St. Paul, Minnesota

Bill Garcia
Paramedic
Cantonsville, Maryland

John Gosford, AS, EMT-P
State Training Coordinator
State of Florida
Crawfordville, Florida

Jeffrey R. Grunow, MSN, NREMT-P
Chair, Emergency Care & Rescue
Weber State University
Ogden, Utah

George W. Hatch, Jr., EdD, EMT-P
Chairman, Emergency Medical Services Department
Houston Community College System
Houston, Texas

Sandy Hunter, MA, NREMT-P
Associate Professor
Paramedic Program
Disney 225
Eastern Kentucky University
Richmond, Kentucky

David M. LaCombe, NREMT-P
Director
National EMS Academy
Lafayette, Louisiana

Baxter Larmon, PhD, MICP
Professor
UCLA Medical Center/Emergency Medical Center
Los Angeles, California

W. Ann Maggiore, JD, NREMT-P
Clinical Faculty
University of New Mexico School of Medicine
Department of Emergency Medicine
Placitas, New Mexico

Gregg S. Margolis, MS, NREMT-P
Associate Director
National Registry of EMTs
Columbus, Ohio

Kim McKenna, RN, BSN, CEN, EMT-P
Chief Medical Officer
Florissant Valley Fire Protection District
Florissant, Missouri

Mickey Moore, AAS, EMT-P
Central Georgia Technical College
Macon, Georgia

Christopher Nollette, EdD, NREMT-P
Director, Emergency Medical Services
Moreno Valley Campus
Riverside Community College
Moreno Valley, California

David Page, MS, NREMT-P
Faculty, Emergency Health Services Department
Inver Hills Community College
St. Paul, Minnesota

George E. Perry, EdD
EMS Coordinator
Martinsburg, West Virginia

Judith A. Ruple, PhD, RN, NREMT-P
Associate Professor
College of Health & Human Services
The University of Toledo
Toledo, Ohio

John J. Shea, NREMT-P
Paramedic Educator
UCLA—Daniel Freeman Paramedic Education
Inglewood, California

Walt Alan Stoy, PhD
Professor
University of Pittsburgh
Center for Emergency Medicine
Pittsburgh, Pennsylvania

Mark Terry, BA, NREMT-P
Battalion Chief—Training
Johnson County MedAct
Lee's Summit, Missouri

Donna G. Tidwell, BS, RN, EMT-P
Director of EMS Personnel Licensure & Education
Tennessee Department of Health, EMS Division
Fairview, Tennessee

John Todaro, REMT-P, RN, TNS
Director of Education
Florida Emergency Medicine Foundation
Orlando, Florida

Kelly Trakalo, BS, RRT
Marketing Director
FISDAP
University City, Missouri

Bruce Walz, PhD, NREMT-P
Chair, Department of Emergency Health Services
University of Maryland, Baltimore County
Baltimore, Maryland

Clifford D. Wilson, AAS, EMT-P
Battalion Chief/Medical Officer
Kitsap County Fire District 7
Port Orchard, Washington

Donna Wilson, EMT-P
MTU Coordinator
Oregon Health Division
Terrebonne, Oregon

Foreword

In the spring of 1995, a group of EMS instructors gathered in a small meeting room during a national conference to discuss the challenges that faced EMS education and the practice of teaching. During the ensuing discussion it became clear that there was a need to create a forum that could address these concerns. Before long, a proverbial hat was passed around the group and enough money was collected that day to incorporate an organization that became the National Association of EMS Educators.

As EMS educators, we like to relate that story because it exemplifies the resourcefulness of teachers. No other group of individuals embodies the spirit of life-long learning like EMS educators.

Many of us will attest to the trepidation we felt when we first began our teaching careers. Some of us were lucky; we had a mentor or coach who could show us the ropes of what it took to be effective in the classroom. Others were able to take formal classes in educational methodology. Many of us learned the hard way—through trial and error. Eventually, through hard work, skill, and a good deal of luck, we became better educators. How often, though, did we wish there was a resource that could serve as a guide to assist us in improving our skills as effective educators.

It's no wonder that EMS educators decided to put pen to paper and create this book. A collaborative effort by members of NAEMSE, *Foundations of Education* represents the Association's mandate—to provide resources and assistance to EMS instructors. This particular resource is the culmination of hours of hard work by many people, all tied to the specific vision of providing a reference book with the tools you need to teach with at your fingertips. *Foundations of Education* provides essential topics in teaching strategies and methodology to assist novice and experienced instructors who have begun to coordinate and direct educational efforts within their organization.

Chapters have been written by contributing authors who are acknowledged experts in their respective specialties. You will hear many different "voices" as you read this book, making the experience richer. These educators provide combined decades of experience teaching on the front lines, and speak from true, hard-earned experience. *Foundations of Education* incorporates historical and current trends that are implemented and advocated by professional educational institutions and organizations.

The book has been laid out in an easy-to-follow format. Part I details the roles and responsibilities of effective EMS educators and lays a foundation for greater understanding of the principles of teaching and learning. Part II offers insight into how students learn and effective ways in which to enhance learning for optimal results. Part III explains the domains of learning and gives educators the tools needed to draft effective lesson plans, goals, and objectives; handle legal issues; and utilize technology to enhance learning. Part IV takes the principles of learning even further, offering proven teaching strategies for individuals, small groups, large groups, distance learning, and in field and clinical settings. Part V delves into the details of student assessment, from choosing the right evaluation method all the way through remediation, if it should be needed. Part VI rounds out the duties of educators, with guidance on office management and budgetary concerns.

Several unique features have been built into the book to assist you in building your foundation as an instructor. Case-in-point boxes illustrate the application of important concepts in a real-world setting, and Teaching Tips offer valuable insight from teachers working in the field. This book serves as the link to applying the concepts of the 2002 National Guidelines for Educating EMS Instructors. Application of these concepts will assist you in enhancing your students' success in the classroom and thus in the care of the patients they encounter.

Ultimately, this book has been written for you, the EMS instructor. Whether you teach EMS at an academic institution, Friday nights at the volunteer station house, or weekends at a community-based function, this book will be the reference that you will want to reach for time and again. We hope you find *Foundations of Education* an invaluable tool for your professional growth as an EMS educator.

Linda M. Abrahamson, BA, RN, EMT-P
NAEMSE President

Arthur Hsieh, MA, NREMT-P
NAEMSE Past-President

Debra Cason, RN, MS, EMT-P
Editor
NAEMSE Past-President

Contents

Instructor Roles and Responsibilities

A career as an educator is one of the most noble and challenging callings in society. Few individuals possess the knowledge, ability, ethics, self-motivation, and communication skills to successfully contribute to a profession in this way. Whereas all educators play pivotal roles in the advancement of a profession, only emergency medical services (EMS) educators face the challenge of teaching the critical content of how to save lives—usually over a short time. Their students not only must understand facts, they must master concepts so they can apply them quickly and accurately in uncontrolled and unpredictable environments. Our goal, therefore, is to teach students the knowledge (what we do with our head), skills (what we do with our hands), and behavior/attitude (what we do with our heart) required of a competent practitioner, as illustrated on the textbook cover.

The EMS educator is the essential facilitator of this complex learning process. As with any challenging journey, the path to becoming an excellent EMS educator begins with the first step. This part of the text outlines the attributes and roles of effective EMS educators, and explains their unique responsibilities. As you gain experience and refine your teaching practice, you may wish to refer back to these chapters later to reflect on your professional growth.

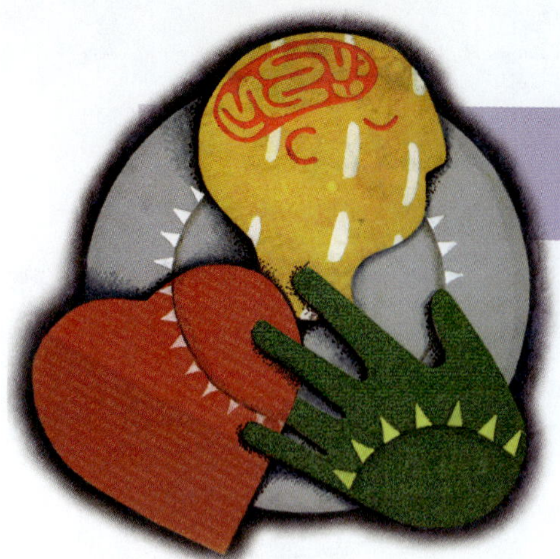

CHAPTER 1

Attributes of Effective Educators

"In a completely rational society, the best of us would be teachers and the rest of us would have to settle for something less!"

—*Lee Iacocca*

An educator begins his or her career with a clean slate, but few give much thought to how they wish to be remembered at the end of their teaching career. Because the first weeks and months are critical in terms of the type of instructor one will become, every new educator should consider the kind of instructor he or she wants to be right from the beginning. In addition, new educators should consider the attributes that can make them effective instructors, as well as extraordinary instructors.

With a clear image of the type of instructor they want to become, new educators can face the many external pressures that come with the job. Otherwise, those external pressures may end up directing the shape and outcome of their career. Emergency medical services (EMS) educators, similar to EMS providers, can choose to lead a career defined by high standards of diligence, caring, compassion, and integrity. This chapter can help educators to identify their teaching philosophy, as well as attributes that contribute to one's becoming an effective educator (Box 1-1). Furthermore, in this chapter, the educator will gain a clear understanding of what it means to be professional, and will learn the consequences of being unprofessional. This chapter also explores specific characteristics and qualities of effective teaching and effective communication, which go hand in hand.

Any discussion of the attributes of effective EMS *educators* should begin with a review of the qualities of effective EMS *providers*. The EMT-Paramedic National Standard Curriculum describes 11 model characteristics that apply to all levels of EMS providers. The EMS instructor should strive to embody these same characteristics, which include the following:

- Integrity
- Empathy
- Self-motivation
- Neat appearance/personal hygiene
- Effective communication
- Self-confidence
- Effective time management
- Teamwork and diplomacy
- Respect
- Patient advocacy
- Careful delivery of services

PROFESSIONALISM DEFINED

In recent years, much attention has been devoted to the issue of professionalism in medical education and practice.[1-8] Certain professional associations, such as the American Medical Association (AMA), have become concerned about how both the body of knowledge and the delivery of medical care have affected the physician's time-honored responsibilities toward patients. Medical educators have also been concerned about the impact a physician's behavior can have on the professional development of medical students and residents, hence the recent call for a renewed focus on professionalism.

Dr Herbert M. Swick proposed a list of nine characteristics that define professionalism.[9] Although Swick's work focused on professionalism as it relates to physicians, many of his thoughts and concepts are applicable to educators in every field. The definition and understanding of professionalism must be grounded both in the nature of the profession (education) and in the nature of the professional field (in this

BOX 1-1 Developing a Teaching Philosophy

David Royse, in his text *Teaching Tips for College and University Instructors*, proposes that all educators should construct a teaching philosophy that represents what is most important to them as educators. In identifying his own philosophy, Royse considered the instructors who had influenced him positively, both personally and professionally, as well as those who had affected him with their poor teaching and interpersonal skills. His philosophy of important issues includes the following:

- Create a sense of community in the classroom. Students learn more and enjoy learning when they feel connected to one another and to the instructor
- Ensure that education is a two-way, interactive process. The instructor is neither infallible nor an authority on all matters
- Give respect to each individual person in the classroom
- Be accountable to the students. Make sure to prepare appropriately and be on time for class, as well as to offer timely, high-quality student feedback
- Make sure that learning is fun. Include humor as part of all classes
- Apply learning to issues and problems in the world today
- Hold lifelong learning as a goal

From Royse D. Teaching Tips for College and University Instructors. Boston: Allyn & Bacon; 2001.

BOX 1-2 Swick's Elements of Professionalism

1. Professionals subordinate their own interest to the interest of others.
2. Professionals adhere to the highest ethical and moral standards.
3. Professionals respond to social needs, and their behaviors reflect a social contract with the communities served.
4. Professionals demonstrate core humanistic values, including honesty, integrity, caring, compassion, altruism, empathy, respect for others, and trustworthiness.
5. Professionals exercise accountability for themselves and for their colleagues.
6. Professionals demonstrate a continuing commitment to excellence.
7. Professionals exhibit a commitment to scholarship and to advancing their field of study.
8. Professionals deal with high levels of complexity and uncertainty.
9. Professionals reflect upon their actions and decisions.

Three Additional Characteristics of Professionalism

10. Professionals create a nonpolitical classroom environment.
11. Professionals respect confidentiality.
12. Professional educators strive to have their students surpass them in both mastery of the content material and actualization of being a professional.

Modified from Swick.[9]

case, EMS). Furthermore, professionalism must be considered on two levels: the individual and the collective.

In addition to those listed in Dr Swick's work, medical professionals must exhibit three characteristics if they are to meet their obligations to their patients (students), their communities, and their profession (Box 1-2).[9]

ELEMENTS OF PROFESSIONALISM

1. Professionals subordinate their own interest to the interest of others

Because most educators have numerous responsibilities, they sometimes confront conflicts of interest in their work. These conflicts may arise, for instance, between the policies and demands of the educational institution and those of the health systems that employ the students. When such conflicts arise, educators must ensure that the students' interests and needs remain paramount. Instructors must constantly advocate for their students. Professionalism in the field of education reflects the educator's willingness to put students' needs before his or her own.

2. Professionals adhere to the highest ethical and moral standards

Because it is believed that professional work has a moral value, educators are compelled to behave ethically in both their personal and their professional lives. Educators must realize early in their teaching profession that they are never "off duty," just as EMTs and paramedics are never truly "off duty" in their communities. An educator's behaviors will be judged against the highest ethical standards, whether he or she is in the classroom, providing patient care, or taking a day off at the beach. The ethics of educators is an important and complex topic that warrants separate discussion. (See "Ethics for the EMS Educator" later in this chapter.)

3. Professionals respond to social needs, and their behaviors reflect a social contract with the communities served

Any profession best meets its obligations when its members attend actively to community and social needs. Sullivan's concept of civic professionalism stresses the importance of social leadership.[10] One way in which EMS educators can begin to fulfill their social contract is to form advisory groups from within the community to help guide educational services. It is not enough that educators think they know what is best for the community they serve; they must actively seek out the opinions of those within the community. This involves gathering information on the scheduling of courses, the number and type of courses offered, and suggested additions and deletions to the curriculum.

4. Professionals demonstrate core humanistic values, including honesty, integrity, caring, compassion, altruism, empathy, respect for others, and trustworthiness

Although most experienced EMS educators agree that it is difficult to write standard learning objectives for social values, no argument has been put forth about their importance as part of the foundation of EMS education. Values such as compassion, altruism, integrity, and trustworthiness are so central to the nature of the educator's work that no educator can be truly effective without holding deeply to such values. Unfortunately, it is possible to turn out students who excel in their skills and knowledge, but who lack social values. The care delivered by these students, once they become practitioners, may be insensitive, overly aggressive, and laden with risk for the provider, the patient, and the employing agency.

TEACHING TIP: Perhaps the best way to impart the values of honesty, integrity, caring, compassion, altruism, empathy, respect for others, and trustworthiness to students is to be a good role model of these values.

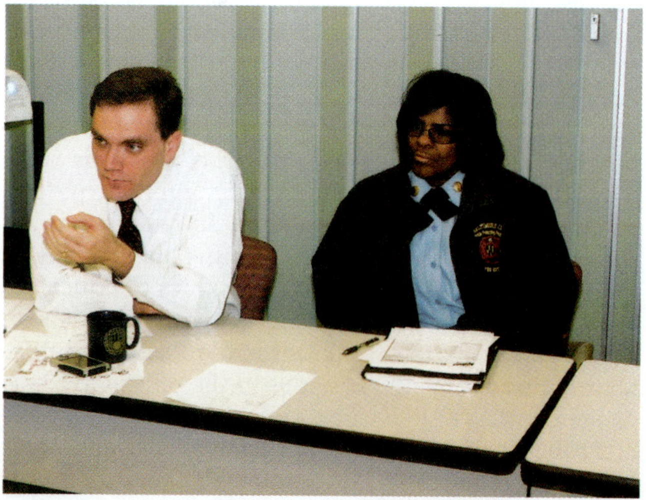

FIGURE 1-1 An advisory group can provide important input for the educational program, thus enhancing the value of the program to the community.

5. Professionals exercise accountability for themselves and for their colleagues

Educators enjoy relative academic freedom and autonomy in the classroom as one of the most highly valued principles of education. However, academic freedom and autonomy do not mean that standards of practice and accountability for performance can be ignored or altered. Educators must adhere to educational and clinical practice standards at the institutional, state, and national levels. The best way to ensure that educators are upholding standards of practice is to have a well-developed peer review process in place.

Several methods are commonly used to develop a peer review process. The key is to have as many different perspectives as possible from which feedback is obtained. Peer review is different from student evaluation. Although student evaluations are an import feedback tool, they come from a relatively unsophisticated audience. Having the head of the department or program sit in on a classroom session and provide feedback is the most common form of peer review. Equally valuable, and sometimes less intimidating, is having a peer instructor provide this service. Note that the instructor doing the peer evaluation does not have to be an expert in EMS, but he or she should be an experienced educator. Another means of procuring peer review is to obtain feedback from state or national testing organizations. Still another type of peer review is feedback that can be obtained from EMS services and other agencies that employ graduates from the course. Last, don't forget to talk with clinical instructors and field preceptors. They are invaluable sources of information regarding student strengths and weaknesses. The ideal would be that all these peer review feedback processes would become formal and routine aspects of every school evaluation process.

6. Professionals demonstrate a continuing commitment to excellence

All professions are based on intellectual work, a specialized body of knowledge, and expertise; thus, the commitment to maintain one's competency within the field is an important professional quality. Demands to stay current with the body of knowledge require educators to maintain the highest standards of excellence through the continuing acquisition of knowledge and development of new skills. This can be challenging in that the amount of new material in every field of science is growing at an exponential rate. In the field of EMS, required periodic refreshers and testing of instructors have been considered means of ensuring that educators remain current.

Subject Knowledge

To fulfill the sixth element of professionalism—that is, *Professionals demonstrate a continuing commitment to excellence*—instructors must stay abreast of any and all sources of valid information and must maintain a current and accurate knowledge base. Several common, appropriate resources for staying up-to-date include fellow instructors, students, other healthcare professionals, patients, periodicals, and conferences and continuing education opportunities.

Fellow Instructors

An instructor should maintain a list of fellow instructors who have special knowledge in a particular area of the curriculum, as well as a list of instructors who have a special gift for presenting information, running labs, or conducting meaningful classroom experiences. These instructors may constitute a personal advisory group, which can help an educator to focus on his or her commitment to personal excellence.

Students

If an instructor has a student with particular expertise in a given area, the instructor might consider using that student as a resource. Of course, it is wise to first mentor the student in the development of the presentation, or to gently ease the student into the presentation by informally asking the student to comment on his or her experience in the given area—with advance permission, of course.

Other Healthcare Professionals

Instructors should maintain a list of other emergency medical technicians (EMTs), paramedics, nurses, physician assistants, and physicians who have expertise in a given area of the curriculum. These people can be contacted as content experts, guest lecturers, lab assistants, or curriculum and exam reviewers.

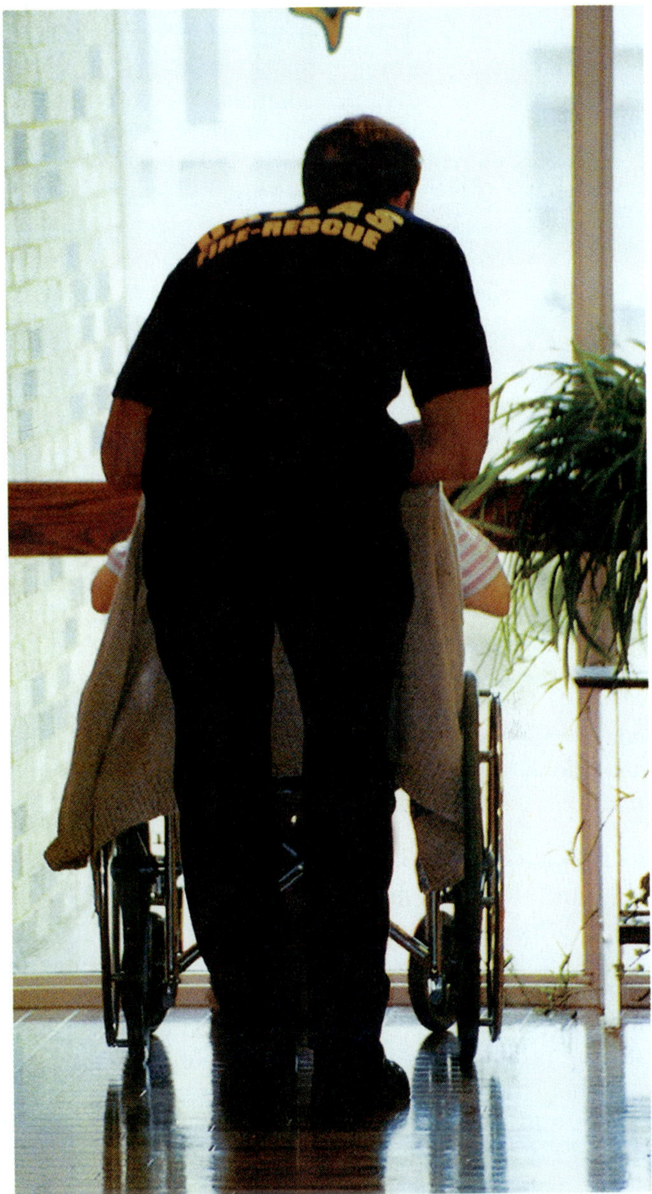

FIGURE 1-2 Instructors should encourage students to learn from their patients.

Patients

Clinicians and educators can learn tremendously from each patient encounter. Often, at their first meeting, patients know more about the pathophysiology and treatment of their diseases than the clinicians do. They certainly know infinitely more about how it *feels* to have a particular disease than any healthcare provider who has not had that disease can possibly know. One can learn a great deal from patients by listening carefully with an open mind (Figure 1-2). Finally, some patients with chronic or unusual illnesses and family members may be open to teaching healthcare professionals about their disease experiences; they may even view the opportunity to come into the classroom or clinic to teach as a welcome sign of respect and a chance to meaningfully contribute.

Periodicals

The EMS educator should subscribe to at least one professional EMS peer-reviewed journal and one professional educational journal. Membership in professional organizations, such as the National Association of Emergency Medical Services Educators (NAEMSE) or the National Association of Emergency Medical Services Professionals (NAEMSP), provides the educator with subscriptions to the official journals of these organizations. To take full advantage of periodicals as a resource for maintaining a current, accurate knowledge base, instructors can encourage their program managers to include in the budget support for memberships in national educational and clinical associations.

TEACHING TIP: Require every student in every course to turn in two articles from clinical or educational peer-reviewed journals. The purpose of this exercise is for students to learn about the professional journals and to get to know where they are located. Also, require students to provide the address of one Web site resource. In addition to the learning opportunity that this activity provides to students, EMS instructors generally receive numerous interesting articles to read, along with 10 to 15 new Web addresses per class.

Conferences

EMS educators have a responsibility to learn current patient care methods and teaching strategies, and conferences provide the perfect learning opportunity. EMS educators should not limit themselves to local, regional, or even state conferences, but should attend national conferences as often as possible. Furthermore, the EMS educator should not limit himself or herself to *EMS* conferences. There are wonderful national conferences on distance education, how to give presentations, technologies in education, testing and measurement, and student counseling (Figure 1-3).

7. Professionals exhibit a commitment to scholarship and to advancing their field of study

In all professions, one of the most basic defining elements of members is the commitment to advance the body of knowledge of that discipline. This commitment to scholarship can be manifested as a desire to share one's knowledge for the benefit of others—whether students, other instructors, or members of the community. All professionals should be strongly committed to supporting research within their area of study. This requires:

- A functional knowledge of research methods
- The ability to conduct literature searches or reviews
- Evaluation of research for use in the classroom
- Presentation of research to students to instill a commitment among the next generation of professionals

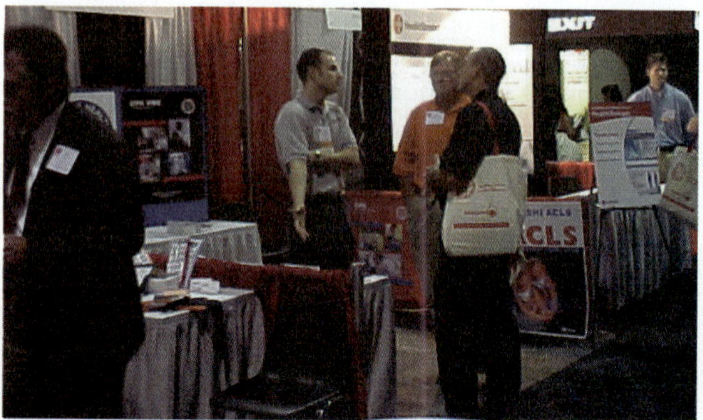

FIGURE 1-3 Instructors can keep abreast of new clinical topics, as well as educational techniques, by networking at conferences.

Without formal and informal forums at which instructors can routinely gather and share knowledge, any profession is severely limited in its ability to advance (Box 1-3).

8. Professionals deal with high levels of complexity and uncertainty

Uncertainty and ambiguity have long characterized the practices of medicine and education. Instructors, similar to healthcare providers, must be able to exercise independent judgment to make appropriate decisions in the face of complex and often unstable circumstances, and usually with incomplete information. Instruction that is simple and repetitive or that does not involve a great deal of judgment does not require the independent decision making that is a hallmark of these professions.[11] Furthermore, instructors who rely strictly on canned curricula and do no more than repeat the work of others without adjusting the material for a given audience, adding personal insights, or developing creative approaches of delivery, fall far short of the term *professional educator*.

9. Professionals reflect upon their actions and decisions

Professional educators must be able to reflect dispassionately on the decisions they have made, as well as on their actions. These self-reflective activities not only improve their knowledge and skills, they also bring balance to their professional and personal lives.

Although the nine *Elements of Professionalism* discussed here are based largely on definitions developed by Dr Swick, the following three additional characteristics are proposed, for the educator's consideration.

10. Professionals create a nonpolitical classroom environment

Instructors must create a safe, nonpolitical environment for their students. Local, state, and national politics have no place in the classroom environment. In fact, all students should be treated with respect, regardless of their EMS service affiliation. Moreover, the roles of the EMS paid provider and volunteer should be equally honored. Certain topics, however, are appropriate for critical, professional discussion, such as different perspectives on rural and urban medical care. When questions arise about sensitive or controversial issues, the professional educator must present all sides of the argument in an unbiased and balanced manner.

11. Professionals respect confidentiality

All healthcare professionals are acutely aware of the issues associated with patient confidentiality. Educa-

BOX 1-3 Bringing Research Into the Classroom

by Liz Criss, RN, MEd, CEN

Bringing research into the classroom can be a challenge. Both instructors and students may view it as an intrusion into their fast-paced, hands-on program. Every instructor needs to be prepared for the barrage of questions and some skepticism, and even hostility that can follow any introductory session on research:

- What does this have to do with patient care in the field?
- Why is this important to me?
- I got into EMS to take care of patients, why do I need to study research?
- When can we get back into the important stuff?

While it may seem like an uphill battle, it is critically important to introduce the reading and interpreting of research so that students might develop an understanding of how the research will affect their clinical practice and their roles as EMS providers. Discussing it in class, or providing it as a homework assignment, might help get the point across about the need for studying research in the EMS classroom. Once the concept has been introduced it might be interesting to use this as a starting point for future discussions. As the students are introduced to new practices or equipment they could be asked to look for any publications on the applicability of the equipment or practice in the out-of-hospital environment. Any documents that are found can be critically analyzed, specifically looking at the population used to test the procedure or equipment. The point of the exercise is not to be disparaging of the procedure or equipment, but rather to learn to critically study the evidence upon which we base practice. This should also help to reinforce the need for ongoing research and the special role that research plays in the future of EMS.

BRINGING RESEARCH ALIVE IN THE CLASSROOM DOMAIN

Throughout our careers many of us have had the opportunity to make a personal discovery, an epiphany of sorts. Think back on one of these events. You may recall that once you made the personal discovery or "the light bulb came on," the information remained with you for years. Since self discovery is an important part of the learning process, the classroom might be the perfect place to create an appreciation for the research process through a variety of hands-on exercises. Since most individuals in EMS are visual learners, preferring to actively participate in the learning process, these self discovery projects could be just the jump start you need for a discussion about research.

This article is designed to provide you with some very simple classroom exercises that can easily be adapted for inclusion into any EMS curriculum. These exercises will allow students to practice team work; perform an "experiment" without realizing it; and have the opportunity to report their findings to the class. Many of these skills will be important to a successful career in EMS. Besides these benefits, this will be a fun break from the routine.

Each of these exercises focuses on use of common EMS equipment. Once you start preparing each of the lesson plans you will find that much of the equipment has not been well-evaluated or continues to be utilized despite its documented limitations. Be patient when you begin implementing these exercises, it may take a little time to get comfortable incorporating these activities into the classroom, but it will be very valuable in the end. Your enthusiasm for the discovery process will do much to keep the students interested.

Each of the exercises uses a similar small group format; therefore, consider rotating group members throughout the program so they have the opportunity to work with different people. After dividing the students, introduce the topic area and ask each group to begin the exercise by setting goals. They can shape their goals in the form of one or more questions, or simply in sentences or phrases. Have them write them down on paper and be sure that the information they collect during the exercise can meet their goals. Provide all the necessary equipment, then step back and watch what happens. Set a time limit for the exercise. An hour or 90 minutes should be adequate. Then reassemble the class and have each group present their findings. Following the group presentations you might consider introducing some of the literature that covers each of these topic areas.

Exercise 1

This first exercise involves comparing different gauge IV catheters and tubing combinations. One group might evaluate the differences between IV catheters using the same type of tubing for each phase of the exercise. One group might compare flow rates through the single most common catheter gauge when used with different types of tubing; this might include blood tubing, standard drip tubing, and mini-drip tubing. Another group might evaluate IV fluid height with and without a pressure bag. Another group might evaluate the effect of flow rate when extension tubing is added. The overall goal of this exercise is to allow the students to have a better appreciation of the dynamics of fluid flow. At the end of the presentations move into a discussion about some patient conditions and when the different combinations of tubing might be beneficial or harmful. This type of concrete information will provide them with a valuable resource later.

Exercise 2

This exercise involves comparing cervical collars. Student groups can compare neck flexion, extension, and lateral motion with different models of collars and/or with correct and incorrect size collars. Some simple tools, i.e., dowel rods, string, and protractors, will be needed for the students to be able to make some measurements. Be sure the student that is chosen

Continued

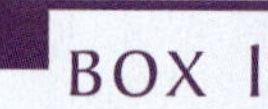

BOX 1-3 Bringing Research Into the Classroom—cont'd

by Liz Criss, RN, MEd, CEN

as the subject does not have neck problems or a stiff neck. For this exercise you may want to set some simple rules like no forcing the head past the comfort level and anyone can ask to be removed as the subject at any time.

To measure the amount of lateral motion place one dowel rod across the shoulders, this will serve as the neutral line, it can be held in place by two of the team members. Tie a piece of string to the center of the dowel rod and hold it straight up the back of the head. Ask the subject to move their head side to side; movement off this center line can then be measured by the protractor. This same process can be used for flexion and extension by placing the dowel rod across the shoulder, front to back, and holding the string along the side of the head, lining it up with the ear. The findings from this exercise may be very valuable in correcting long standing use or misuse of cervical collars. Consider having each group do the same experiment, this could lead very nicely into a discussion about some simple statistics that are important in research.

Exercise 3

This third exercise allows the students to practice both standard and creative ways to immobilize a patient on a backboard. For this exercise you will need to provide a variety of strapping supplies and a digital camera, to let them document their various procedures and also to assist them in presenting their findings. Be sure the student that is selected can safely lie on the board during the training sessions. Some of the goals the students might want to consider in this exercise include checking each strapping technique for neutral alignment of the head or the stability of the strapping technique when the board is lifted or tilted or even something as simple as how long did the strapping take. The findings in this exercise could be used as a starting point for discussing the limited amount of literature surrounding spinal immobilization. This exercise may also serve to correct some long term issues.

As you can see, including "research" into the classroom may not be as painful for either you or the students as you may have once thought. With some creativity and a little bit of planning you can include hands-on exercises into many of the aspects of the EMS curriculum.

From NAEMSE, Domain, Fall 2003-Winter 2004.

tors must be equally sensitive to these issues when they discuss their students with colleagues. Information on individual student performance, personality, and strengths and weaknesses should be considered strictly confidential. The professional educator has a special responsibility to refrain from sharing this information inappropriately.

12. Professional educators strive to have their students surpass them in both mastery of the content material and actualization of being a professional

A key requirement of being a professional is the understanding that it is a dynamic process. Being a professional is not an end point or a destination. Being a professional means that one is on a lifelong journey as a learner and practitioner, and it is the educator's mission to impart this understanding to students.

ETHICS FOR THE EMS EDUCATOR

EMS educators are members of two professions: teaching and healthcare practice. To fulfill the second element of professionalism—Professionals adhere to the highest ethical and moral standards—they must comply with the requirements and standards of each. EMS educators who are EMS providers are subject to the laws of professional ethics that are in force within the jurisdictions and services in which they work. In addition, as members of the teaching profession, all EMS educators are subject to the regulations of the institutions or facilities at which they teach.

EMS educators undoubtedly serve as important role models for students in that the EMS classroom experience is frequently the student's first exposure to the EMS profession. Therefore, EMS educators must understand the importance of ethical standards of behavior. They should have a strong sense of the special obligations that come with serving as an educator, especially since their responsibilities frequently extend beyond the classroom to out-of-class activities with students, both in the community and in other professional activities. They should also recognize their responsibility to serve students and to help students achieve their goals. This responsibility for moral integrity and dedication to the welfare of students must originate within the educator.

The following good practices concerning ethical and professional responsibility can assist new instructors and remind experienced ones of the basic ethical and professional code of their profession. This is by no means to be considered a disciplinary code, although the norms of conduct included are relevant when questions concerning propriety arise in a particular institutional context. The primary purpose, however, is to provide general guidance to EMS educators concerning their ethical and professional responsibilities to students, to colleagues, and to the profession and the general public.

Responsibilities to Students

Because of their inevitable function as role models, educators should be guided by and adhere to ethical and professional standards. As educators, scholars, counselors, mentors, and friends, EMS educators can profoundly influence students' attitudes concerning professional competence and responsibility. EMS educators should help students recognize the responsibility of EMS providers to advance the delivery of emergency medical services for individual persons and for the community at large.

Educators should aspire to excellence in teaching and to mastery of the theories and practices of the subjects they teach. Furthermore, they should prepare conscientiously for class and employ teaching methods appropriate for the subject matter and objectives of their courses. Similarly, classes should always be convened as scheduled or, when impossible, rescheduled at a time that is reasonably convenient for students; if needed, an alternative means of instruction should be provided.

Educators should provide a class syllabus or handbook that clearly outlines the objectives and requirements of a course, including applicable attendance and grading rules. Further, the educator should review these with the class, ensuring that each student fully understands. It is even advisable to have students sign a statement acknowledging receipt of the handbook/syllabus and acceptance of its contents.

A primary obligation of the educator is to treat students with politeness and respect. Educators can do this by creating a learning environment that fosters a stimulating and productive debate in which the pros and cons of important issues are fairly acknowledged and discussed. Allowing students to explore new ideas without fear of censure or criticism within the learning environment is essential to the free exchange of ideas. Educators should nurture and protect intellectual freedom for their students and colleagues.

The Ethics of Student Evaluation

Educators have a fundamental obligation to fairly, honestly, and constructively evaluate student work. This is a crucial aspect of respecting and nurturing students.

Exams and assignments should be conscientiously designed to meet the expectations of student performance, and evaluation materials should match learning objectives and stated goals. Moreover, student work should be evaluated with impartiality. The instructor may enhance impartiality by blinding the review of student material. Thus, the student is not identified until after the review has been completed. Another way to achieve impartiality with essay-type exams is by using a template with important points that must appear in the student's written work.

The standards for assigning grades should be consistent with standards recognized within the facility or institution. Students should clearly understand the basis on which grades are assigned, and instructors should offer an explanation if students ask why they received a certain grade. In addition, instructors should conduct grading in a timely fashion.

The Ethics of Counseling

Educators should make themselves reasonably available to counsel students about academic matters, career choices, and professional interests. Furthermore, they should make every reasonable effort to offer timely and accurate information.

In counseling students, educators must make every effort to hold student information confidential. They should not disclose any information unless required to do so by institutional rule or applicable law. Before providing counseling, educators should inform students of the possibility of such disclosure.

Educators should strive to be as fair and complete as possible when communicating evaluative recommendations for students. If information disclosed in confidence by the student to the educator makes it impossible for the educator to write a fair and complete evaluation/recommendation without revealing the information, the educator should inform the student and refuse to provide the evaluation/recommendation unless the student consents to full disclosure.

The Ethics of Diversity

Educators must make the learning environment a hospitable community and comfortable setting for all students. Discriminatory conduct based on such factors as race, color, religion, national origin, sex, sexual orientation, disability or handicap, age, or political beliefs is unacceptable in the education community. It is important for educators to be sensitive to the harmful consequences of instructor or student conduct, or comments in classroom discussions or elsewhere that perpetuate stereotypes or prejudices.

The Ethics of Personal Relationships With Students

Educators should not use their role or position of authority to induce a student to enter into a sexual relationship, or to subject a student to a hostile academic environment based on any form of sexual harassment. Sexual harassment is sex discrimination that involves unwelcome advances, requests for sexual favors, and other verbal or physical conduct of a sexual nature.

Sexual relationships between an educator and a student who are not married to each other or who do not have a preexisting relationship are also inappropriate. Whenever an educator has professional responsibility for a student, such as in teaching, evaluating, supervising, or advising the student as part of a course, this conduct is inappropriate.

Even when an educator has no professional responsibility for a student but maintains a relationship with that student, the educator should be sensitive to the perceptions of other students. Students may perceive that a student who has a sexual relationship with an instructor may receive preferential treatment from other instructors within the institution.

An educator who is closely related to a student by blood or marriage, or who has a preexisting close relationship with a student, generally should avoid roles involving professional responsibility for that student.

Ethical Responsibilities as Professional Educators

The community of EMS educators has a basic responsibility to refine, extend, and transmit knowledge regarding the teaching and practice of emergency medical services. EMS educational institutions and programs also have a responsibility to maintain an atmosphere of freedom and tolerance in which knowledge can be sought and shared. EMS educators are obligated, in turn, to make the best and fullest use of that academic freedom to fulfill their responsibilities to enrich the profession and practice of EMS education.

As previously discussed, educators have a responsibility to be current in the knowledge of the subjects that they teach. In teaching, as well as in research, writing, and publication, the scholarship of others is indispensable to one's knowledge and growth. To stay current in the EMS field requires continuous study and lifelong learning. To this extent, the Educator must remain a student. Moreover, educators have a responsibility to engage in their own research and publish their conclusions. In this way, educators participate in an intellectual exchange that tests and improves their knowledge of the field, to the ultimate benefit of their students, the profession, and society.

The educator's commitment to truth requires intellectual honesty and open-mindedness. Although an educator should feel free to criticize another's work, distortion or misrepresentation of a colleague's work is always unacceptable. When another person's scholarship—whether that of another educator or that of a student—is used in the preparation of classroom materials or in the writing of articles, this should be acknowledged. Significant contributions by others to presentations or articles require acknowledgment every time the ideas are used or transmitted. Appropriate ways to achieve this acknowledgment include shared authorship, attribution by footnote or endnote, and discussion of another's contribution within the main text or within the presentation.

An educator has a responsibility to preserve the integrity and independence of research and to promote the development of new knowledge. Sponsored or compensated research activities or presentations should always be acknowledged with full disclosure of the personal interests. Conflicts of interest should be acknowledged and brought forward for discussion among educators and students. It is best to err on the side of conservatism when one is addressing conflict of interest situations. If an instructor believes there might be a conflict, there probably is, so it is wise to disclose the possibility to others with whom or for whom he or she is working.

Ethical Responsibilities to Colleagues

Educators should treat colleagues and staff members with politeness and respect. Additionally, they should comply with institutional rules or policies requiring confidentiality concerning oral or written communications. Such rules and policies typically exist with respect to personnel matters and evaluations of student performance.

As is the case with students, sexual harassment or discriminatory conduct involving colleagues or staff members on the basis of race, color, religion, national origin, sex, sexual orientation, disability or handicap, age, or political beliefs is unacceptable.

Ethical Responsibilities to the EMS Community and the General Public

An EMS educator occupies a unique role as a bridge between the EMS professional community and students who are preparing to become members of that community. EMS educators must accept the responsibilities of their professional status. At a minimum, they should adhere to the Code of Rules of Conduct of state EMS divisions. EMS educator or provider conduct that warrants discipline should be a matter of serious concern to the EMS educator's school and to the general public.

One of the traditional obligations of EMS educators is to engage in uncompensated public service. As role models for students and as members of the EMS profession, EMS educators should strive to fulfill this responsibility. They can meet this obligation in a variety of ways, including direct patient contact through public aid programs, lecturing in continuing EMS education programs, educating public school pupils or other public groups concerning the EMS system, and teaching community health and safety programs.

Conclusions Regarding Ethics

This chapter serves to assist new educators and to remind experienced ones about the basic ethical and professional code of their profession. The educator must understand what constitutes good practice in terms of ethical and professional responsibility. Additionally, EMS educators must recognize their responsibility to serve students and to help students achieve their goals. This responsibility to serve students requires moral integrity and a dedication to providing what is in the best interest of the student.

Every EMS educator has the responsibility to adhere to the code of the profession and to be aware of the ethical and professional conduct requirements of the system in which he or she is teaching. It is important for EMS educators to remember that they have an ethical responsibility to students, colleagues, the EMS profession, and the general public. Because it is paramount that the professional EMS educator should uphold high standards within the profession, breeches of ethical conduct should not be taken lightly.

CREATIVITY IN TEACHING

According to Thomas L. Schwenk and Neal Whitman, all effective instructors have one attribute in common—they present creative lessons that stimulate their students and make learning easier.[12] An educator can achieve this kind of creativity by starting with the lesson plan. As the educator develops a lesson plan, he or she should ask if there is something he or she can do to make the learning more creative.

Creativity is defined as any activity that is novel and useful and results in contributions to human experience. Novel approaches in the classroom may involve the use of interesting modalities of communication, the application of inventive or unorthodox teaching techniques, and the provision of memorable and meaningful educational experiences through graphic demonstrations or imagery. Useful approaches may include providing correct, up-to-date, and relevant information, along with opportunities to develop good problem-solving skills and good patient care attitudes. If these qualities are combined into a grid, four possible types of instructor are revealed (Figure 1-4).

Creative educators are both novel and useful. They reveal the "inner relevance" of what they teach.[13] Creative instructors exhibit three characteristics:

1. They are selective in choosing their teaching methodologies.
2. They pay attention to delivery.
3. They teach beyond the printed material, beyond the textbook.

	USEFUL	NOT USEFUL
NOVEL	Creative teacher	Charlatan
NOT NOVEL	Pedantic bore	Old goat

FIGURE 1-4 Types of instructors.

Charlatan

Instructors can be charlatans—that is, persons who claim knowledge or skill that they do not possess—when they focus more on being novel, entertaining, and well-liked than on being useful. Students generally love charlatans. As a result, all will appear to be going well until students have to sit for the state or national exam. That's when students will discover that their instructor has not adequately prepared them for the exam.

One sign that an instructor is a charlatan is that he or she excessively uses "war stories." Additionally, charlatans rarely have prepared teaching materials and rely more on personal interaction than on content. Moreover, charlatans can be spotted by the fact that they rarely take responsibility for their students' failures—failure is always someone else's fault.

Pedantic Bore

It is certainly better to be a pedantic bore than a charlatan—at least students receive useful information from a pedantic bore. Rarely is anyone who is interested in teaching EMS a born and unredeemable pedantic bore. Pedantic bores are made, not born. The primary reason that educators may be boring is that they truly find the content material boring, or they may be so overbooked that they are simply trying to survive (Figure 1-5).

TEACHING TIP: Instructors should not attempt to lecture on something they don't really own. If the instructor has enough time to really prepare to present a topic, he or she will tend to get pretty excited and will really start to employ the creative process.

Becoming More Creative

By acting more creative, an instructor can actually become more creative.[14] Instructors shouldn't be afraid to try new methods in the classroom, or even to fail. Creativity may be viewed more as a process than as a product.[15] In fact, the four stages of this process have

CASE IN POINT

Two months in advance, an instructor of a paramedic class recruited one of the best trauma surgeons from the regional Level I Trauma Center to present the topic of chest trauma, one of the most important lectures for a paramedic class. She sent him a copy of the course schedule and learning objectives for the lecture, so that he would know exactly where the students were in their learning process when he arrived. She also invited him to review the test questions that she had on the topical material, as well as to write any questions that he felt were important to include. She then sent a reminder 30 days in advance, offering to print any handouts and to make sure that any ancillary audiovisual presentation materials were "loaded and ready to go." His office confirmed his appointment, saying that he would bring anything he needed with him.

The surgeon arrived on time and in good spirits. His lecture was entertaining and filled with valuable surgical tips and anomalies. He spoke of heroic saves in unusual cases, and tragic deaths due to occult injuries. He brought alive the imagery of the heroic trauma team working feverishly to save the lives of those who arrive *in extremis*—those whose only chance to survive was granted them by the speedy and competent work of the paramedics. The class gave him a warm applause and stood in line to speak with him after the lecture.

The instructor sat and listened in dismay. The guest surgeon ignored the content objectives. She would have to squeeze another 1-hour lecture into the already overflowing course schedule. He overlooked certain key things in his lecture, like the assessment and treatment of injuries such as traumatic asphyxia, tension pneumothorax, hemothorax, aortic rupture, and flail chest. He had been entertaining and charming, but if the students took the National Registry exam based on his lecture, they were certain to fail. Nowhere in the National Registry do they discuss the surgical removal of a pulmonary embolism, or attempts to surgically intervene in a patient with Boerhaave's syndrome, or of racing against time in surgically correcting a dissecting aortic aneurysm that is proximal to the renal artery. However, the students loved the lecture and the hour they spent with such a prestigious instructor. His evaluations were wonderful.

been identified as preparation, incubation, illumination, and verification.

Stages of Creativity

In the *preparation stage*, the instructor investigates the subject, deciding on what he or she wants students to value or know. It is often very helpful for instructors

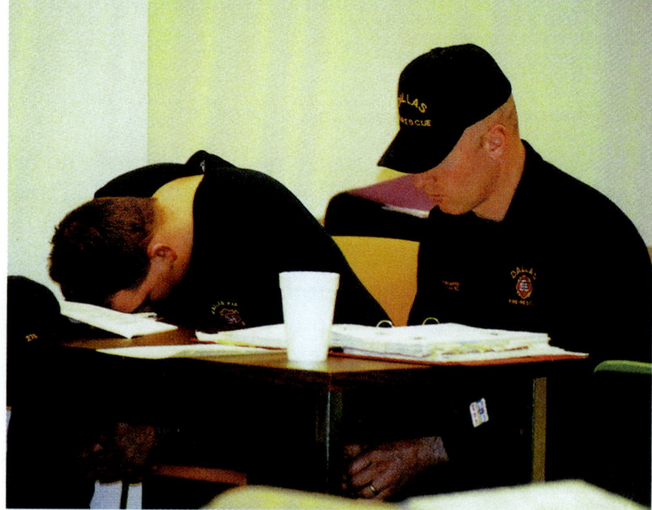

FIGURE 1-5 A clue that the class is boring is a student who has fallen asleep.

to brainstorm with other instructors at this point. The more possibilities one explores, the more likely one is to discover effective and creative approaches to presentation.

During the *incubation stage*, the instructor does not devote conscious thought to teaching the assignment, but continues to work at the subconscious level. Not allowing oneself time for the incubation stage of the process defeats the whole process of creativity. The educator must allow time for doing the subconscious and deliberative creative work, and this process cannot be rushed. Instructors who chronically overbook themselves can expect to do less than their best work.

In the *illumination stage*, the creative instructor becomes aware of how the topic can be presented. It is at this point that the organization of the content is combined with a plan on how to present it.

In the *verification stage*, the instructor teaches, and the validity of the instruction is tested. At this point, the reflective educator should contemplate whether or not he or she had the desired impact on his or her students.

TEACHING TIP: The number one way educators sabotage themselves is by not allowing themselves sufficient time to prepare. When they don't schedule adequate time to be creative, update their material, or simply review their lesson plans before presenting, they give students less than their best.

Positive Attributes

Along with being creative, other basic positive qualities contribute to one's becoming an effective instructor. Chickering and Gamson reviewed 50 years of research on effective teaching. They identified seven common principles of good teaching practice, which were later validated by additional research findings. They concluded that effective teaching involves the following[16]:

- Frequent student-faculty contact
- Encouragement and cooperation among students
- Use of active learning techniques
- Prompt feedback
- Emphasis on time on task
- Communication of high expectations
- Respect for diverse talents and ways of learning

Negative Attributes

The positive attributes of effective instructors have been described throughout most of this chapter; however, it is equally important here to point out certain negative attributes that can define an instructor. Provided in the following paragraphs is a brief list of characteristics that generally are considered to be negative characteristics within the classroom environment. The educator who becomes familiar with these styles of teaching will likely have greater success in avoiding them.

Dominating instructors have difficulty organizing and running discussions. They demonstrate low levels of participation in student activities, especially if they don't learn to control this negative characteristic.

Noncurrent (out-of-touch) instructors have difficulty clarifying issues, beliefs, and problems. These instructors also tend to have problems explaining, informing, and demonstrating.

Egocentric instructors **(instructors who believe the world revolves around them)** have difficulty referring students to other people and offices. They try to be their students' only source of information. In addition, these instructors find it almost impossible to defend other faculty, course directors, or agencies. They lay blame for any problem in the course to some external source, rather than taking responsibility.

Burned-out instructors find it nearly impossible to motivate or encourage students.

Curriculum-based versus student-based instructors (i.e., instructors who place more importance on the curriculum than on the student) find it very difficult to clarify questions and to construct tests. These instructors have trouble getting into a student's head and seeing the class from the student's perception.

BOX 1-4 Keeping Your Career Batteries Charged

by Melissa Alexander

Ever wonder about those people in EMS education whose careers follow a path not unlike that of a well-known television commercial rabbit playing his little bass drum? Meanwhile, is your career at a standstill (you know, like the bunny with Brand X batteries)? How does one survive and grow in a career in EMS education? Building a career in EMS education is not essentially different than building a career in any other discipline. The first step, of course, is to have a clear picture of what a "successful career" means to you. Setting goals is essential, but not enough in itself. What does it take to achieve career goals?

Experienced career advisors suggest that once you have determined your goals, the following behaviors are important to achieving them: producing quality work, cultivating your image, learning the power structure of your organization, acquiring command of valuable resources, staying visible, not staying too long in a job that's not meeting your needs for career growth, finding a mentor, supporting your boss, staying mobile, thinking laterally, focusing on life-long learning, and developing a network of colleagues. The remainder of this article focuses on the specific use of these concepts in the field of EMS education.

PRODUCING QUALITY WORK

Quality work is absolutely necessary, but not sufficient for career growth. Mediocre work may allow some to attain a degree of advancement, but his or her weaknesses will eventually cut short the opportunities to advance. What is "good work" in EMS education? Examples of good work include excellence in teaching, excellence in scholarly work (publications, research, etc.) and excellence in service to the profession through involvement in professional organizations.

CULTIVATING YOUR IMAGE

The way in which others in your organization and in the profession perceive you is critical to your opportunities for advancement. And while it should go without saying, appearance is an important part of your professional image. The expectation for the degree of formality of dress is a function of organizational culture. While khakis and a polo shirt may be acceptable at certain times and places, take note of how those whom you consider successful in the field dress and carry themselves. Image also refers to your professional substance and comportment. Practice the qualities for which you want to be known. Additional items of which others take note when assessing your image include things such as grammar and the presence or absence of distracting mannerisms.

LEARNING THE POWER STRUCTURE

As an astute reader, you know this means "politics." Organizational charts depict the organization's official power structure. But, as you have most likely learned from experi-

Continued

ence, most organizations have an "unofficial" power structure consisting of individuals who are influential, but not necessarily because of their job title. These people may possess personal power within an organization stemming from debts owed to them by others in the organization. Knowledge of the organizational power structure allows you to function more successfully within an organization.

STAYING VISIBLE

Often, his or her supervisor only indirectly, at best, knows the quality of work of an educator. Working autonomously has its rewards, but in order to maintain a presence, and thus be thought of when projects and opportunities arise, you will need to make your accomplishments known to your supervisor and influential others, without bravado. This can be accomplished, for example, by giving progress reports on projects. Being seen at social functions, professional conferences, and meetings is important as well. Your attendance not only makes you visible, but portrays your support of the organization. These functions can include everything from an afternoon tea reception for the dean to going to company picnics to showing up for your community college's athletic events. The important thing is, if you have an opportunity to be seen and portray a positive image, take it.

NOT STAYING IN A JOB THAT ISN'T MEETING YOUR CAREER NEEDS

If you aren't getting the opportunities you need in your current position, start looking for a position with more to offer. Staying in an unsatisfactory position for a prolonged period of time indicates a lack of initiative. When interviewing for jobs, ask specifically about opportunities for career growth and professional activities. Is the company or institution you're looking at on the cutting edge, or is it a place that doesn't encourage risk-taking and creativity? What is the program's reputation in the EMS community and EMS education community? Find out as much as you can about the organizational culture and whether or not it will be a good "fit" for you professionally and personally.

FINDING A MENTOR

Learning can be a great experience, but life's hard lessons are best learned vicariously. A mentor is someone who is experienced, influential, and well respected in the field. Find someone in EMS education whose work you admire and who can give you guidance and support in your own career. Mentors are important in providing you with contacts and opportunities in the field. You may or may not find a suitable mentor within your place of employment. You can also find a mentor through professional organizations.

SUPPORTING YOUR BOSS

Your success, at least in the short term, depends on your relationship with your immediate supervisor. It is your supervisor who assesses your performance and makes decisions regarding promotion, opportunities, pay increases and retention. If your boss is well respected in the field, being supportive of him or her will help you be recognized, as well. Conversely, if your boss lacks power in your organization or in the field (either regionally or nationally), or is perceived as being incompetent, evaluation of your performance by your boss is not likely to be meaningful to others. If an imminent change in departmental structure is not likely, consider changing positions.

STAYING MOBILE

The best opportunities don't often happen in our own backyards. The number of great positions available at any given time in EMS education is small. In recent years, there has been a leveling off in the number of new programs. Being willing to move to where the opportunity presents itself makes it more likely that you will find an appealing position.

THINKING LATERALLY

Promotion up the ladder is not the only way to advance your career. Additionally, there is an inverse relationship between the rank of the position and the number of positions available, creating a "bottleneck" effect. Lateral moves, such as from a proprietary company or a municipal agency, to a college or university can enrich your experience portfolio. You may find a niche in a different type of organization, or find that you prefer doing continuing education to doing primary education. Advancing up the ladder can also distance you from the educational process as administrative duties increase.

FOCUSING ON LIFELONG LEARNING

Make yourself a valuable commodity by stocking your skills bag with expertise demanded by the marketplace. As the base of general knowledge continues to expand, it becomes harder and harder to be a generalist, either as a clinician or an educator. Select two or three areas of interest and become an expert in them. Read professional journals to keep abreast of changes in the field. As EMS and EMS education become more complex, the demand for educators with undergraduate and graduate degrees is increasing. Many programs in adult education offer the opportunity to develop projects for credit that are also directly related to the job, making more efficient use of your time as both a student and working adult.

DEVELOPING A NETWORK OF COLLEAGUES

Having a network of contacts has many benefits. Often, the best jobs are those that you learn about by word of mouth. Having a variety of contacts in the local health care and educational communities makes you valuable to your employer. It makes you a person who can get things done. The more people you know in the field, the more opportunities you will have for collaboration and involvement in meaningful projects.

SUMMARY

There is more to being successful than just "doing a good job." Career advancement does not happen by luck or chance for most people, but through opportunities they as individuals have created through the careful artistry of career development. Keep your career batteries charged so you can keep going, and going, and going, and . . .

From NAEMSE, Domain, Fall 2001.

TEACHING TIP: The best ways to avoid developing negative teaching characteristics are the following:

- Equally balance decisions between what is good for the course and what is good for students
- Be a student. This, more than anything else, helps instructors to see things from the student's perspective
- Remember that students need different levels of support at different times in the class
- Be constantly alert to pressures in one's outside life that may creep into the classroom
- Don't overcommit. It is better to say "no" to teaching a class than to teach it poorly

SUMMARY

To teach effectively, educators must decide what kind of instructor they want to become; they must possess a teaching philosophy; and they need to be able to identify attributes of effective teachers. A clear understanding of the definition and characteristics of being *professional* can help to clarify one's long-term career goals of becoming an effective, and maybe even an extraordinary, educator. Having a good grasp of how being professional also means being ethical and striving for excellence helps to guide educators along their journey. Moreover, an understanding of the concepts of *novel* and *useful* teaching strategies can help instructors to focus on what they need to be doing along the way. Finally, periodic review and contemplation of the attributes of an effective instructor—and the negative characteristics—helps one to develop into the best instructor that one can become.

REFERENCES

1. Blumenthal. The vital role of professionalism in health care reform. *Health Aff.* 1994;13(Part I):252-256.
2. Cruess. Professionalism must be taught. *BMJ.* 1997;315: 1674-1677.
3. Hensel, Dicky. Teaching professionalism: passing the torch. *Acad Med.* 1998;73:865-870. Abstract.
4. Relman. Education to defend professional values in the new corporate age. *Acad Med.* 1998;73:1229-1233. Abstract.
5. Reynolds. Reaffirming professionalism through the education community. *Ann Intern Med.* 1996;120:609-614.
6. Swick. Academic medicine must deal with the clash of business and professional values. *Acad Med.* 1998;73:751. Abstract.
7. Swick, Simpson. Fostering the professional development of medical students. *Teach Learn Med.* 1995;7:55-60.
8. Wynia, Latham, Kao, Berg, Emanuel. Medical professionalism in society. *N Engl J Med.* 1999;341:1612-1616.
9. Swick. Toward a normative definition of medical professionalism. *Acad Med.* 2000;75:612-616.
10. Sullivan. *Work and Integrity: The Crisis and Promise of Professionalism in America.* New York, NY: Harper Collins; 1995.
11. Southon, Braithwaite. The end of professionalism? *Soc Sci Med.* 1998;46:23-28.
12. Schwenk TL, Whitman N. *The Physician as Teacher.* Baltimore: Williams & Wilkins; 1987.
13. Kestin. Creativity in teaching and learning. *Am Sci.* 1970;58:250-257.
14. Stein. *Stimulating Creativity.* Vol 1: Individual Procedures. New York, NY: Academic Press; 1974.
15. Whiting. *Creative Thinking.* New York, NY: Reinhold Press; 1958.
16. Chickering AW, Gamson ZF. Seven principles for good practice in undergraduate education. *AAHE Bulletin.* 1987;39:3-7.

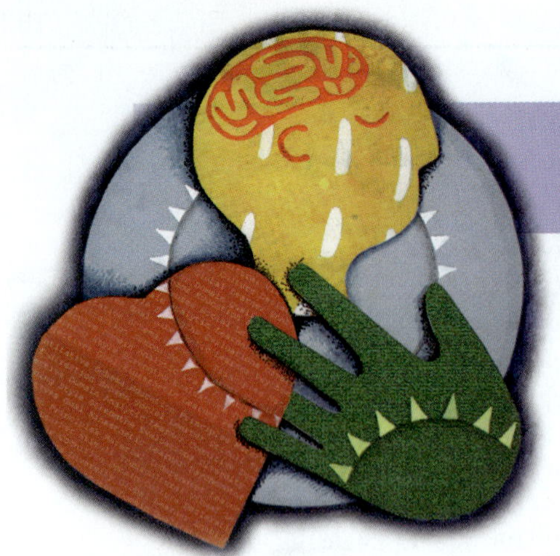

CHAPTER 2

EMS Educator Roles

"We teach to change the world. The hope that undergirds our efforts to help students learn is that doing this will help them act toward each other and their environment with compassion, understanding, and fairness."

—Brookfield, 1995

The role of the educator encompasses more than simply teaching students in the classroom setting. The educator must have a thorough understanding of the scope of his or her responsibilities, which this chapter examines. One of the main responsibilities is teaching with a team mentality. Although an educator may spend considerable time as the only instructor in the classroom setting, a team approach to teaching enriches the adult learning environment. To facilitate this, it is important to identify the names and roles of other persons who constitute the instructional team. For the purpose of this chapter, the following definitions are used.

Primary instructor: A person who possesses the appropriate academic or allied health credentials, an understanding of the principles and theories of education, and the required teaching experience necessary to provide quality instruction to students.

Secondary instructor: A person who possesses the appropriate academic or allied health credentials and an understanding of the principles and theories of education, and who may have *limited* teaching experience. Secondary instructors are responsible for assisting primary instructors and providing instruction to students. In some situations, they may be responsible for lab exercises in which students practice psychomotor skills. The secondary instructor may even conduct classes on specific topics within his or her realm of expertise. The teaching skills that the secondary instructor possesses determine his or her specific responsibilities within the classroom.

RESPONSIBILITIES OF THE PRIMARY INSTRUCTOR

The primary instructor may be called upon to provide leadership or supervision over a series of courses, or even over an entire EMS education program. Additionally, he or she may be called upon to provide the coordination of courses within a program.

Frequently, primary instructors are responsible for documenting student progress and course work progression. They have a responsibility to provide timely feedback to students concerning their progress toward successful completion of the course. In some circumstances, this feedback (with the students' written permission) may be shared with other persons, such as students' employers or sponsors.

Course coordination, an important role of many primary instructors may include coordinating visiting faculty and guest lecturers and scheduling and supervising secondary instructors. Moreover, the primary instructor may guide the development, maintenance, and assignment of clinical rotations and pre–hospital internship experiences.

The primary instructor may also be chiefly responsible for the development of policies and procedures for courses or for the program. These policies govern such activities as the selection and screening of students, the practices of student discipline, and the evaluation of outcomes.

Additionally, the primary instructor is often asked to identify sources of disciplinary problems and to suggest solutions. In such situations, he or she must be able to work closely with the medical director, school or facility administrator, other faculty, and students to resolve problems in the classroom or clinical setting.

Furthermore, primary instructors are frequently involved in the provision of remedial instruction. They must be able to assess both students and situations to identify the causes of problems; then, they must develop workable strategies to help students to succeed.

RESPONSIBILITIES OF THE SECONDARY INSTRUCTOR

Similar to the role of primary instructor, the secondary instructor's role is often defined by the scope of assigned responsibility in the classroom, lab, hospital, or field. The two main responsibilities of secondary instructors are to provide instruction to students and to support primary instructors. Secondary instructors generally possess an entry level teaching competency and are not expected to perform with the same proficiency as an "experienced" instructor. Because the primary instructor often sets the tone for the class, the secondary instructor must be aware of curriculum expectations, acceptable presentation styles, and rules and regulations pertinent to the class. The optimal relationship between the primary and the secondary instructor is one in which mentoring and professional growth take place for both individuals (Figure 2-1).

In summary, the primary instructor is responsible for the largest part of the classroom experience. Together, primary and secondary instructors are expected to deliver the curriculum, mentor and support each other, and ensure that the program and the students continually strive to meet high standards. The breadth of responsibility assigned to both levels of instructors reinforces the need for participation in a program of teaching instruction before one enters the field of education.

STUDENT EXPECTATIONS OF EDUCATORS

Erving Goffman wrote extensively about student expectations of educators and the ways that educators can sabotage themselves by failing to meet these expectations. The following information about role expectations is adapted from his work.[1]

Students have certain basic expectations of their instructors. Since every new and seasoned educator was once a student and likely returns to that role time and again, it would seem that he or she would have a solid understanding of student expectations. However, when one is taking on the role of educator, it is always helpful to be reminded of, and to keep in mind, certain basic expectations that students have (Table 2-1).

The educator's level of experience, training, and position give the educator a different worldview than that of his or her students. In accordance with this, educators are generally expected to suppress their feelings and to convey a professional demeanor that is stoic, pleasant, and welcoming. This is similar to the expectation that the caregiver will comfort a dying patient by touching the patient's hand and saying something such as, "We are going to do everything that we can to take good care of you."

Educators have many modalities for expressing themselves and conveying their role, including the words they speak, facial and postural signs, tone of voice, and inflection. This expressive repertoire also includes the insignia of office or rank, uniform or clothing, age, and grooming. Just as the EMT dresses in uniform for quick identification and acceptance by patients, so should the EMS educator dress for respect and professionalism.

Students expect educators to have the ability to communicate the course content. Educators can spoil the impression that they want to make by forgetting content, appearing nervous or self-conscious, or giving

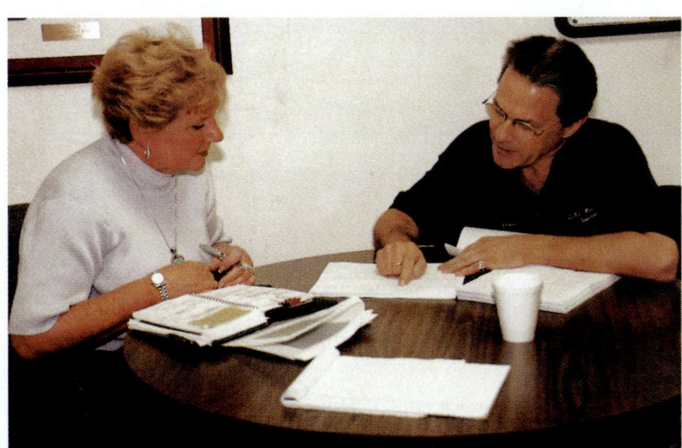

FIGURE 2-1 Mentoring a new instructor is a rewarding experience for both primary and secondary instructors.

TABLE 2-1 Student Expectations

Professionalism	A calm, pleasant, and stoic demeanor A positive and welcoming attitude Appropriate appearance and conduct, even in settings other than the formal classroom or learning laboratory
Competence	Ability to clearly communicate content and ideas, expressing complex and difficult concepts in ways that make them understandable and memorable Ability to demonstrate skills
Investment in student success	Positive, encouraging attitude that shows that learning can be achieved

way to inappropriate outbursts of laughter or anger. Additionally, students expect their instructors to provide them with a simplified view of the course and material up front.

Educators can sabotage themselves in a number of ways in trying to establish their role and authority within the classroom. Most notably, students sense when an educator is not personally invested in student success, and they may react negatively to this perceived indifference. Moreover, students neither expect nor need their educators to be on the same social plane that they are on. Thus, an educator's appearance and manner should set him or her apart from students. Confusion is likely to occur if instructors *appear* to have greater professional status than their students but *act* in an equalitarian, intimate, or even apologetic manner.

Students expect educators to behave as educators at all times. Educators are never offstage when students are present. Educators must be aware of the regions in which they perform their roles. Front regions, such as classrooms and offices, include areas where educators perform formal roles for the observation of their students. But even in back regions, such as hallways, faculty lounges, and out-of-class settings, where educators may wish to relax and express their "true feelings," they must remember that they are always subject to student expectations and are never truly offstage. The *Case in Point* at right demonstrates how a primary instructor and a teaching assistant violated the boundary expectations between students and instructors.

CASE IN POINT

The paramedic class invited its instructors to the post-midterm exam party. The primary instructor and his teaching assistant went to the party, believing in collegiality and bonding with students. It seemed like a good way to relieve stress and build a closer relationship with the class.

However, one student began drinking straight shots of whiskey between beers and started to become visibly intoxicated. Two other students were becoming argumentative over a personal matter. The lead instructor maintained his composure and suggested that they hold off on any arguments while the party was going on. The two students looked at him and saw his look of disapproval. They resented his interference but ceased their argument, respecting his role as instructor. A third student, an attractive young woman, began openly flirting with the teaching assistant, who was flattered and enjoyed the attention. After all, it was just a harmless party. It was time to relax.

Everyone left an hour later and drove home. None should have been behind the wheel of an automobile. Fortunately, there were no accidents, and no tickets were received.

Three days later, the lead instructor was called into the Dean's office and was confronted about the party. "I understand that you went out and socialized with the class after the midterm exam. Is that correct?"

"Yes, it is," the lead instructor responded, growing nervous. "Is something wrong? Did something happen?"

The Dean leaned forward with hands on his desk and spoke in a very deliberate and controlled voice. "Yes. Something happened. You drank socially with some underage students. You got into an argument. You have a complaint filed against you and your teaching assistant for inappropriate conduct. You have very likely compromised your ability to lead this class any further. At minimum, you have compromised your ability to keep this class on a professional plane. You will need to write a letter of explanation to be considered by the faculty review committee. I do not know what the outcome will be."

No formal action was ever taken. The verbal warning was sufficient. It was a hard lesson. The educator is always on stage and is never on the same social plane as the students.

EDUCATOR RESPONSIBILITIES

Many new educators assume that the bulk of their time will be spent in preparing and delivering lectures. The reality is that educators have many additional duties and must have the skills and characteristics to adapt to these other responsibilities. Although it is true that whenever an instructor teaches a new class, he or she can expect to dedicate considerable time and effort toward the preparation and delivery of course materials, this "advance" work will decrease each time the class is taught. Additional administrative duties and responsibilities will generally increase and expand and will increasingly consume a large part of the educator's time.

Preparing for the Class

Good teaching appears effortless. This is true in performances in sports, the arts, and clinical care. Professional competence is smooth and seamless. Amateurish performances appear jerky and look extremely difficult. How do those professional athletes, musicians, and clinicians make their performances look so easy? They prepare in advance with countless hours of practice and preparation. To achieve the appearance of effortless and smooth instruction, the educator needs to prepare a game plan and build a resource collection well in advance of the first class session.

CASE IN POINT

It was just another day of the week. The ECG rhythm class was from 8 AM to 10 AM. The materials and handouts were ready. The lab was scheduled from 10 AM to NOON, so equipment had to be set up early that morning, a task that the teaching assistant handled. A curriculum committee meeting was planned to take place over lunch. The state conference would be held in 3 months, and the objectives, description, and handouts were needed by next week, so the literature search and slide presentation outline had to be done this week. Cardiac Case Scenarios were this afternoon, and these needed to be pulled from last year. The Cardiac Module exam was Friday, and it still had to be finalized and printed. At least 20% of the questions needed to be "switched out," and another 20% had to be modified so that the security and integrity of the exam could be maintained and the finer points of the exam kept up-to-date. Student evaluations from the Respiratory Module had just been received, so the evaluation summary had to be completed and reviewed. Two students failed the Respiratory Modular exam and needed to be counseled to pass the retest. It had to be made clear that they could not fail any other exams, or they would be dismissed from the course exam. The county EMS Council met that evening to discuss the latest legislative initiative to cut funding. It was a critical meeting that could not be missed. The local EMS chief had just called to say that one of the internship students did not know the local protocols and was rude about it when confronted. The student was sent home and was not welcome back. A vendor stopped in to demonstrate the latest in spinal immobilization equipment.

It was 7 AM, and the alarm had just gone off. It was just another day in the life of an EMS educator.

Developing adjunct materials to stimulate class discussion and learning

It is helpful for the instructor to have preplanned scenarios, discussion topics, and quizzes that have been developed and made available well before the first class meets. These adjunct materials should support and coordinate lessons that are being taught. Audiovisual materials, for example, can be used to support lectures and presentations, but they may take a surprising amount of time to develop. The Internet is an excellent source for images, but use of these images requires that the educator must have the resources to scan existing photographs and convert slide images. Creating a file of supporting classroom activities for each block of course material is time intensive but worthwhile.

Ordering and operating equipment

A surprising amount of time and effort can go into ordering, maintaining, and cleaning equipment. Anything that can be done to help minimize this work, time, and energy spent will be helpful. For instance, an instructor may set up a routine for periodic ordering of new supplies and equipment; assign students to help clean, repair, and move equipment and supplies on a schedule; and acquire adequate room to store, organize, and maintain the equipment (Figure 2-2).

Developing class materials and handouts

Nearly every organization or institution of higher education gives educators preparatory time to develop class materials and handouts, usually at least in a ratio of 3:1 for each hour of instruction. Tasks associated with developing and maintaining class instructional materials and handouts should take much more time than it takes to deliver the material. It is essential that the educator schedule sufficient time for this work every semester. For the first time that one is teaching a class, a good rule of thumb is to schedule at least three times as much time for preparation as for instruction. After the first time, it may be sufficient to schedule 1 hour of preparation for each hour of instruction. However, instructors who teach the same lecture with the same materials year after year eventually find themselves the object of student scorn. Updates and revisions are essential, particularly in the healthcare field.

Participating in professional activities

It is critically important that educators participate in professional activities outside the educational organization. Professional associations and conferences provide an excellent way for educators to stay current

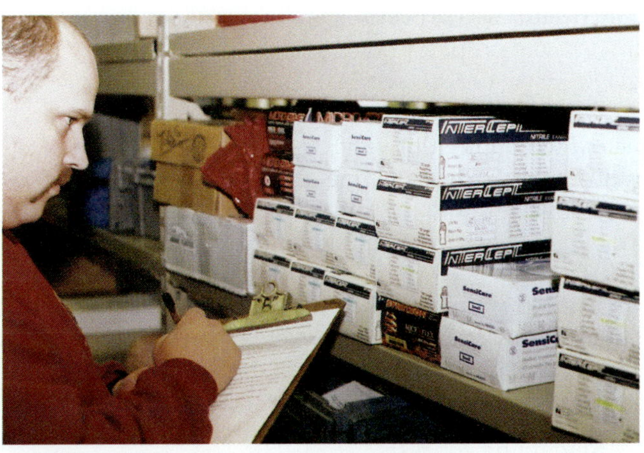

FIGURE 2-2 The instructor may need to assume responsibility for ordering equipment and supplies.

both in content-related areas and in new teaching methods and strategies. In addition, professional networking can contribute significantly to a program's success through the sharing of resources and ideas. Every EMS educator should consider joining local, state, and national EMS educator associations.

Teaching the Class

Organizing and leading discussion sessions

It is important that a portion of each class be devoted to discussion of the curriculum. Two of the most valuable and effective ways of achieving this are (1) to start each lecture or session with a brief overview of the learning objectives, and (2) to follow each session with a brief summary of the key learning points. (See Part IV, Delivering the Message, Chapters 12-18, for a more in-depth look at teaching methods.) As has been mentioned previously, developing an engaging discussion that prompts students to share their ideas and views is a time-consuming but worthy investment of time.

Explaining lab procedures and assignments

In EMS clinical education, practical sessions, or "labs," should account for approximately half of the total amount of time spent in the course. These should include practical skills workshops, patient assessment exercises, and patient care scenarios. Developing labs is just as time intensive as developing lectures. Preparing for invasive labs, such as intravenous and medication administration workshops, generally takes much more time than inexperienced educators may think it would take. Be sure to allow enough time to obtain and set up the necessary equipment and supplies, and to schedule and brief any secondary instructors. If secondary instructors are paid employees, then additional recruitment and hiring time may be needed. The hiring and orientation process can take months in some cases.

Making and grading tests

The development of valid tests is a highly specialized skill. A great deal of time, energy, and expense goes into ensuring that a test is valid. (See Part V, "Evaluation," for more information on evaluation.) Most EMS educators develop a bank of test questions and answers from which to generate their tests. Although this saves considerable time, even these tests need to be updated and validated.

Reviewing for tests

It is common in EMS education for educators to conduct review sessions before tests are given. However, students rarely come to these review sessions prepared with questions. To avoid teaching directly to the test, the instructor might consider preparing a number of challenging applied patient problems for students to discuss. In this way, the instructor will be able to give the students a thorough review without giving away the specific material included on the test.

Evaluating student performance

It is time consuming for the educator to develop fair and effective criteria for grading student performance. Developing grading criteria is more of a process than a single event, and the educator should never stop trying to improve the evaluation process. Good educators have multiple performance references to use in evaluating their students' performance—attendance, participation, test scores, practical skills scores, projects, and scenario testing, for example. Developing, reevaluating, refining, recording, and providing feedback on these different reference points takes time and effort.

Using feedback to improve

No matter how expert one's course coordinator, no matter how competent the medical director, no matter how talented the cadre of educators, students will likely find fault with some aspect of the program. It is the educator's responsibility to anticipate a certain degree of criticism and discontent, and to maintain a positive and constructive attitude that preserves the learning community. Spending time listening to constructive criticism communicates an important sense of caring. Students are typically focused on their singular critical and immediate task—passing the course. Rarely will they be able to comprehend the larger issues associated with curriculum development, course coordination, and limits on the instructors and the educational program. In spite of this, the instructor can typically obtain helpful information that may lead to improvements in course delivery, clinical assignments, and internship experiences.

Teaching procedures

When a competent instructor demonstrates and explains procedures, most students readily comprehend them and feel comfortable with what they have seen. However, that does not mean that most students will be able to do the procedure themselves. Teaching students a procedure requires that each step be broken down, demonstrated, and explained, followed as soon as possible by student performance of each step with careful monitoring and coaching. Once students master the steps, they should be coached through several complete sequences. Finally, they should be given the chance to perform the skill in the context of patient care scenarios.

Administrative Tasks and Duties

Holding instructor meetings

Departmental meetings are a necessary part of staying connected with the broader picture (Figure 2-3). The educator should eagerly participate in faculty meetings, as curriculum development and educational design are best accomplished collaboratively. Sharing information about student progress and performance is also important, so that problems can be identified and a plan of action initiated. Additionally, clinical issues or procedures may need to be reviewed together to promote instructor consistency.

Developing a budget

Education is a business. Facilities, instructional materials, and instructors cost money. Sources of revenue are required to fund an educational program. Thus, developing and maintaining a budget is a significant part of the education administrator's responsibilities. This often means seeking out external sources of funding, such as grants and donations.

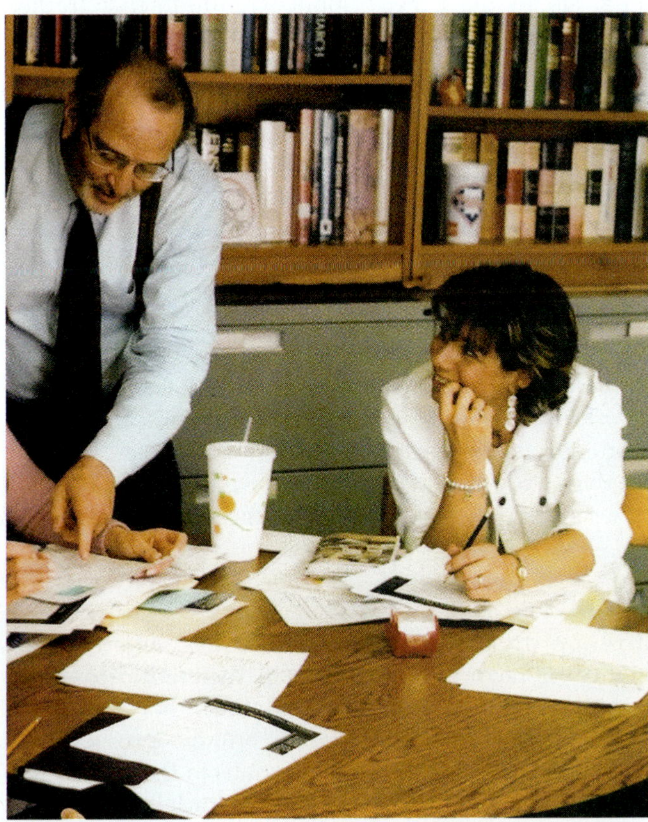

FIGURE 2-3 It is important to hold faculty meetings to discuss important topics, such as student progress, curriculum development, and exam item development.

Evaluating personnel

Scheduling times for evaluating and providing frequent feedback for educators and any educational support personnel is a vital and necessary part of the EMS education administrator's job. The administrator's role includes working with primary and secondary instructors to ensure that they are developing appropriate skills as educators. It may also be helpful for the administrator to periodically clarify job responsibilities.

Maintaining departmental records and reports

Records of enrollment, curricula, counseling, schedules, attendance, grades, attrition, and successful completion are all critical to the educational institution. These constitute fundamental legal documentation. Reports to various agencies are also required and may seem endless. The Committee on Accreditation of EMS Professions (CoAEMSP) requires an annual report from accredited programs to document their evaluation of the program's success toward achievement of program goals and objectives. These documents are also significant in helping with and supporting future decisions, such as justifying the hiring of additional staff or the purchase of more equipment.

Attending committee meetings

In addition to the vital role of teaching, most educators in academic institutions are expected to improve the overall environment of the organization and the community. This includes serving on a variety of educational committees whose work can range from long-term curriculum development, to admissions, to handling of student grievances.

Attending advisory committee meetings

All EMS educators should form either a formal or an informal advisory committee. An advisory committee should be representative of the community in which the EMS program operates. Individual persons involved in an advisory committee typically include representatives of employers of graduates, hospital personnel, regulatory agency representatives, graduates, members of the local medical community, and consumers. Program personnel, such as program director or course coordinator and medical director, as well as program faculty, are also included but may be *ex officio* members. Specifically, the goal of the advisory committee is to provide feedback on the program and on how it is meeting the community's EMS educational needs. Difficult program decisions such as admission requirements and effective evaluation criteria are often less contentious with advisory committee involvement.

Participating in state and local rule-making committees

Educators who do not participate in their EMS regulatory committees at the local, state, or national level lose their ability to effectively voice their concerns and opinions on many vital issues. It is imperative that educators be involved in these issues and decisions; seemingly insignificant issues can result in the need for additional resources or instructional time in an already overbooked schedule. Additionally, EMS providers and regulators may inadvertently overlook important educational issues when changing rules or adding medical drugs or procedures.

Maintaining clinical expertise

A difficult task, particularly for full-time educators, is maintaining clinical competency. Although educators can attend classes or read journals to keep abreast of new technology and cutting edge content, clinical skills may be more time-consuming to maintain. Often, the educator must work or volunteer part time for an EMS service to maintain patient care skills. Some academic institutions encourage instructors to work clinically by having a 35-hour work week or a 9-month contract. When possible, some educators participate actively with students in hospital and field settings, thus maintaining a level of clinical interaction.

STUDENT ISSUES

Holding Conferences

Some students, particularly those who are not progressing satisfactorily, need one-on-one time for feedback, tutorial help, and counseling (Figure 2-4). Each student should, at minimum, have the opportunity to talk with the primary instructor privately at the course midpoint to discuss his or her progress. If the student is progressing satisfactorily, this meeting can be brief. On the other hand, if the student is failing to meet minimum class standards, the educator must be prepared to give the student specific information pertaining to his or her performance deficits, along with concrete examples of how to improve this performance. Records of these meetings must be placed in students' files.

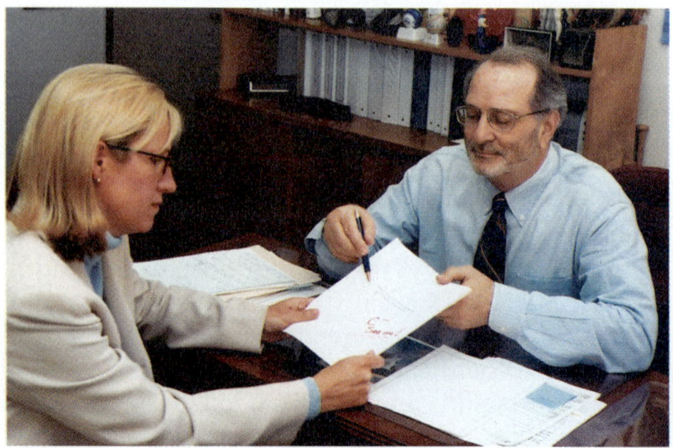

FIGURE 2-4 Student-teacher conferences provide students with valuable feedback about their performance.

Referring Students to Other People and Offices

Another role of the educator is to refer students to appropriate counseling resources or potential employers. The educator might refer a student to a career opportunity, to remedial classes, or for diagnostic testing, as might be the case with a student with a suspected learning disability.

Motivating Students to Complete Class Assignments

Some students do not require motivation to complete class assignments on time, but many do. The educator must take time and energy from his or her already busy schedule to devise strategies that encourage students to meet performance requirements, rather than simply nagging them to do so. Enforcing deadlines and dealing with students who do not meet deadlines, however, requires even greater time and energy. Educators can include two items in the curriculum to assist this effort. First, every assignment and due date should be printed on the course syllabus that is distributed and reviewed on the first day of class. Second, the consequences of missing the deadlines must be spelled out. Many educators are very clear about the assignments in their syllabus but do not explain the consequences of failing to complete assignments, making a faulty leap in logic that suggests that students will intuitively understand the ramifications. Finally, every student must be treated in the same way. If one student receives extra time to complete an assignment, then all other students in the class must receive the same.

Writing Letters of Reference

It is appropriate for students to request letters of reference or recommendation from their educators. An instructor may wish to set guidelines that determine what type of recommendation will be provided. A good place to publish these criteria is in the course syllabus. Some common requirements for letters of reference include a student's taking more than one course with the educator, earning above average grades (generally a B or better), exhibiting positive professional learning attitudes, not having disciplinary problems, and doing something to contribute positively to the class or program (e.g., helping with a research project or guest lecturing).

Counseling Students on Personal Issues

Because the educator instills respect and trust, some students will approach him or her for personal advice and guidance. Sometimes, even when they are not seeking advice and guidance, they may bring their personal issues to the instructor. Most educators spend a small part of their week dealing with personal issues of their students. It is paramount that the educator respect the student's feelings and confidentiality in these matters. It is also critically important that privacy is provided for these discussions. Developing a list of community resources and having them readily available for making referrals is also essential. Common issues that can be expected include pregnancies, work terminations, evictions, physical abuse, personal illness, illness of a loved one, loss of financial aid, substance abuse, harassment from other students, learning disabilities, and conflicts in schedules. Knowing the institution's policies and resources on these issues will go a long way in helping the educator to determine what role to have in these issues. It is also critically important that the educator know the responsible professional limits and liabilities of acting in the role of counselor. The profession of counseling is now licensed in most states, and several levels of professional counseling licenses are available, including Licensed Mental Health Counselor and Licensed Professional Clinical Counselor. An educator who means well might offer counseling and comfort to a student who later attempts suicide or commits some violent act; the educator could be liable for practicing as a counselor without a license.

Advising Students on a Career

In most cases, students take EMS courses in hopes of obtaining a job. A vital part of the EMS educator's job is developing contacts within the local EMS community to help place students. Hosting career days is another way some schools meet this need. Educators must stay current on various job requirements, salaries, and employment practices.

Tutoring Students

A few general approaches can be taken to providing remedial tutoring. One is to set aside time on a regular basis each week. A second, ideal approach is to seek available tutorial resources within the institution or larger community. A third approach is to assign tutorial responsibilities to a secondary instructor, if there is one.

Some precautionary notes apply to providing tutoring, however. The first is to be careful to set limits on the time that services will be provided, as some students have a need that is impossible to fill. If unlimited tutoring is offered, some students will take up that offer. Not only will the educator's time be drained, but the student may still fail, and the failure becomes the responsibility of the educator. A second cautionary note is that it is best to tutor only in open groups, never by private or exclusive appointment.

Encouraging Class Groups

Nearly every class hits a slump at some point. This usually occurs about three quarters of the way through the class. Remember that a major role of the educator is that of coach. Many educators find that they give motivational talks to nearly every class at some point.

Clarifying Issues, Beliefs, and Problems

No matter how brilliant the lectures, no matter how well crafted the syllabus, key points and policies must be reiterated multiple times. This is a matter of human nature. There is no point in being despondent over the need to do this.

TEACHING TIP: Anything worth saying is worth repeating three times—especially to tired, overloaded, overwhelmed students.

COMMON ROLE ADJUSTMENTS

Overall, the educator is expected to handle the teaching load and to continue on the path toward growth and scholarly excellence. Perhaps the most challenging aspect is balancing one's professional and personal lives. The second most challenging aspect is keeping one's clinical skills sharp.

The roles and expectations of the beginning EMS educator are new and very different from those of the EMS care provider. These new roles and expectations are more than just an extension of those clinical roles. They require a new set of assertive behaviors, for the power structure and length of relationships with students are completely different from those between care provider and patient. These new roles and expectations challenge and test the educator's teaching abilities.

One of the first and most important challenges facing the new educator is that of establishing authority and credibility in the classroom. After establishing authority, the educator must be able to exercise that authority prudently. This textbook and other education literature can offer effective guidelines for establishing and exercising authority as an educator; however, there are no foolproof guidelines that apply in every situation. Each class, as a group, and each educator, individually, are unique.

Four characteristics of the educator help establish authority in the classroom: experience, expectations, knowledge, and goals.

Experience Versus Authority

In general, an older educator relies more on teaching experience than on the authority of a title or position. Often, new educators learn the hard way that the title of *instructor* does not automatically impart esteem or credibility in a class. New instructors often learn that humility and deferential behaviors are typically more powerful with students than is authoritarian bluster. The educator's ability to deal with the thousand and one challenges of teaching far outweighs any badge of authority that goes with the title *instructor*. This same phenomenon can be seen in the streets, where respect for EMS caregivers is earned through competent performance.

CASE IN POINT

The new EMS educator recently hired by the local community college had 10 years of experience in EMS and had been a practicing paramedic for 7 of those last years. She was highly respected for her clinical skills, and she had a great personality to go with it. She was perfect for the instructor position at the local community college. Today was her first day in class.

She was a little nervous as she walked into class as lead instructor for the first time and faced 23 students. She was more nervous than she had ever imagined she could be, realizing that she was now responsible for maintaining course continuity, covering the entire curriculum, covering for guest lecturers who did not show up, resolving disputes, counseling, providing discipline, developing and administering exams, and assigning grades. It hit her for the first time—what it meant to be the lead instructor—just as she introduced herself in her new role.

With genuine humility, a professional demeanor, and a little humor, she won over the class. She began, "Hello, this is my first day of class. You have a lot to teach me. I hope that we enjoy our journey of learning together. We're going to begin by introducing ourselves to one another. I'll start by telling you a little bit about my background, and why these folks asked me to come here to be your lead instructor."

Expectations Versus Discipline

Seasoned educators inspire students to follow and obey them simply by their professional demeanor—the way that they impart their knowledge and understanding. It is this expectation of leadership and performance more than any badge of authority that will maintain order and discipline in the classroom. The seasoned instructor rarely needs to resort to disciplinary action for misconduct in the classroom. Setting high professional and academic expectations early in the course will prove to be a valuable strategy in avoiding the use of unnecessary discipline. Most caregivers have witnessed similar scenarios in the field. Crews may naturally follow a senior paramedic or EMT whom they respect, regardless of rank or title; other supervisors or chiefs become frustrated when they are unable to lead their subordinates.

TEACHING TIP: Remember that it is always better to set high expectations at the beginning of a class, then be willing to back down a little, than to try to raise expectations later. Students will continually surprise their instructors, if given the chance to strive for high goals.

Knowledge Versus Insignia

No title, rank, or uniform will make up for a lack of content knowledge. It is hopeless for an educator to hide behind a title or position when faced with a question to which he or she does not have an answer. Seasoned educators know that students will ask questions they cannot answer. They expect these questions and honor them. Indeed, no EMS educator or any educator in any profession is expected to know every answer to every possible question. Educators who feel confident are not intimidated or threatened by questions that they cannot answer. When a question arises that they cannot immediately answer, they feel confident in telling students that they will get back to the class with the answer as soon as possible. It is also acceptable to inquire whether another student has the answer, or to assign a student to research the answer and report back to the class. Immature educators—those not yet confident in their authority or abilities—will often make up an answer or try to deflect the question. Both of these strategies leave students frustrated, and the educator's authority is undermined as a result.

TEACHING TIP: An effective strategy in dealing with difficult questions is to address them on the first day of class. The instructor might say that occasionally students will ask a question that he or she won't be able to immediately answer. When that happens, the instructor will write the question in the corner of the blackboard, and it will stay there until, together, they find the answer to the question

This approach does three things. First, it validates the students' right to ask questions. Second, it keeps the instructor off the pedestal of "infallible." Last, it keeps the educator honest and reliable in the promise to find answers to student questions.

Goals: Firm Grasp Versus Cookbook

Experienced EMS providers know what they want to accomplish for each patient, and they generally know several ways to go about it. The same is true for experienced educators. What worked in one class may not work in another. It is more important that educators have their own teaching philosophy and a clear understanding of what students need to learn than merely a series of lesson plans in cookbook fashion. The instructor should keep the educational goals in mind, and should constantly ask whether what he or she is teaching today brings him or her closer to those goals.

SUMMARY

It is paramount that educators are well grounded and comfortable in the content that they are expected to teach. Many other issues will place demands on their time and energy, and they cannot be weak in content areas. Educators also must realize that teaching is a team sport; new instructors should actively seek out resources outside the classroom to help them address some of the issues that may otherwise overwhelm them. Secondary instructors can be a valuable addition to any class, but they may not know intuitively what to do. When an educator works with secondary instructors, the time taken to mentor them will be returned many times. Finally, new educators must seek a balance between teaching obligations and personal commitments, as well as the need to maintain current clinical skills. Attention to this balance must be a high priority and should begin on the first of day of class.

REFERENCE

1. Goffman, Erving. *Presentation of Self in Everyday Life.* New York: Anchor Books; 1959.

PART II

The Student

Emergency medical services (EMS) students are as different from one another as are the patients they will eventually treat—from working adults looking for a second career to high school students who are still discovering their own selves. They come from a wide variety of backgrounds with varying levels of knowledge and life experience. Yet, each must grasp concepts and apply information that is often expected of physicians, anesthesiologists, social workers, and even race car drivers.

This part of the text provides valuable information about the general attributes of today's EMS learners. Educators will find that an understanding of the basic principles of education, including information about their students' various learning styles and factors of a supportive learning environment, will help them to meet their teaching goals and ultimately, to produce effective, well-rounded EMS personnel.

Remember, EMS students rarely present in a classic "textbook" fashion. They are human, with all their glorious strengths and weaknesses. They deserve all your knowledge, wit, and respect—and, in turn, you will receive theirs.

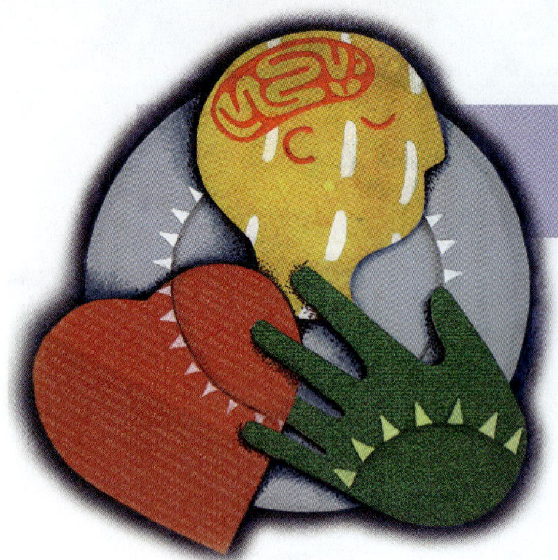

CHAPTER 3

Principles of Adult Learning

"Theories and goals of education don't matter a whit if you do not consider your students to be human beings."

—Lou Ann Walker

The emergency medical services (EMS) educator needs to become familiar with the principles of adult learning, since the typical EMS student is an adult. The learning styles, needs, responses, and expectations of adults differ from those of younger learners. Even when educators teach first responder or EMT courses to adolescents in high school, the instruction and learning follow more adult principles than those involved in teaching children.

An educator can develop certain techniques that enhance student comprehension and information retention by striving to understand and incorporate certain basic principles regarding adult learning into his or her teaching strategies. Even in the environment of ever-evolving educational theory, several concepts regarding adult learning are commonly accepted and useful in application.

This chapter is an overview of what is known about how adults learn and how they retain information, which will help educators to clarify the educational needs of adult learners. The most logical place to start such a discussion is with the basic concept of adult learning, or *andragogy.*

PEDAGOGY VERSUS ANDRAGOGY

In 1968, Malcolm Knowles introduced the concept of andragogy—the art and science of teaching adults. He used the term *andragogy* to separate adult learning principles from those centered on children, or pedagogy.[1] Andragogy is based on certain basic assumptions, which are examined here.

Autonomy and Self-Direction

Adults expect and enjoy independence, or a certain amount of autonomy, in what they learn and how they learn it. They like to have control, and they feel comfortable taking control of their learning. Moreover, for adults, learning is a process of sharing with the instructor, as well as with other students. The instructor, however, is responsible for facilitating and encouraging the student's self-direction, as opposed to simply supplying students with facts. Brookfield suggests that direction and guidance from the educator are essential because many adults actually need help in determining their learning needs.[2]

Adults approach education with the expectation of learning new skills and knowledge, and they focus on the final goal. Ultimately, they want to be well prepared to practice competently and to pass the state or national exam. In light of this, the adult is less tolerant of wasted time and tasks that have no apparent value. In fact, educators should expect more criticism from the adult learner than from the younger learner, especially when the student feels that his or her expectations are not being met.

Problem-Centered Orientation

Adults are relevancy oriented, which means they need to know *why* they are being told to learn something before they are open to learning it. Therefore, educators must ensure that learning is problem-centered, rather than subject-centered. For example, the paramedic student may not value the knowledge of human physiology until it becomes relevant to a specific medical condition that he or she will treat in the field.

Life Experience

By the time a person reaches adulthood, he or she has naturally accumulated many enriching life experiences. This gives the adult learner the advantage of being able to relate new facts and concepts to real life experiences—a fact that enriches and reinforces the adult learning experience. Because adult EMS classes typically include students with wide-ranging levels of expertise and educational backgrounds, the instructor can draw upon the adult learner's experiences and incorporate them into his or her instruction. In this adult learning model, all members of the class share information and experiences with one another. In fact, in some areas of the curriculum, students may have more information and experience than the instructor does. With this in mind, the educator should strive to ensure that class communication is multidirectional and is more of a dialogue than a lecture.

Goal Orientation

Adults are pragmatic. In other words, they want to be able to apply the information they learn immediately, or at least have some understanding of how their learning will be of direct benefit to them. Adults generally do not tolerate studying anything that they cannot apply to tasks they expect to perform. Moreover, adults appreciate an educational program that is organized with clearly defined course components that can help them to achieve their goals.

Although Knowles himself and others[2-5] have recently questioned the validity of the differences between andragogy and pedagogy, the previously mentioned attributes of adult learners can at least aid the educator in developing teaching techniques that will motivate adults to learn. Currently, learning is viewed as a continuum from childhood into adulthood; this is why the validity of different adult and child learning processes has been questioned. Rather, there seems to be a transition from approaching education from a childlike perspective (teacher-centered) to approaching it from an adult perspective (student-centered and self-directed). This transition point varies from individual to individual, and there is no discrete point at which it occurs—that is, no magical evolution takes place between high school graduation and higher education.

Other Characteristics of Adult Learners

Adult learners typically display characteristics that can be divided into two broad categories: physiologic and psychosocial. Although adults are much more diverse than children are physiologically, sociologically, and psychologically, general characteristics and central tendencies are presented here; the educator must keep in mind the individual variations.

PHYSIOLOGIC VARIABLES

Physiologic variables in adult learners specifically relate to how changes in vision, hearing, energy, and health affect learning. These variables involve the natural process of maturing.

Lighting

Instructors must provide adequate lighting to ensure that older students can view presentations and take notes. Long courses that rely heavily on audiovisual projections for most presentations can tax the eyes of the mature learner. This is particularly true for adults older than 35 years of age, yet many modern techniques of presentation fail to take this into account.

Task Performance

Although the adult's capacity to learn can remain essentially unchanged with age, the older learner has slower reaction times and less efficient senses on which to depend for learning, such as sight and hearing. In addition, the older learner may have reduced energy levels and diminished attention level as a result of fatigue (Figure 3-1).

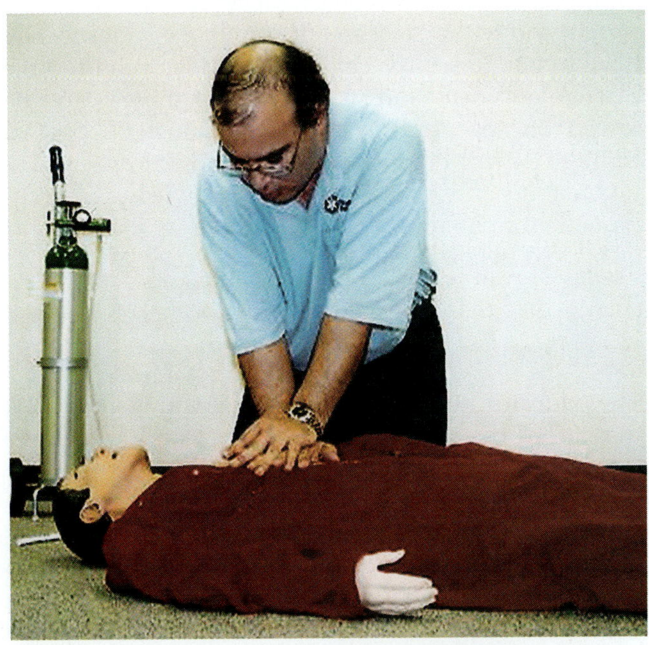

FIGURE 3-1 An older learner may become fatigued more easily than a younger student and may have slower reaction times.

Adjustment to External Temperature Changes

For an adult to learn successfully over an extended sitting period, a comfortable temperature and environmental setting is required. This is important to note because sometimes it is necessary to teach in the bay of the fire station. Anytime a room can be made comfortable with adequate temperature control, this will add significantly to the adult's ability to learn.

Distractions

For some students, pagers and cell phones may be a way of life. However, what may be only a minor nuisance or no nuisance at all to a younger learner can become an intolerable distraction to the adult learner. The educator can help to create a productive environment for adult learning by asking students to turn off pagers or to place them on vibrate. Other distractions include televisions, office and radio chatter, and emergency apparatus coming into and out of a station. The educator must be aware of these environmental distractions and must work to minimize them as much as possible.

PSYCHOSOCIAL VARIABLES

The psychosocial variables of the adult learner include the differences between adult and child learning behavior. For instance, adult learners may have firmly established attitudes, beliefs, and values, and they may be more rigid in their thinking than younger learners. Through years of living, adults have acquired a set pattern of behaviors, along with set ideas about what is right and wrong, fact and fiction. These patterns may have to be "unset" or challenged for learning to take place. New ideas and ways of doing things can't be forced on the adult learner; they must be proved through logic and good science. The adult learner must understand and believe the new knowledge or technique before he or she will be willing to abandon his or her old beliefs.

Success

The educator must strive to create learning situations that afford the greatest potential for learning success; this includes taking special care not to embarrass the adult learner. When adult learners are placed on the defensive, they are less likely to be open to learning and are more likely to be protective of their thoughts and feelings; they may perceive the classroom as an unsafe learning environment. The saying "praise in public and criticize in private" clearly applies to the adult learner.

Respect

Returning to school is often a momentous decision for the adult learner, and attendance often represents a considerable investment. Having made this important and commendable decision, the adult learner expects—and deserves—to be treated with respect. The resourceful educator draws upon the wealth of knowledge and experiences that these learners bring with them to enrich the class for all students.

Critical Thinking Skills

The adult learns best by adding new information to an already existing framework, and has greater difficulty remembering isolated facts. The educator can determine what approach will be most effective in developing and presenting course material by knowing the educational and professional backgrounds of students. With this knowledge, the educator can add new information to the students' existing framework—or expertise.

TEACHING TIP: The educator should get to know his or her students' backgrounds, so he or she can better integrate new ideas with those ideas students already know. Linking new information to old is a particularly effective way to aid information retention in the adult learner.

Practical Limitations and Considerations

The adult learner has competing responsibilities, and the EMS instructor who does not consider these factors risks losing very good students (Box 3-1). These limi-

BOX 3-1 Principles for Teaching Adult Learners

With adult learners, instructors should:

- Involve students in the planning process
- Actively engage students in the learning process
- Incorporate a variety of teaching methods to meet the needs of students with a variety of learning styles
- Focus on "real world" problems
- Emphasize how the learning can be applied
- Practice information quickly after it is presented
- Relate the material to the learner's past experience
- Allow debate and challenge of ideas
- Listen to and respect the opinions of learners
- Encourage learners to be resources to the instructor and to one another
- Use students to evaluate learning
- Give learners control
- Reinforce positive behavior whenever possible

tations and considerations may involve scheduling challenges, scarce time, financial stresses, conflicts between job and family responsibilities, and transportation problems. It is important that the educator respect the challenges that each student faces (Figure 3-2).

MOTIVATION

Adults typically have different motivators for learning than do younger students. The instructor can apply an important classroom management and performance enhancement tool by understanding what motivates students, because motivation creates the desire to learn. By knowing what motivates students, the instructor can understand student behavior and choose relevant motivational tools. For example, if a student who is trying to support his family on his EMT wages is reminded that the top five students in his paramedic class will be guaranteed interviews for openings at the county ambulance service, he may be strongly motivated to succeed in the program. Furthermore, understanding one's own motivation for personal excellence in *teaching* is vital to maintaining high-level activity and instruction in one's classroom.

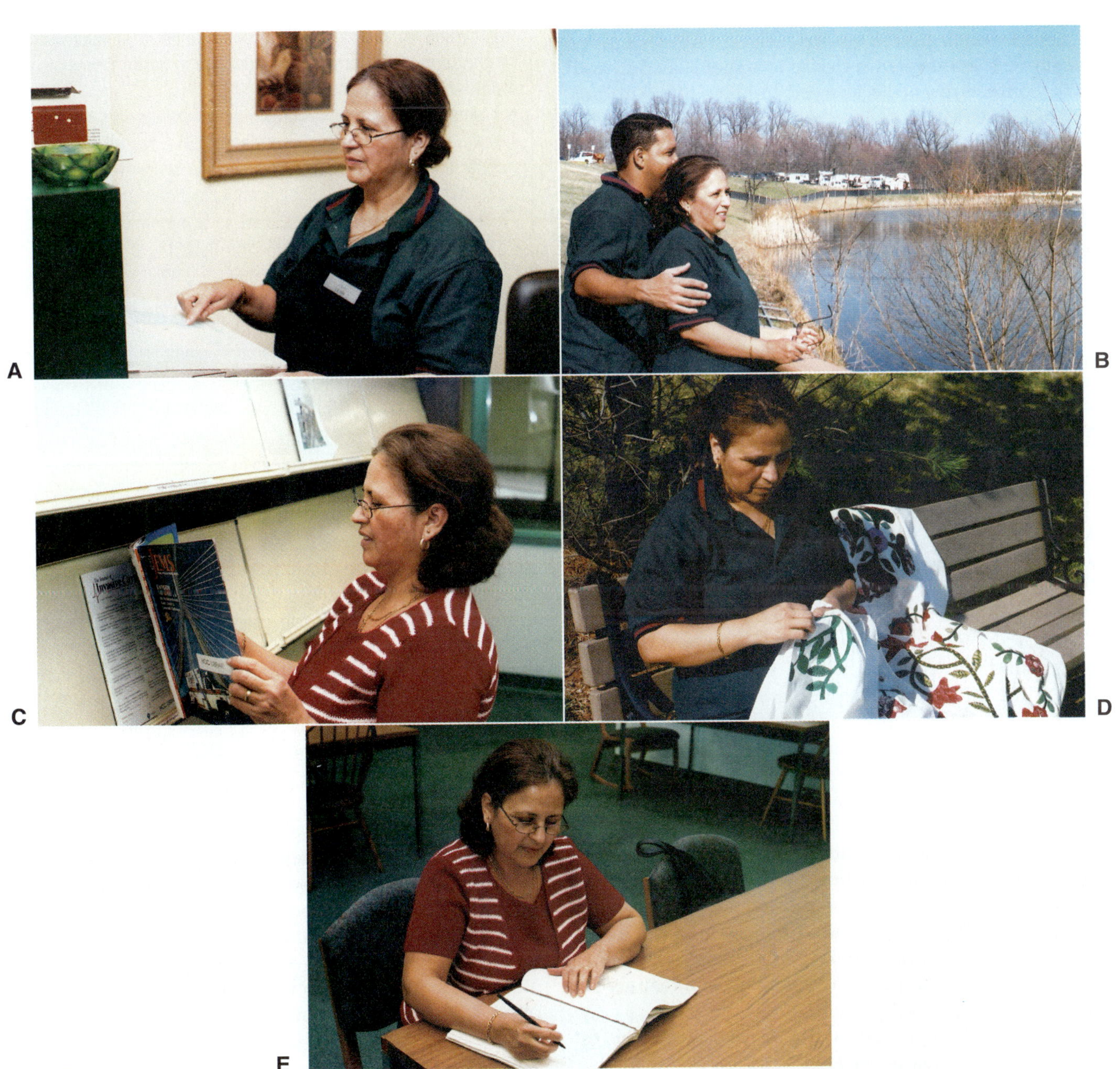

FIGURE 3-2 Teaching adults means teaching people with varied life experiences and responsibilities.

TEACHING TIP: Active listening is a great way to receive information and is a skill that few instructors master. During class, it is easy to divide attention between several students at once, but that is not always effective. The instructor should monitor how actively and attentively he or she listens to students. Active listening may help the instructor to identify what motivates his or her students.

Intrinsic and Extrinsic Motivators

Motivators are divided into two groups: intrinsic (internal) and extrinsic (external).[6] Intrinsic motivators are internal drives for behavior, such as a desire to help others or to serve the community, a need for personal or professional growth and development, a need to boost one's self-esteem, a desire to achieve, and a need to be competent and to succeed in one's life. Another intrinsic motivator is to make or maintain social relationships or to relieve boredom. Adults are usually more highly motivated by these intrinsic factors than by extrinsic factors.

In contrast, extrinsic motivators come from outside of the individual person. Examples of extrinsic motivators include the possibility of a promotion, a bonus, additional vacation time, or the need to find or maintain a job.

Once an instructor knows and understands his or her students' motivators, he or she can use language, examples, and incentives relevant to each student's motivators.

CASE IN POINT

A construction company foreman is confident and competent at his job. The other workers look up to him, and he prides himself on being an excellent contractor and manager. His group is enrolled in a mandatory first aid class as part of their company's safety program. The instructor is dreading teaching this group because she is concerned that they will not be interested in the material. However, she learns before the class that the foreman has a strong will to succeed, in addition to a healthy ego and a desire not to "look bad" in front of his subordinates.

The instructor knows that she has a useful tool by which to motivate this group by identifying the foreman as the team leader and encouraging and supporting his learning. By helping *him* to succeed, she will ensure that he will stay motivated to master the material, while simultaneously motivating the others who respect him to perform well also and learn the information.

Additionally, the instructor uses examples that are relevant to the students' experiences. She describes accidents and injuries that could occur on a construction job site. When teaching spinal immobilization, she uses the example of a roofer who falls while laying shingles. When teaching hemorrhage control, she uses the example of a framer who cuts himself while using a power saw. The students are able to see the relevance of the class to them personally, and they are more motivated to pay attention and practice the skills presented in class. In fact, several students pursue supplemental learning beyond the classroom by attending additional classes in construction site safety.

Maslow's Hierarchy

A discussion of motivation would be incomplete without including Maslow, one of the most referenced authors on human motivation. Maslow worked on his "hierarchy of needs" theory over a period of years (1943, 1954, 1971), making alterations as he sought to understand the subject. In fact, the hierarchy varies depending on the exact period in which he completed his research. His theory has influenced many fields, including education, and can be helpful to the instructor as he or she seeks to identify and understand students, their needs, and what motivates them.

Maslow, a humanist, believes that a person strives for a higher potential and desires to reach higher levels of his or her calling, to become a fully functioning person—or, as Maslow describes it, to achieve "self-actualization." Moreover, individual persons can grow and actualize their potential in the right environment, but in a less-than-healthy environment, individuals do not grow to meet their potential.

Maslow's theory consists of a hierarchy of levels of *basic* human needs, then *higher* needs, or "growth" needs, which can be attained only when the more basic needs have been met. At the lowest level of the hierarchy, basic needs include physiologic needs, such as oxygen, food, water, and a reasonably constant body temperature. An individual who is deprived of any of these basic physiologic needs would be controlled by these needs and would desperately seek to attain them. Until these needs are satisfied, an individual cannot move to the next level.

Safety and security needs, the next level in the hierarchy, describes the ability to be free from fear of physical danger and of deprivation of the basic physiologic needs, as well as self-preservation. These needs include feeling secure about maintaining property and a job to ensure food and shelter. Safety needs are usually insignificant for adults until an emergency or a social structure disruption occurs, such as war, 9-11, or the Oklahoma City bombing, for instance. Children, on the other hand, often feel the effects of insecurity and need to feel safe.

The next level is the need for love, affection, and "belongingness." Maslow explains that individuals strive to overcome loneliness and separation from family, friends, and society. This level of need includes not just receiving love and affection, but also giving love and affection. If there is difficulty attaining this sense of belongingness, individuals may substitute achievement.

The next and final level of Maslow's hierarchy of basic needs includes esteem needs. An individual has the strength and motivation to strive to fulfill this need only when the more basic needs have been met. Humans must have a stable, high level of respect for themselves and respect from others. Becoming competent and gaining recognition (validity from others) produces feelings of self-confidence, power, and usefulness to society. As with the other levels of need, individuals may not always seek to fill these needs through constructive behavior, but sometimes through disruptive or immature actions.

Once all these basic needs have been met, an individual, according to Maslow, is ready to pursue the higher level, or "growth," needs. Although Maslow initially identified only self-actualization needs, after more study, he identified four specific levels: cognitive needs, aesthetic needs, self-actualization needs, and self-transcendence needs. Again, each of these levels of need is attempted only after the lesser need has been achieved. Cognitive needs include knowing, understanding, and exploring. Aesthetic needs include order and beauty. Self-actualization is reaching one's potential, or, as described by Maslow, "What a man can be, he must be." This is an intrinsic motivation; it is not related to what others think is important. Self-transcendence is a connection to something beyond the ego; it involves helping others to find self-fulfillment and to reach their potential.

Instructors must be able to talk to students and must attempt to understand life events that may impact their motivation. A student's inability to pay attention to studies or immature behavior may be linked to basic unmet needs. An instructor may be assisted in understanding and addressing the specific needs of students by considering Maslow's hierarchy and determining where students stand within this hierarchy (Figure 3-3).

Barriers to Learning

Not all learners come to the classroom adequately motivated. The phrase "barriers to learning" can be used to describe conditions or situations in which motivation is lacking. Common barriers include family and career responsibilities that result in lack of time,

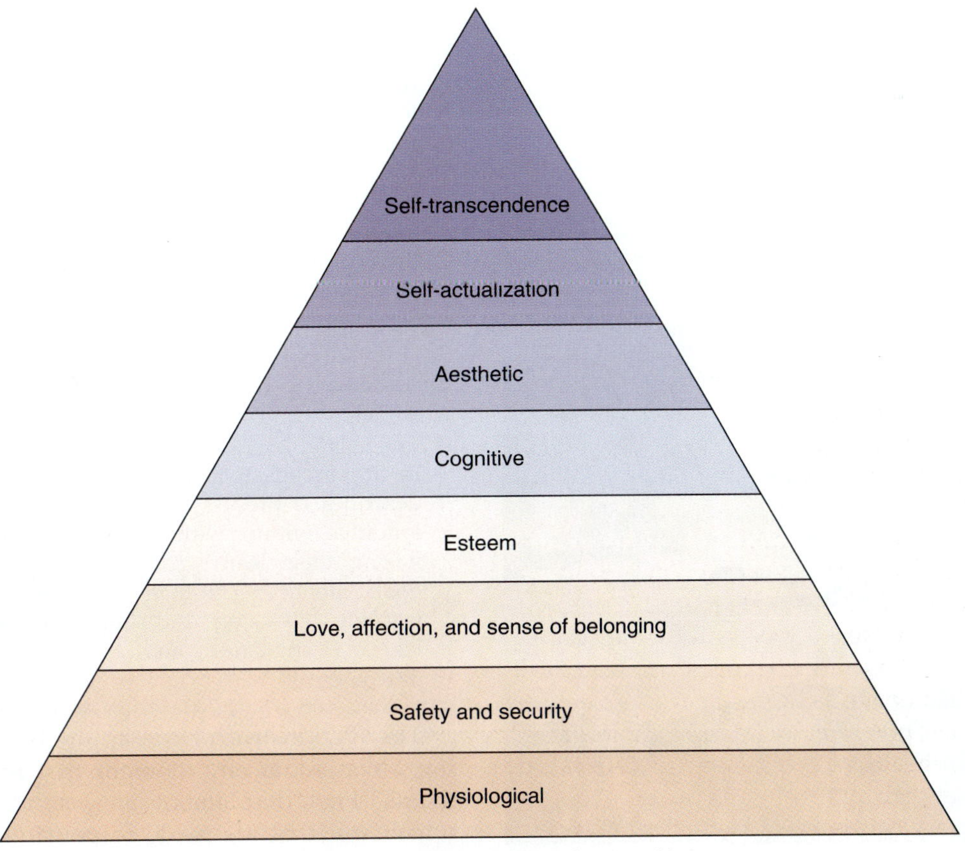

FIGURE 3-3 Maslow's hierarchy pyramid.

money, or confidence. Additionally, scheduling problems, bureaucracy ("red tape"), and problems with childcare and transportation are often difficult barriers to overcome (Figure 3-4). Lack of confidence can also be a significant barrier to learning, as can resentment or disinterest due to required, or involuntary, education.

Educators should understand that such barriers exist, and that they may be able to effect positive change in students through their role as mentor, guide, and advocate. The educator must strive to decrease barriers whenever possible and must encourage learners to explore ways to overcome their personal barriers. Encouraging attention to intrinsic motivators (e.g., success, helping others) may also be helpful. These barriers might otherwise limit students' ability to grow as prehospital EMS providers and to become lifelong learners.

SELECTED LEARNING THEORIES

This section examines several selected theories of learning and offers practical lessons that educators can gain from these theories. Although dozens of theories, preferences, and concepts are associated with learning in educational psychology, four of the more common types have been selected for discussion here. These include Self-Directed Learning, the Theory of Margins, Transformational Learning, and Context-Based Learning.

Self-Directed Learning

The theory of self-directed learning involves many related concepts, such as self-planned learning, self-teaching, autonomous learning, and independent study. Distributed learning and distance education are also frequently used modalities for self-directed learning.

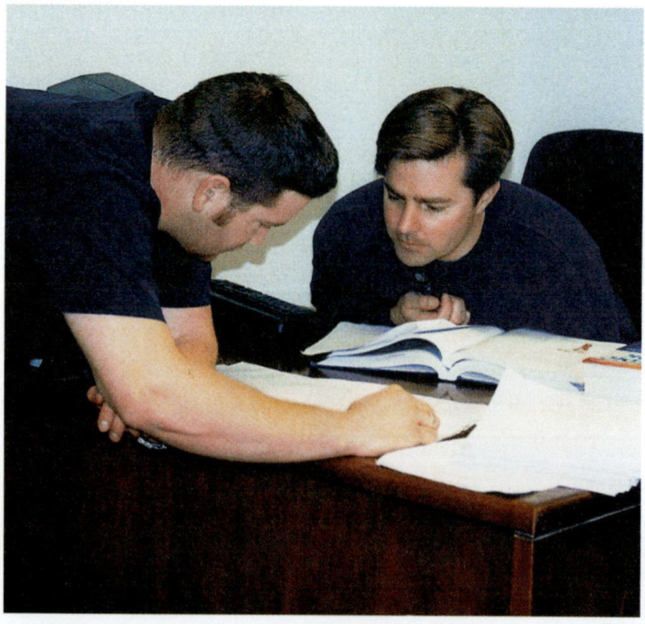

FIGURE 3-4 Scheduling problems and bureaucracy can be significant barriers to learning.

Self-education has been described as nothing more than the manner in which information is acquired—that of learning without an instructor present.[8] However, the absence of an instructor, althouth it is an important characteristic of self-directed learning, is only *one* of several characteristics of self-directed learning. At least three additional characteristics are particular to self-directed learning, namely:

- A longer learning time period
- A wider range of studies
- A higher level of subject mastery and critical thinking

Self-direction in learning comes from a lifelong learning perspective. Kidd supports this view in the following passage: "It has often been said that the purpose of adult education, or of any kind of education, is to make the subject [student] a continuing, 'inner-directed,' self-operating learner."[9]

Self-direction in adulthood is a process in which the learner assumes primary control of what he or she desires to learn. Moore describes a self-directed learner as an individual who can:

> Identify his learning need when he finds a problem to be solved, a skill to be acquired, or information to be obtained. He is able to articulate his need in the form of a general goal, differentiate that goal into several specific objectives, and define fairly explicitly his criteria for successful achievement. In implementing his need, he gathers the information he desires, collects ideas, practices skills, works to resolve his problems, and achieves his goals. In evaluating, the learner judges the appropriateness of newly acquired skills, the adequacy of his solutions, and the quality of his new ideas and knowledge.[10]

A related view of self-directed learning that stresses the phases of a leaning process has been offered by Knowles:

> In its broadest meaning, "self-directed learning" describes a process in which individuals take the initiative, with or without the help of others, in diagnosing their learning needs, formulating learning goals, identifying human and material resources for learning, choosing and implementing appropriate learning strategies, and evaluating the learning outcomes.[11]

The EMS instructor can apply this theory by creating a classroom environment that includes two elements. First, implement an *institutional* process in which students are made responsible for identifying their learning needs and deciding on the strategies they plan to use to reach them. Then, promote self-directed learning from the point of view of an *internal* process. In other words, the student is encouraged to set his or her own goals in terms of learning outcome. By doing so, students take responsibility for their own learning.

For example, the instructor might plan an activity on the first day of class that requires students to immediately assume responsibility for their own learning. He or she could assign students to define their career choice (EMT-Basic, EMT-Intermediate, or EMT-Paramedic) by investigating a variety of resources and to write a paper with their definitions, observations, and findings. Instructors who ensure that students have initial success with their self-directed assignments can help to motivate them in their studies, and in the process, can help them to become lifelong learners.

CASE IN POINT

The EMT instructor looked at the curriculum requirements for the EMT Basic course and tried to imagine how to possibly cover all of the material adequately. He thought there was no possible way to have the students learn to be proficient in their skills and understand what they were doing, and still cover every topic during class. Yet he realized that they were all very motivated adults. He concluded that surely they could learn much of this on their own. With that in mind, he devised a self-learning plan that would help to improve his class in several ways.

First, he took the required bloodborne pathogens and Health Insurance Portability and Accountability Act (HIPAA) of 1996 materials that had been added to the curriculum and placed them into a self-directed learning module that had to be completed and passed (by a written test) before students could even register for the courses. This would be his first "commitment filter" because competition to get into the class was so strong.

Second, he took the medical terminology, hazardous materials, and weapons of mass destruction (WMD) modules, and from these, he created self-directed learning modules that had to be completed by students during class at specific points in the schedule. The medical terminology module was required within 1 week of the start of class. The hazardous material module was required to be completed by the fourth class. Completion of the WMD module was required by the end of the program, but it had to be submitted before students could take the certification exam.

By shifting this content to self-learning modules, the instructor increased contact hours for content related to patient care skills and materials that the students would use on most of their EMS calls. He ended up with a better-prepared, less frustrated, better-performing class.

Theory of Margins

The theory of Power-Load-Margins, commonly called the *Theory of Margins*, provides a model for looking at how much ability (*power*) a student has compared with how much learning the student needs to accomplish (*load*). *Margin* is the difference between "power" and "load." This theory is one way of describing the pressures placed on an individual during the learning process. In general, the less margin an individual has, the more likely he or she is to succeed.

Research behind the theory

Howard Y. McClusky, an experimental psychologist, examined adult learning and introduced the Theory of Margins in the early 1960s, after several years of research.[12] He believed that the theory was relevant for understanding adult lives, especially as adults age and the various demands and pressures placed on them increase.

According to McClusky, the key factor of adult life is the *load* that the adult carries in living, along with the *power* that is available to that person to carry the load.[13] He described *load* as the self and social demands required by a person to maintain a minimal level of autonomy; *power* as the individual's resources, abilities, possessions, and position on which he or she can draw to cope with the load; and *margin* as the difference between the "power" and the "load." The more margin a person has, the more likely it is that he or she can deal with the load, because he or she has greater reserve capacity. A student with an overwhelming load, caused by the need to work a full-time job and take care of children and possibly an ill parent, might have no margin for handling even the most minimal academic load.

McClusky further divided load into two groups of interacting elements: external and internal. The *external* load consists of tasks involved in normal life requirements (e.g., family, work, and community responsibilities). *Internal* load consists of life expectancies developed by the people themselves, such as aspirations, desires, and future expectations. Power consists of a combination of such external resources and capacities as family support, social abilities, and economic abilities. It also includes various internally acquired or accumulated skills and experiences that contribute to effective performance, such as resiliency, coping skills, and personality.

Practical application of the theory

Instructors can affect their students' margins in both positive and negative ways. McClusky's Power-Load-Margin theory can be applied to the degree that instructors contribute to the depletion of margin in adult students.[14] Day and James at the University of Wyoming,[15] in a series of interviews with adult students, found numerous examples of instructor-generated load that they clustered into four areas: attitude, behavior, task, and environment (Box 3-2).

One of the most surprising findings of this research was that the attitudinal and behavioral dimensions of the instructor-generated load were identified more than three times as often as the task dimension. In other words, adults adjust their margin to deal with the expected task demands assigned to them by the instructor better than they do with interpersonal issues. Unexpected demands, such as instructor attitude and behavior, create barriers to the student's ability to satisfactorily complete a learning objective.

Day and James identified several ways in which instructors can minimize the effects of instructor-generated load.[15] These techniques include the following:

1. Recognize and understand that the concept of margin exists in adult students.
2. Understand that the concerns of students do not center merely on the content of the course.
3. Recognize that an instructor can contribute to the load in learners, and that he or she does so through behavior, learning environment, attitude, and the structure/content of the class.
4. Address the issue of margin during the first class.

The Theory of Margins provides a framework for discussion of how much work a given EMS course typically requires, and of how much time a student has to devote to the course. In addition, it gives both the instructor and the student a conceptual model by which to discuss how illness, personal problems, and work and family problems can add up to an unmanageable situation. Perhaps the most powerful component of this model is the way that an educator's attitude, lack of organization, or use of busywork can dramatically narrow a student's "margin," thus reducing his or her performance and chance of success in a class.

BOX 3-2 Examples of Instructor-Generated Load[6]

Instructors attributed greater margin to students:

Attitude

- Instructor treats learner as an inferior person
- Instructor ignores learner's opinion
- Instructor is too impatient
- Instructor is too rigid

Behavior

- Instructor has distracting mannerisms
- Instructor mumbles or is difficult to understand
- Instructor is disorganized
- Instructor avoids eye contact

Task

- Instructor gives inappropriate assignments
- Instructor's guidelines for evaluation/grades are unclear
- Instructor gives busywork
- Instructor allows too little time to complete assignments

Environment

- Learning environment is too hot or too cold
- Lighting is poor
- Desks and chairs are uncomfortable
- Noise or other distractions can be heard from neighboring classrooms

CASE IN POINT

An EMS instructor was teaching first responder as a contract course to a group of government workers. The course was being conducted on-site, and students were being detailed from their offices to the class. The class was meeting for 7 hours each day over a 7-week period. By the fourth week of class, the instructor noticed that several students frequently returned late from lunch, or not at all, for the second half of the day. He knew that none of those students would be eligible to take the state certification exam because of their absences. On questioning the students, the instructor discovered that most participants were supervisors or upper management personnel who could not afford to take the entire workday away from their offices, even though the highest administrative level required the training course. Students agreed that they could come for half-day sessions and were willing to do so, as they really did enjoy the course and valued what they were learning. The instructor proposed that the program should meet for half-day sessions for the remainder of the time. He was also able to convince the administration to allow him to offer two mornings of makeup sessions, so all the absent students could make up the classes they had missed. In this manner, he was able to have all students complete the training program. He and the administrators agreed that future contract courses would be offered as only half-day sessions.

This instructor applied the Theory of Margins by increasing the power the students had (by responding to their need and allowing them to help devise a solution) and decreasing their load, thus increasing their margin.

Transformational Learning

The theory of transformational learning emerged with the work of Jack Mezirow,[16-18] and it is defined as "learning that initiates and creates deep and lasting personal changes," sometimes known as a *paradigm shift*.[19] In transformational learning, acquisition of specific knowledge and skills is often secondary to the deeper and lasting change in perception and thought. Although EMS educators may rarely intentionally seek out transformational learning opportunities for their students, such experiences often appear unexpectedly. Many instructors can recall times when a student approached them at some point during or after the class and said, "You've changed my life. Now I know what I want to do."

CASE IN POINT

A student came into her instructor's office frustrated and ready to quit. She told the instructor that she couldn't do the drug calculations no matter how hard she tried. The instructor, similar to every paramedic program instructor who has taught drug calculations, sat and listened attentively. Yes, drug calculations are one of the most challenging tasks for some students to learn, and some students *never* master the calculation skills that are essential to be a paramedic. However, this was a very bright student who had a block for some reason; she *believed* that she simply could not learn these calculation tasks.

The instructor thought about the student's background and about why she might not be learning the skill. He realized that she was a licensed cosmetologist, a beautician who ran her own business. He looked at her and said, "Don't you have to calculate your business expenses every month? Project the supplies you need and order them? Calculate how much they will cost? Calculate the costs of your utilities, lease, taxes, and other business expenses? Don't you have to anticipate how many customers you will have, how long it will take you to serve each one, and schedule them?" He continued, "How is all of that any more complicated than drug calculations? Isn't it all the same, except for changing dollars to milligrams, and ounces to bottles, instead of milligrams to kilograms?"

Suddenly, the student's face changed. She smiled. Her eyes lit up. She said, "I got it!" She left the office, passed her pharmacology tests with high scores, and became a practicing paramedic. Today, she is also a critical care nurse. She had a *transformational learning experience* that occurred unexpectedly in one brief moment—just by being asked the right questions at the right time.

Research behind the theory

Transformational learning is based on the concepts of *meaning perspectives*, or one's overall worldview, and *meaning schemes*, or smaller components that contain specific knowledge, values, and beliefs about one's experiences.[16] A number of meaning schemes work together to generate one's meaning perspective. Meaning perspectives are shaped during childhood and youth, and they form the basis for a person's view of the world from his or her perspective. They operate as perceptual filters that determine how an individual will organize and interpret the meaning of his or her life experiences.

Meaning perspectives naturally change and evolve as the number and depth of life experiences increase. However, there are occasions when significant events occur that may induce powerful emotional responses within the individual. These life-changing events may include intensely personal issues such as divorce, death of a loved one, health crises, financial upheavals, or unexpected job changes, or they may involve large-scale incidents such as disasters and accidents. When these events occur, the individual must assess the information and decide whether it fits within his or her current meaning perspective. No transformative learning occurs as long as the information fits comfortably. However, if the event is so significant as to create upheaval and conflict in what one believes, a transformative learning experience may occur, as the new information shifts the meaning perspective to a new position.[18]

Practical application of the theory

Although transformational learning has powerful potential for enhancing and accelerating a student's self-actualization processes, an EMS instructor must consider some important points in attempting to understand these processes. Baumgartner advises instructors to consider ethical questions that may arise in the planning and delivery of transformational learning.[20] Baumgartner also discusses the dynamics and the balance of power in the classroom, emphasizing the necessity of a trusting and caring relationship between students and instructors. Students who see the instructor as an authority figure may be reluctant to challenge conventional values, beliefs, and interpretation of facts. Thus, Baumgartner recommends that educators must have a formal code of ethics and a forum for adult educators in which mutual support and exploration of the dynamics of transformational learning are encouraged.

Transformational learning can frequently elicit strong emotional responses from both the student and the instructor, often unexpectedly. Because of his or her powerful potential, the instructor should take the time to deal with transformational learning moments when they occur. For example, a class discussion about medical maladies among the homeless leads to a larger discussion of the exact nature of homelessness itself. The instructor gives a research assignment to a group of interested students, instructing them to find relevant information about the topic. As the students research the topic, several of them find the information to be very powerful and alter their preexisting thoughts regarding the homeless. As a result, they feel better prepared and more empathetic to the homeless patients they contact in the field.

CASE IN POINT

The EMT course covered the topic of child abuse and neglect. During the lesson, the instructor noticed that one student was withdrawn and very quiet. This was out of character for the student. The instructor approached the student during the break to see if he was ill, or if something was bothering him. The student related a story from his own childhood. He explained how his best friend had been the victim of child abuse. He told how he had watched his friend endure several years of abuse, and that he had been sworn to secrecy. Because they were both young children at the time, he thought that he was doing the right thing by not telling. He spoke of the feelings of loss when his friend moved away suddenly and he never heard from him again. He told the instructor how this experience had caused him to want to become an EMT, so he could help other children in similar situations. The instructor urged the student to share his story with the rest of the class, and when the break was over, he did. All students were riveted during his story, and one other student shared a similar experience with the class. This led to a much deeper discussion of the topic than could have been possible from the instructor's lecture alone. The whole class could clearly see how this experience had transformed the life of the student involved.

Context-Based Learning (Situated Cognition)

Context-based learning, or *situated cognition*, assumes that information is more easily learned if it is taught within the environment where it will actually be used by the student.

Research behind the theory

Lave and Wenger claim that learning normally manifests as a function of the activity, context, and culture in which it occurs—*the situation*.[21] This contrasts with most traditional classroom learning activities, which are often presented in an abstract form and out of context. In context-based learning, social interaction is a critical component of situated learning. Students become involved in a "community of practice." The community is made up of experts and novices. Experts are identified as individuals with real life experience that reflects the content, whereas novices are those who wish to learn the content but lack or have minimal practical experience. The community, which comprises both experts and novices, embodies certain beliefs and behaviors.

Situated learning is usually unintentional (incidental), rather than deliberate. Lave and Wenger call the process "legitimate peripheral participation." Content is learned, and value is assigned to it when it is within the same environment as individuals who have mastered the content.[22]

Practical application of the theory

To apply this principle, the instructor should try to make each case scenario and workshop as realistic as possible. This can be achieved through carefully crafted scenario scripts and a realistic environment. If a lab can be made to appear like a home living room or a real motor vehicle collision, then learning will be enhanced.

Lave and Wenger provide an analysis of situational learning in five different settings: Yucatan midwives, native tailors, Navy quartermasters, meat cutters, and alcoholics.[22] In all cases, the researchers observed a gradual acquisition of knowledge and skills as novices learned from experts in the context of everyday activities. In EMS, students who have opportunities to observe and practice their skills in real life environments and to interact with field providers benefit greatly. Although formalized internships may not be practical for every EMS class at every level of training, the opportunity for students to participate in patient scenarios in a nontesting format may provide a reasonable alternative (Figure 3-5).

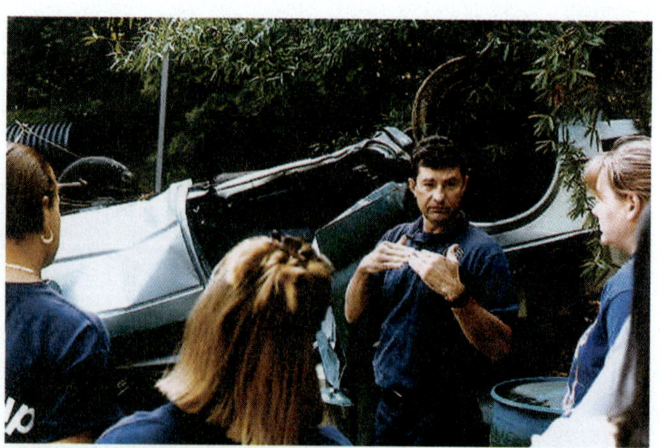

FIGURE 3-5 Students who participate in real life environments are more likely to be successful learners.

CASE IN POINT

The students were nearing the end of their didactic training and were beginning to transition into the "pulling it all together" phase of the program, during which they would spend time in the field setting with preceptors from the ambulance service. The primary instructor, clinical coordinator, medical director, and field preceptors were meeting to finalize the details of their rotations. The primary instructor was nervous because he felt the students' skills were weak, and that this would reflect poorly on his teaching abilities. This was his first time as the primary instructor. During the final practical skills evaluations, several students scored as "marginal" or "average," and one even failed the evaluation totally and would have to complete a remediation cycle before he would be allowed to attend any clinicals. The clinical coordinator reminded everybody that the students were novices, and that the preceptors needed to work closely with them to develop their skills in all three domains of learning: cognitive, affective, and psychomotor. After the first couple of weeks of clinical rotations, the primary instructor noticed that the students were performing very well on in-class scenarios and simulations. He could not understand why they had suddenly improved so dramatically in their performance. During a mentoring session with the program medical director, he began to understand how the theory of contextual learning was affecting his students' performance. He even decided to try and include more practical application exercises in his future courses.

SUMMARY

In conclusion, principles applied in the teaching of adult learners are not the same as those used for teaching children. The differences must be taken into account if success is to be achieved with the adult learner. The educator must also become familiar with the physiologic and psychological variables common to adult learners. Moreover, the four major theories of adult learning highlighted in this chapter and the corresponding examples will aid educators in applying them in practical ways to help students succeed. EMS educators will have a greater capacity for tailoring classroom activities effectively and successfully when they attain a fuller understanding of how adults learn.

REFERENCES

1. Knowles M. *Andragogy Not Pedagogy!* New York, NY: Associated Press; 1968.
2. Brookfield S. Developing critically reflective practitioners: a rationale for training educators of adults. In: *Training Education of Adults: The Theory and Practice of Graduate Adult Education*. New York, NY: Routledge; 1988.
3. Imel S. *Guidelines for Working With Adult Learners*. ERIC Digest #77. Syracuse, NY: ERIC Clearinghouse on Adult Career and Vocational Education; 1988.
4. Imel S. *New Views of Adult Learning*. Trends and Alerts No. 5. Syracuse, NY: ERIC Clearinghouse on Adult, Career and Vocational Education; 1999.
5. Brookfield SD. *Understanding and Facilitating Adult Learning. A Comprehensive Analysis of Principles and Effective Practice*. Milton Keynes: Open University Press; 1986.
6. Mendler A, Moody R. *Motivating Students Who Don't Care: Successful Techniques for Educators*. National Educational Service; 2001.
7. Krzyzewski M, Phillips D. *Leading with the Heart: Coach K's Successful Strategies for Basketball, Business, and Life*. Warner Books; 2000.
8. Brockett and Hiemstra. *Self-Direction in Adult Learning: Perspectives on Theory, Research and Practice*. London and New York: Routledge; 1991.
9. Kidd. *How Adults Learn*. New York Association; 1973.
10. Moore A, et al. EMS stress training concept "Kobayashi Moru" scenarios. Domain 3. National Association of EMS Educators; Spring 2003.
11. Knowles M. *Andragogy Not Pedagogy!* New York, NY: Associated Press; 1968.
12. McClusky H. The course of the adult life span. In: Hallenbeck WC, ed. *Psychology of Adults*. Chicago: Adult Education Association of USA; 1963.
13. McClusky H. Education for aging: the scope of the field and perspective for the future. In: Grabowski SM, Mason WD, eds. *Learning for Aging*. Washington, DC: Adult Education Association of the USA; 1974:324-355.
14. McClusky H. An approach to a differential psychology of the adult potential. In: Grabowski SM, ed. *Adult Learning and Instruction*. Syracuse, NY: ERIC Clearinghouse on Adult Education (ERIC Document Reproduction Service No. ED 045 867); 1970.
15. Day and James. Margin and the adult learner. *MPAEA Journal of Adult Education*. 1984;13:1-5.
16. Mezirow J. A critical theory of adult learning and education. *Adult Education Quarterly*. 1981;32:3-24. [Retrieved September 24, 2001 from ERIC database EJ253326.]
17. Mezirow J. Transformative learning: theory to practice. *New Directions for Adult and Continuing Education*. 1994; 74:5-12.
18. Mezirow J. Transformative learning: theory to practice. *New Directions for Adult and Continuing Education*. 1997; 74:5-12.
19. Clark. Transformational learning. *New Directions for Adult and Continuing Education*. 1993;57:47-56.
20. Baumgartner. An update on transformational learning. *New Directions for Adult and Continuing Education*. 2001; 89:15-24. [Retrieved September 24, 2001 from http://www.esd.edu/~knorum/learningpapers/transform.htm.]
21. Lave J, Wenger. *Cognition in Practice: Mind, Mathematics, and Culture in Everyday Life*. Cambridge, UK: Cambridge University Press; 1988.
22. Lave J, Wenger. *Situated Learning: Legitimate Peripheral Participation*. Cambridge, UK: Cambridge University Press; 1990.

SUGGESTED READINGS

Anderson JA. Cognitive styles and multicultural populations. *Journal of Teacher Education*. 1988;39:2-9.

Boud D, et al, eds. *Reflection. Turning Experience into Learning*. London: Kogan Page; 1985.

Jarvis P. Learning. In: *ICE301 Lifelong Learning*. Unit 1(1). London: YMCA George Williams College; 1994.

Kolb DA. *Experiential Learning*. Englewood Cliffs, NJ: Prentice Hall; 1984.

Kolb DA, Fry R. Toward an applied theory of experiential learning. In Cooper C, ed. *Theories of Group Process*. London: John Wiley; 1975.

Schwenk, Whitman, Brigham Young University. *The Physician as Teacher*. Baltimore: Williams and Wilkins.

Tennant M. *Psychology and Adult Learning*. 2nd ed. London: Routledge; 1997.

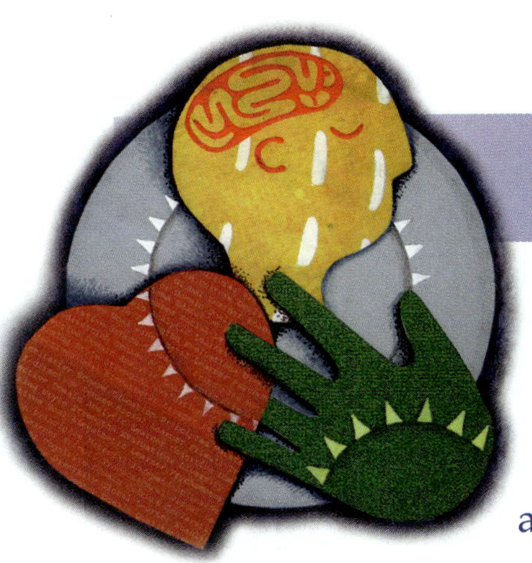

CHAPTER 4

Learning Styles

"Any training that does not include the emotions, mind, and body is incomplete; knowledge fades without feelings."

—*Anonymous*

When an educator walks into a classroom, he or she faces a group of learners—each with specific levels of intelligence, experience, aptitude, maturity, and interest. The educator's job is to convey knowledge, skills, and attitudes to each student. In doing so, one of his or her greatest challenges is to determine the most appropriate means or process for facilitating that learning. In addition, the educator must strive to make learning a meaningful, pleasant, and rewarding experience for the learner—one that promotes knowledge acquisition and retention. Therefore, the educator must appreciate that each learner has a unique means of taking in, processing, and retaining knowledge and skills. This is referred to as a *learning style.* This chapter explains how educators can identify different types of learners according to their learning style, and how they can use that information as a tool for enhancing learning and for guiding instruction.

LEARNING AND THE SENSES

The senses are the main conduit through which a learner experiences and interacts with the learning environment. The types and numbers of senses involved in learning experiences determine how individuals learn and what they retain. It is generally understood that seeing is the main sense of learning, accounting for 83% of learning experiences; hearing accounts for 11%, followed by 3% for smell, 2% for touch, and 1% for taste.

When sensory stimulation involves more than one sense, learners retain information better. Up to 90% of information can be retained when a learner says what he or she is doing while performing an activity—just saying something aloud improves retention by 70%. The combination of seeing and hearing, such as with an illustrated lecture, improves retention by 50%; seeing alone provides 30%, hearing 20%, and reading 10% toward retention. This sensory involvement explains why it is common practice to supplement instruction with visual and auditory aids, such as slides and audiotapes. The educator must reach out to learners through as many senses as possible, in attempting to appeal to individual learning styles.

WHAT IS A LEARNING STYLE?

Learning styles involve the use of a schema. *Merriam Webster's Dictionary* defines *schema* as:

1. A diagrammatic presentation; broadly, a structured framework or plan.
2. A mental codification of experience that includes a particular organized way of perceiving cognitively and responding to a complex situation or set of stimuli.

If a person is given a list of things to remember, for instance, a shopping list, he or she can use a schema to help remember the list. The person can make the list into a story, relate it to a song, or develop a visual map or mental picture. One can even develop a routine of physical movement to help recall the items. The nature of the schema chosen may be directly related to the person's learning style or preference. For example, the person who develops a mental picture likely has a preference for visual learning; the person who uses a song prefers auditory learning; and the person who develops a pattern of body motions tends toward kinesthetic learning. Because learning involves the intake, processing, and recall of information, presenting information in a way that is consistent with a learner's style makes the teaching-learning process more effective and efficient.

BOX 4-1 Types of Learners

- Auditory
- Visual
- Kinesthetic
- Analytic
- Global
- Social
- Independent

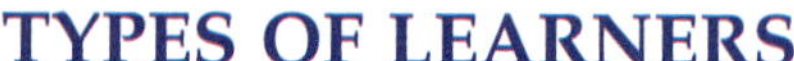

TYPES OF LEARNERS

This section describes auditory, visual, kinesthetic, analytic, global, social, and independent learners, as well as strategies for facilitating their learning experiences (Box 4-1).

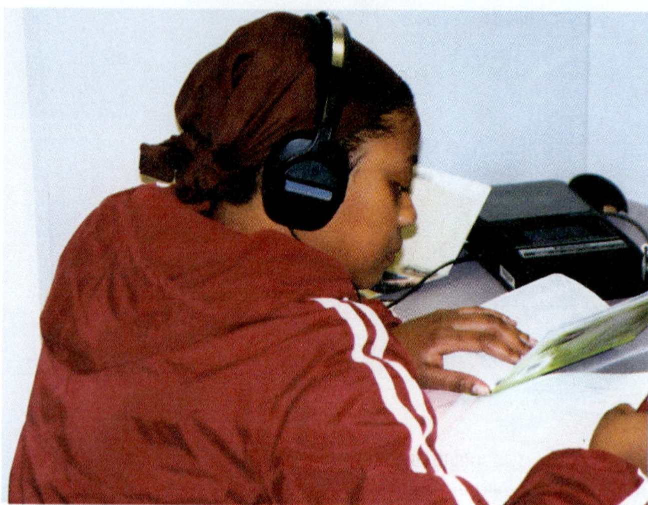

FIGURE 4-1 Auditory learners may benefit from hearing a previously recorded base station report.

Auditory Learners

Persons who learn best by hearing information are considered auditory learners. They benefit from oral presentation of information, discussion, listening, and verbalizing. They are comfortable listening to a taped lecture or an audiotape. Auditory learners can be reached through the use of phrases such as, "I hear you," and, "Listen up, class." These learners absorb didactic material best when it is taught through lectures, oral presentations, and class discussions.

When learning new skills, auditory learners must hear the instructions and any noise or tones produced by the equipment. When electrocardiogram (ECG) recognition is used as an example, this student would be best taught speaking out the rhythms, such as, "Beat, beat, complex, beat, beat, complex" for a second-degree block. He or she would also be inclined to "talk his or her way through" the ECG strip analysis process. In practice, an auditory learner would want to turn on and listen to the cardiac monitor tone while treating a patient (Figure 4-1).

TEACHING TIP: For auditory learners, *say* everything. For example, in addition to listing the steps of a procedure on a blackboard, say the steps aloud. Also, encourage auditory learners to audiotape lectures and other presentations and to play them back when studying.

Visual Learners

Persons who need to see what they are learning are considered visual learners. They benefit from the visual presentation of material and learn best when they can look things up, write things down, and watch the performance of a skill. Educators can help these learners "see" the words by using, for example, handouts, videotapes, slides, overheads, illustrations, posters, radiographs, and moulage. These individuals may speak in terms of "seeing you around" and "try to picture this." Returning to the ECG example, visual learners will need to study an ECG strip and perhaps mark intervals to help determine the rhythm. They will tend to watch the monitor whenever possible (Figure 4-2).

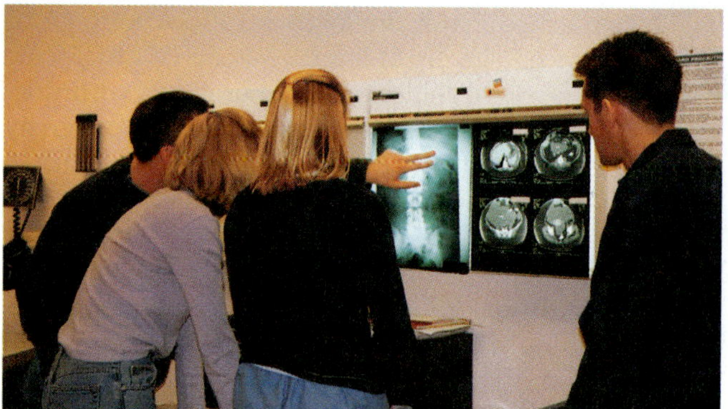

FIGURE 4-2 Visual learners may benefit from relating anatomy classes to x-rays.

TEACHING TIP: Always ensure that visual aids (e.g., slides, overheads, flipchart notes) are correct. The visual learner will remember the information as he or she saw it the first time.

Kinesthetic Learners

Persons who learn with their bodies are considered kinesthetic learners. They prefer to associate movement and tactile experiences with learning. Educators can enhance learning for kinesthetic learners by pro-

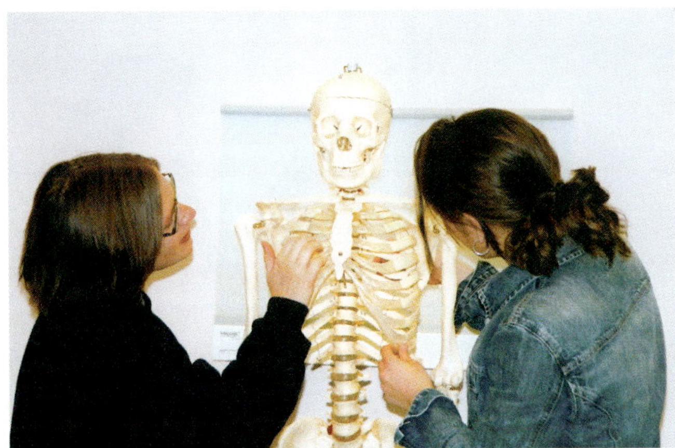

FIGURE 4-3 Touching and feeling things such as a skeleton can help the kinesthetic learner to understand and retain information.

viding opportunities for students to take things apart, make things work, and use their hands for tactile stimulation (Figure 4-3). For example, when teaching the anatomy of the heart, the educator could pass around an anatomic model so students can feel the structure. Kinesthetic learners may speak of "catch you around," or, "let's get going." Laboratory sessions, scenarios, and role playing are all effective learning activities for kinesthetic learners. They can also benefit from "air writing," in which terms, formulas, and other key statements are written in the air with the hand or finger.

TEACHING TIP: When skills are taught, a kinesthetic learner will benefit from having the technique demonstrated on him or her. This type of learner discovers a great deal by *feeling* the procedure applied to him or her.

CASE IN POINT

During an ECG interpretation lesson, the educator notices a paramedic student struggling with the material. The student has been studying strips and rereading textual material, but continues to misinterpret rhythms. Because this particular student tends to be physical (i.e., very active, uses hands to gesture when talking), the educator decides to implement strategies used for kinesthetic learners. He works with the student to trace ECGs with her fingertips, then to tap out the rhythms of various tracings with her feet. After running through several strips, the student seems to experience a breakthrough in understanding. She even begins to use her arms and legs to mimic a tracing in an impromptu "dance," which the class enjoys.

Analytic Learners

Persons who are logical thinkers, who process information logically, sequentially, and in small parts that build toward a whole, are considered analytic learners. They are often described as "left-brained." Using the analogy of "the forest from the trees," the analytic learner separates the forest from the trees. He or she will look at every tree in the forest before feeling certain enough to conclude that it is a forest.

Analytic learners work comfortably by following a protocol or algorithm. They are well served by lectures that follow outlines, reading assignments, and multiple-choice questions on exams. They typically enjoy spelling, numbers, thinking, reading, analysis, and speaking. According to the ECG example, the analytic learner will look at an ECG strip and immediately begin a systematic analysis: Is it regular or irregular? Fast or slow? Is there a P wave?

When learning a skill, analytic learners will benefit from detailed steps of the procedure provided in written and visual materials. These students are most comfortable mastering steps and specific information, and they need encouragement to learn judgment and global, applied concepts.

Structure, in terms of both educational process and material presented, is important to analytic learners. They may get frustrated, for example, to discover inconsistency between what is said in class and what their books say, or between what is taught and what they have been taught in the past. They may also be uncomfortable with learning that is out of sequence, or when the order of learning has been changed or rearranged. For the analytic learner, it is important to present a consistent message.

TEACHING TIP: When a guest lecturer or secondary instructor is used, it is important to ensure consistency with the material and approach to which students have become accustomed. Analytic learners, in particular, will have trouble processing any differences. Make sure, for example, to supply the guest educator with objectives to teach from, as well as an awareness of any controversial or potentially problematic content areas. If possible, observe the class, so you can clarify points or fill in gaps later.

Global Learners

Persons who think in terms of the big picture and who need to see the whole before the parts are considered global learners. They are often described as "right-brained." Returning to "the forest from the trees" analogy, the global learner will look at several trees, quickly declare it a forest, and then begin to see individual trees.

These learners tend to be creative, artistic, imaginative, emotional, and intuitive. They may be less likely to follow protocol, preferring to treat patients based on outcome, rather than on process. Global learners can also process information simultaneously; thus, they may easily move back and forth between activities and tasks. A common example of the global learner is the student who can be engaged in a task while giving instructions to others or interacting with students who are doing other tasks.

When teaching the global learner, it is important for the educator to start with an overview of the lesson, so the student knows where he or she is going. These students are most comfortable focusing on the global concepts and intuition, and they need encouragement to learn specific steps and the theory behind applications.

TEACHING TIP: Global learners can quickly become frustrated if paired with an analytic partner, and vice versa. However, they may complement one another in the total learning experience. The educator can work with students who approach material differently by helping them to understand the differences and to value both approaches.

Global learners enjoy working in teams. If the pace of instruction lags or is too tedious, they may become bored or distracted because they have already moved ahead to the conclusion. Techniques appropriate for these learners include mental imagery, drawing, maps, metaphors, and experiential learning.

TEACHING TIP: Skills practice provides an opportunity for the educator to incorporate varying sensory activities and social interactions. However, specific strategies are needed to address the needs of analytic and global thinkers. Some ideas for reaching these students include:

- Use of scenarios rather than simple practice of an isolated skill
- Use of algorithms or protocols that students can follow
- Proper balance between procedure and desired result (Are other methods acceptable to accomplish the desired outcome?)
- Having students put skills in context by relating activity to patient assessment findings

Social Learners

Persons who process information best when engaged in multiple tasks in busy environments with other learners are considered social learners. They tend to enjoy study sessions, group projects, and cooperative learning. Educators should provide opportunities for group work in class, classroom discussions, study groups, and skills groups. For social learners, background noise in the classroom or practice area, such as music or a radio, is not necessarily distracting and can even be helpful.

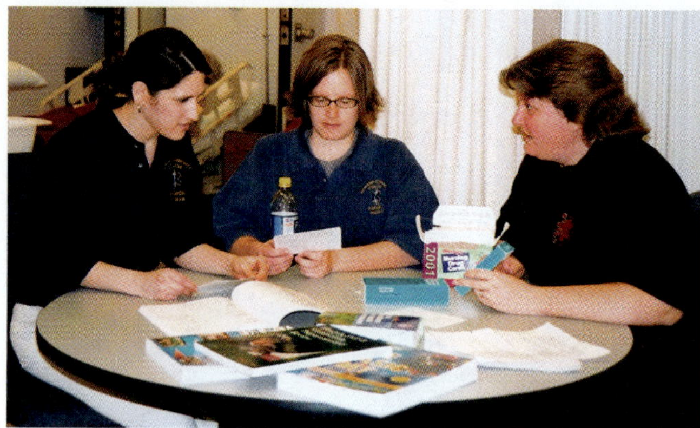

FIGURE 4-4 Social learners usually enjoy group projects and teamwork activities.

Independent Learners

Persons who prefer to process information independently, isolated from other learners, are considered independent learners. They will seek quiet, undisturbed study environments. They react well to reading assignments, written exams, and reports. Independent learners may feel uncomfortable in "touchy-feely" classroom situations led by an educator who encourages social interaction through group exercises and projects. The response and demeanor of independent learners should not be mistaken by the social educator as lack of enthusiasm or disdain for the content; rather, the student may be uncomfortable with the presentation style.

TEACHING TIP: When students are placed into groups, it is important for the educator to mix social and independent learners within groups. Otherwise, some groups will be gregarious, whereas others may be inhibited.

ADDRESSING VARIOUS LEARNING STYLES

Learning styles are multidimensional, that is, they involve sensory input, context, and environment. Because of this, the learning styles of students vary both within individual students and within the group. An educator may have to simultaneously reach learners who are visual, analytic, and independent, as well as those who are kinesthetic, global, and social—and all variations in between.

An important point to remember is that adult learners, although they have a learning preference, can adjust to other learning styles and use different styles for learning different types of material. Adults are capable of learning in almost any situation. However, the efficiency and enjoyment of the learning process for each student will vary, depending on how closely it matches his or her preferred learning style. For example, a visual learner may be required to listen to an audiotape as part of a class assignment. Although he or she may not find this experience as pleasurable as seeing an illustrated lecture on the same topic, and may need to listen to the tape repeatedly to master the material, the student can ultimately learn from the exercise.

Educators commonly remark that they have students who are "book smart" but can't seem to grasp practical skills. Other learners can memorize a long list of facts but can't seem to put them all together to develop a coherent plan of patient care. In such cases, the problem is not that these learners lack intelligence; rather, they learn some material more easily when it is presented in a style that matches their learning preference. Likewise, students may struggle with material that is presented in a style that is not congruent with their preferred method of learning.

In addition to learners who have a preference for sensory processing of new material, some regard as important the context in which information is presented. For example, some learners can easily grasp theoretical concepts presented verbally or in writing, whereas others can learn the material only when it is presented through concrete examples.

ASSESSING STUDENTS' LEARNING STYLES

Before developing an instructional plan that addresses variations in student learning styles, the educator must assess the learning styles of the persons in the group. Because those who pursue a particular profession often have similar learning styles, an assessment can allow the educator to focus on the predominant learning style of the group of students.

An educator can assess students' learning styles informally in various ways, including talking with them and getting to know them; observing their behavior individually and in groups when different teaching strategies are employed; and analyzing their success in learning and retention, given different teaching strategies. For example, when an educator is talking with a student, if the student uses gestures or moves about, the educator can assume that the student is a kinesthetic learner. If the educator notices that a student speaks the words to himself while reading, then the student most likely is an auditory learner. If, after material is presented by lecture only, the student does more poorly on a quiz than he or she had done with previous material presented via video, the student is probably a visual learner. Educators can also assess students through a formal assessment process, or a standardized test, which can occur as part of a program entrance exam process, or at the beginning of an individual course.

Remember that standardized tests are designed to assist the learner and the educator in evaluating the potential for academic and clinical success. These assessment methods should not be used as "gatekeepers" to determine which students will be allowed into a particular course. The educator is also cautioned against using test results to "prejudge" learners. Many factors beyond learning style preference, such as innate intelligence, motivation, and previous learning success, contribute to learning and student success. Finally, even if the class appears to have a dominant learning style, the educator must continue to vary the instructional approach to stimulate as many senses as possible.

Although many standardized tests for learning styles exist, those that are most commonly used in health professions education include the Learning Styles Inventory, the Health Occupations Basic Entrance Test, and the Myers-Briggs Type Indicator.

Learning Styles Inventory

The concept of determining an individual's learning style was pioneered by Kolb, with the introduction of Kolb's Learning Style Inventory.[1] The inventory is completed by answering a series of questions that identify a person's preference for learning in four areas: concrete experience, reflective observation, active conceptualization, and active experimentation. Kolb refers to these four areas as learning cycles. By adding together scores for the various learning cycles, four types of learners are identified. The *converger* has dominant abilities in abstract conceptualization and active experimentation. A converger favors the practical application of ideas. The *diverger* is the opposite of the converger (concrete experience and reflective observation) and has strong imaginative abilities. A combination of abstract conceptualization and reflective observation defines the *assimilator,* who is apt at creating theoretical models. And the *accommodator* is an individual who adapts to the circumstances at hand, usually through plans and experimentation, and represents the union of concrete experience and active experimentation.

In addition to Kolb's Inventory, other measures of assessing learning style have been developed. The Learning-Style Model by Rita Dunn and Kenneth Dunn is one of the most researched and tested learning style inventories.[2] This model breaks learning styles down into five stimuli that are made up of several elements (Table 4-1). The learner completes a Learning Style Inventory, which asks questions related to the five stimuli and their elements. From the

TABLE 4-1 The Learning-Style Model[2]

Stimuli	Elements
Environmental	Lighting
	Sound
	Temperature
	Seating arrangement
Emotional	Motivation
	Persistence
	Responsibility
	Structure
Sociologic	Alone or with peers
(i.e., how people learn)	Authoritative adult or collegial colleague
	Variety in learning or routine pattern
Physiologic	Perceptual skills
	Time-of-day energy levels
	Intake (eating)
	Mobility
Psychological	Hemispheric
	Impulsive or reflective
	Global or analytic

information gleaned about the elements, a learner can categorize his or her preference for learning in terms of the five main stimuli. This inventory gives the learner more information about how he or she *likes* to learn than is provided by the cognitive information–processing model of Kolb, which tells the learner *how* he or she learns. The Dunn and Dunn model also provides more information on learning preferences that is of value to the educator.

Health Occupations Basic Entrance Test

The Health Occupations Basic Entrance Test (HOBET) is a diagnostic test used to assess an applicant's academic and social skills preparation.[3] The computerized version is known as the C-HOBET. The test evaluates several areas that are essential for academic success:

- Essential math skills
- Reading comprehension for science textbooks
- Reading rate
- Critical thinking appraisal
- Test-taking skills
- Stress levels
- Social interaction profile
- Learning styles

Applicants are compared either individually or as a group with national scores. Test results allow applicants to identify areas of weakness before they enroll in course work. Thus, the student enters the classroom aware of his or her individual weaknesses and can seek strategies to improve success in these areas. The educator is also aware of the student's strengths and weaknesses and can adjust the instructional method accordingly.

Myers-Briggs Type Indicator

The Myers-Briggs Type Indicator (MBTI) is designed to determine a person's personality type.[4] It is based on the theory of personality characteristics and types developed by the psychoanalyst Carl Jung in the 1900s. The MBTI determines preferences on four dichotomies:

1. **Extraversion–Introversion:** Describes where people prefer to focus their attention and get their energy—from the outer world of people and activity, or their inner world of ideas and experiences
2. **Sensing–Intuition:** Describes how people prefer to take in information–focused on what is real and actual, or on patterns and meanings in data
3. **Thinking–Feeling:** Describes how people prefer to make decisions—based on logical analysis, or guided by concern for their impact on others
4. **Judging–Perceiving:** Describes how people prefer to deal with the outer world—in a planned, orderly way, or in a flexible, spontaneous way

Combinations of these preferences result in 16 personality types, which are represented by a four-letter acronym. For example, "Type INTJ" would be an introvert who uses intuition and thinking, as well as judging, to define his or her personality. The MBTI is useful in that it identifies differences among "normal" individuals that can lead to conflict and stress with individuals who are of different types. Strategies for addressing and avoiding these conflicts are provided. Various versions of the MBTI exist, including short versions that can be taken online. However, to be most useful, test results should be interpreted by professionals who have been trained in the administration and use of the MBTI.

ASSESSING THE EDUCATOR'S LEARNING STYLE

In addition to the impact of individual styles on a student's learning experience, the effects of the educator's personal learning style must also be considered. Educators tend to teach the way they like to learn; thus, an educator runs the risk of focusing on a particular method of instruction and possibly neglecting the needs of learners who require an alternative method of instruction.

Educators may also have difficulty understanding "problem" students owing to a difference in learning styles between the learner and the educator. For example, a learner may seem disruptive because he fidgets or moves about during class, but in actuality, he is a kinesthetic learner who feels confined in a strictly visual and auditory classroom.

Educators can use any of the common learning inventories previously mentioned to determine their own personal styles. Some educational institutions and instructor training programs have developed "teaching style inventories" that are based on learning style theory and research. The Myers-Briggs Type Indicator is a useful tool for determining differences between educators and students. For example, an instructor who is an extrovert may be perceived by an introverted learner as overbearing. Because of diversity within the classroom, it is important for educators to know their own learning styles and to make strong efforts to reach out to learners who use different styles or approaches to learning.

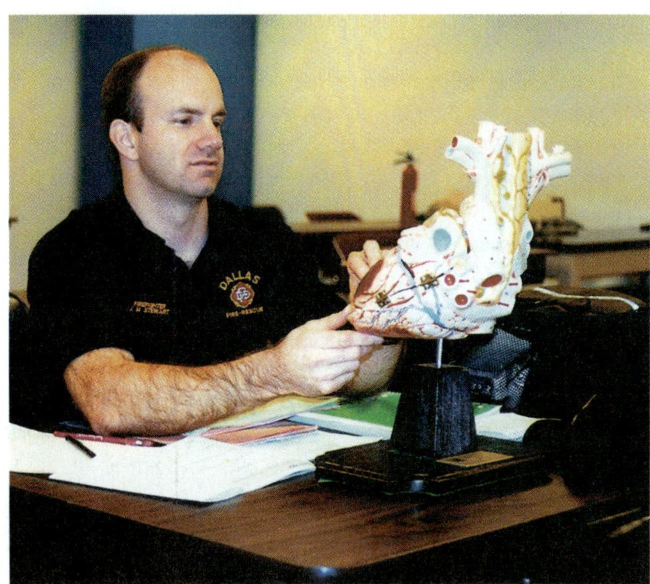

FIGURE 4-5 Diverse instructional methods can help ensure that each student has the opportunity to efficiently comprehend material.

USING LEARNING STYLES TO ENHANCE TEACHING

It has been said that, "Variety is the spice of life." The same holds true for the classroom, especially when it comes to supporting the various learning styles of students. The simplest way for an educator to reach most learners is to vary teaching styles throughout the course and within each lesson. Variety does not necessitate jumping around and changing techniques just for the sake of change; however, a concerted effort should be made to present material in different ways to reach more learners through different senses.

The educator can use a basic instructional format, such as lecture, and supplement it with aids and activities that appeal to other learning styles. The illustrated lecture is a good example. With this method, the educator lectures (auditory) and uses projected media or writing boards (visual) or models (kinesthetic) to emphasize key points. Something as simple as a handout of the lecture outline can provide additional stimulation to help learners perceive and retain information. Workgroups can be formed or discussion begun to explore new material or solve problems; this meets the needs of social learners. Scenarios, because of their broad perspective, appeal to both global and analytic learners.

Reaching out to learners with varying learning styles is an achievable goal when the educator has a solid understanding of learning styles, basic principles of adult learning, and the various teaching strategies that are appropriate for different material and situations. Even traditional classroom activities can assist educators in providing varied presentations of the same material.

Use of diverse instruction methods ensures that each student will receive at least a small portion of the lesson through his or her preferred method of learning (Figure 4-5). This prevents disillusionment and frustration on the part of the learner. In addition, it provides an opportunity for the learner to more efficiently and enjoyably comprehend the presented material. For some students, these periods of "learning comfort" (i.e., times when the material is presented in a manner consistent with the student's preferred learning style) may prevent inappropriate classroom behavior. By periodically spacing changes in presentation style throughout a lesson, the educator is able to refocus learners and stimulate their interest.

Diversity in presentation style also helps learners develop alternative learning styles and sensory preferences. For example, a visual learner may find use of an auditory mnemonic helpful. Or, an auditory learner can benefit from "going through the motions" of a procedure with the hands before taking a test. Because teamwork is so important in healthcare and in emergency medical services (EMS) in particular, practical sessions in which learners work in teams will promote the development of social learning preferences in independent learners. Similarly, algorithms will help global learners to become more analytic. Most learners are able to adapt to different learning styles.

MULTIPLE INTELLIGENCES

Thus far, this chapter has described a traditional approach to learning styles, which have been discussed in terms of perception, receipt of information, and processing of information. But is there more to learning and the broader idea of intelligence? Some researchers think so. Howard Gardner of Harvard

CASE IN POINT

An educator is planning a lesson on musculoskeletal injuries to meet the EMT objective—"List the major bones or bone groupings of the spinal column, the thorax, the upper extremities, and the lower extremities." How might the educator enhance his or her traditional lecture to meet a variety of learning styles? Here are some ideas he or she might incorporate:

- As the opening attention getter, play the song, "Them Bones" (". . . the thigh bone is connected to the hip bone . . ."). Ask students to follow along by touching each of their own bones as the song progresses
- Show a human skeleton, and review aloud the functions and types of bones, asking students to point to their own bones as types are mentioned
- Using slides, illustrate the key points of the lecture, with important points bolded and color-coded
- When discussing bone structure, pass around a model of a vertebra for students to examine and touch
- When introducing new terms, ask students to repeat the term aloud as a class
- Using blocks of wood of varying sizes with a hole in the center, have students label each appropriately sized block as a vertebra, then place it on a wire coat hanger to build a spinal column
- Break the class into small groups, and give each group the assignment of developing a poem, song, or mnemonic for remembering the major bones of the body
- Pass around a model of a joint for students to examine and manipulate
- Show a short video clip, perhaps of an orthopedic operation, that shows a joint or bone type
- Show orthopedic x-rays for guided review
- Present a display with models or diagrams that explain the physics of joint movement and muscle involvement. This could include mathematical equations that explain the forces involved
- During presentation of new material, make sure to relate the new to the old and to the overall context of the lesson

University has proposed that individuals have varying degrees of ability in eight areas, which he refers to as *intelligences*.[5] These intelligences are grouped into three broad categories: object-related, object-free, and person-related (Table 4-2).

Each individual person has varying strengths of each intelligence, and each person combines these intelligences in a personal way that defines his or her overall intelligence. For example, a person may have the ability to play the piano beautifully but may struggle in mathematics. Another individual may be adept at understanding himself or herself but weak at understanding others. These are examples of different intellectual strengths or combinations of strengths possessed by individuals.

TABLE 4-2 Multiple Intelligences[5]

Category	Type of Intelligence	Meaning
Object-related	Logical–mathematical	Ability to work with equations and expressions, to think and process information in a logical way
	Spatial	Ability to think in three dimensions, to use and manipulate images, to apply graphic information
	Bodily–kinesthetic	Physical ability; ability to manipulate objects
	Naturalist	Understanding of natural and man-made systems; ability to identify and classify
Object-free	Linguistic	Ability to use words for thinking and expression
	Musical	Sensitivity to pitch, melody, rhythm, and tone
Person-related	Interpersonal	Ability to relate to others
	Intrapersonal	Ability to understand oneself and direct one's life

Similar to the more traditional concept of one intelligence, Gardner's multiple intelligences follow a developmental sequence and emerge at different times in a person's life. They also consist of a series of subintelligences. Overall, Gardner's theory provides an expanded view of what it means to be human.

For the educator, curricula should be developed that combine all eight intelligences. Just as it is important in the more traditional approach to learning styles to vary the presentation of material, so too should the educator plan activities that help the learner to develop his or her dominant intelligences. See

BOX 4-2 Instructor's Lesson Guide

Course: EMT-Intermediate

Session Reference: 6-5
Topic: Heart blocks
Level of Instruction: Cognitive
Time Required: 3 hours
References: EMT-I National Standard Curriculum

Preparation

Attention: Instructor provided
Motivation: Instructor provided
Objective: At the conclusion of this lesson, the student will be able to identify the three degrees of cardiac conduction blocks, given a real or simulated ECG tracing, without assistance, to a written test accuracy of 75%
Overview:

- Anatomy and physiology of the heart
- Supraventricular conduction system
- 1st-degree block
- 2nd-degree blocks
- 3rd-degree block

Learning Activities

Linguistic

In pairs, students read, discuss, and question textbook information.

Visual-Spatial

Learners identify on a heart model the location of the sinoatrial (SA) and atrioventricular (AV) nodes, the internodal pathways, and the nodal blood supply

Musical

Learners compose a percussion piece that mimics the flow of the electrical pulse through a heart with each of the blocks.

Intrapersonal

Individually, learners identify life events that involved a delay or blockage of communications with another person.

Mathematical-Logical

In small groups, learners develop flow charts of the conduction pulse moving through the heart.

Bodily-Kinesthetic

Using paper and soda straws, as well as glue and scissors, learners construct models of the heart's conduction system.

Interpersonal

Learners role-play patients with each degree of heart block and share symptoms with each other.

Naturalist

Learners create lists of events in nature that are similar to the underlying pathophysiology of heart blocks.

Summary

Review

- A&P of the heart
- Supraventricular conduction system
- 1st-degree block
- 2nd-degree blocks
- 3rd-degree block

Modified from Campbell, Campbell, and Dickinson, 1999, p 270.

Box 4-2 for an example of a lesson plan designed to teach ECG recognition through the multiple intelligences approach. Box 4-3 presents Lazear's multiple intelligences toolbox that contains strategies for each of the eight intelligences.

SUMMARY

Each learner brings to the classroom a preference for the way he or she perceives, receives, and processes information. To maximize learning, the educator must be aware of these differences, must employ a variety of teaching strategies, and must provide a variety of learning activities that will reach all students. Similarly, educators must be sensitive to the fact that they, too, have a preference for learning that influences their teaching style and their interaction with students.

The traditional approach to learning styles has been to describe them in terms of sensory perception and social interaction. New theories, such as Gardner's multiple intelligences, are expanding the view of learning styles and challenging educators and curriculum developers to introduce new and varying ways of presenting material.

BOX 4-3 Multiple Intelligences Toolbox

Logical/Mathematical

- Abstract symbols/formulas
- Calculation
- Deciphering codes
- Forcing relationships
- Graphic/cognitive organizers
- Logic/pattern games
- Number sequences/patterns
- Outlining
- Problem solving
- Syllogisms

Musical/Rhythmic

- Environmental sounds
- Instrumental sounds
- Music composition/creation
- Music performance
- Percussion vibrations
- Rapping
- Rhythmic patterns
- Singing/humming
- Tonal patterns
- Vocal sounds/tones

Bodily/Kinesthetic

- Body language/physical gestures
- Body sculpture/tableaus
- Dramatic enactment
- Folk/creative dance
- Gymnastic routines
- Human graph
- Inventing
- Physical exercise/martial arts
- Role playing/mime
- Sports games

Verbal/Linguistic

- Creative writing
- Formal speaking
- Humor/jokes
- Impromptu speaking
- Journal/diary keeping
- Poetry
- Reading
- Storytelling/story creation
- Verbal debate
- Vocabulary

Interpersonal

- Collaborative skills teaching
- Cooperative learning strategies
- Empathy practices
- Giving feedback
- Group projects
- Intuiting others' feelings
- Jigsaw
- Person-to-person communication
- Receiving feedback
- Sensing others' motives

Intrapersonal

- Altered states of consciousness practices
- Emotional processing
- Focusing/concentration skills
- Higher-order reasoning
- Independent studies/projects
- Know thyself procedures
- Metacognition techniques
- Mindfulness practices
- Silent reflection methods
- Thinking strategies

Visual/Spatial

- Active imagination
- Color/texture schemes
- Drawing
- Guided imagery/visualizing
- Mind mapping
- Montage/collage
- Painting
- Patterns/designs
- Pretending/fantasy
- Sculpting

Naturalist

- Archetypal pattern recognition
- Caring for plants/animals
- Conservation practices
- Environment feedback
- Hands-on labs
- Nature encounters/field trips
- Nature observation
- Natural world simulations
- Species classification (organic/inorganic)
- Sensory stimulation exercises

REFERENCES

1. Kolb DA, Rubin IM, McIntyre JM. *Organizational Psychology, A Book of Readings.* 3rd ed. New Jersey: Prentice-Hall; 1979:543-549.
2. Dunn RS, Dunn KJ. *Teaching Students Through Their Individual Learning Styles: A Practical Approach.* Reston, Va: Reston Publishing Company; 1978.
3. HOBET. Shawnee Mission, Ks: Educational Resources Incorporated.
4. Myers IB. *Gifts Differing.* Palo Alto, Calif: Consulting Psychological Press; 1980.
5. Gardner H. *Frames of Mind: The Theory of Multiple Intelligences.* New York, NY: Basic Books; 1985.
6. Lazear D. *Eight Ways of Knowing: Teaching for Multiple Intelligences.* 3rd ed. Arlington Heights, Ill: Skylight Professional Development; 1999.

CHAPTER 5

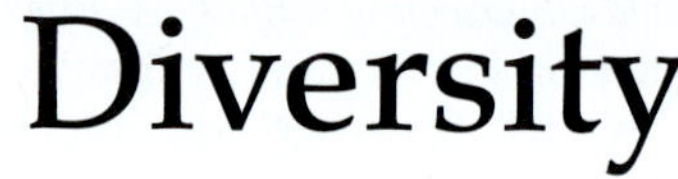

Diversity

"Tolerance implies no lack of commitment to one's own beliefs. Rather it condemns the oppression or persecution of others."

—*John Fitzgerald Kennedy*

Individuals view life through a unique set of perspectives, shaped by years of accumulated experiences and interactions with the world. They absorb and reject the thoughts, opinions, and ideas of others as they see fit. Within the emergency medical services (EMS) classroom, it is important that educators allow and even encourage the presentation of conflicting viewpoints. Instructors have the ability and power to provide the information and setting necessary to promote better awareness and understanding of diversity among students, both within the classroom and later outside of the classroom, when students enter the field as interns and finally as practitioners.

The United States consists of one of the most diverse populations of people, ideas, and cultures in the world. Most people have heard the United States referred to as a "melting pot." Population data bear that out, reflecting great diversity in age, race, and religion throughout the country.[1,2] Many EMS instructors and providers understand the complexities involved in caring for patients and working in a diverse society. However, EMS could improve the elements of diversity seen in its curricula and in its practitioners. The Longitudinal Emergency Medical Technician Attribute and Demographic Study (LEADS) indicated that approximately 70% of the Registry is male and 90% is white.[3] A separate analysis of Registry data from 2001 revealed that approximately 17% of registered emergency medical technicians (EMTs) (of all levels) identified themselves as members of an ethnic minority group.[4]

Because there appears to be a disparity between the diversity of the general population of the nation and that of EMS, it is important that the instructor work toward including elements of diversity throughout the curriculum. This chapter cannot and should not serve as the only guide in that effort. It will, however, identify key concepts (1) to better prepare EMS providers to treat patients within a diverse population, and (2) to improve diversity within the profession, beginning with a culturally aware educational environment (Figure 5-1).

INSTRUCTOR, KNOW THYSELF

All human beings are susceptible to having biases. This is not a value statement; it is simply fact. The 2003 *Merriam Webster Dictionary* defines *bias* as "an unreasonable judgment." For example, an instructor may *unreasonably* believe that all women are too weak to perform many of the tasks commonly required in EMS. That instructor might be seen often rushing to assist the female students in the class, regardless of their capabilities or requests not to be "treated special" during lifting and carrying exercises. This instructor's judgment is obviously not based on any reasoned discourse.

Biases can take many forms. Examples include biases against particular ethnicities, genders, ages, socioeconomic classes, religions, political persuasions, and sexual orientations. The *Case in Point* on p. 54 gives an example of a person who held multiple biases, which created a negative synergistic effect on his attitude and behavior toward others. In this case, the instructor has a bias against a Latina woman's ability to understand and excel in math.

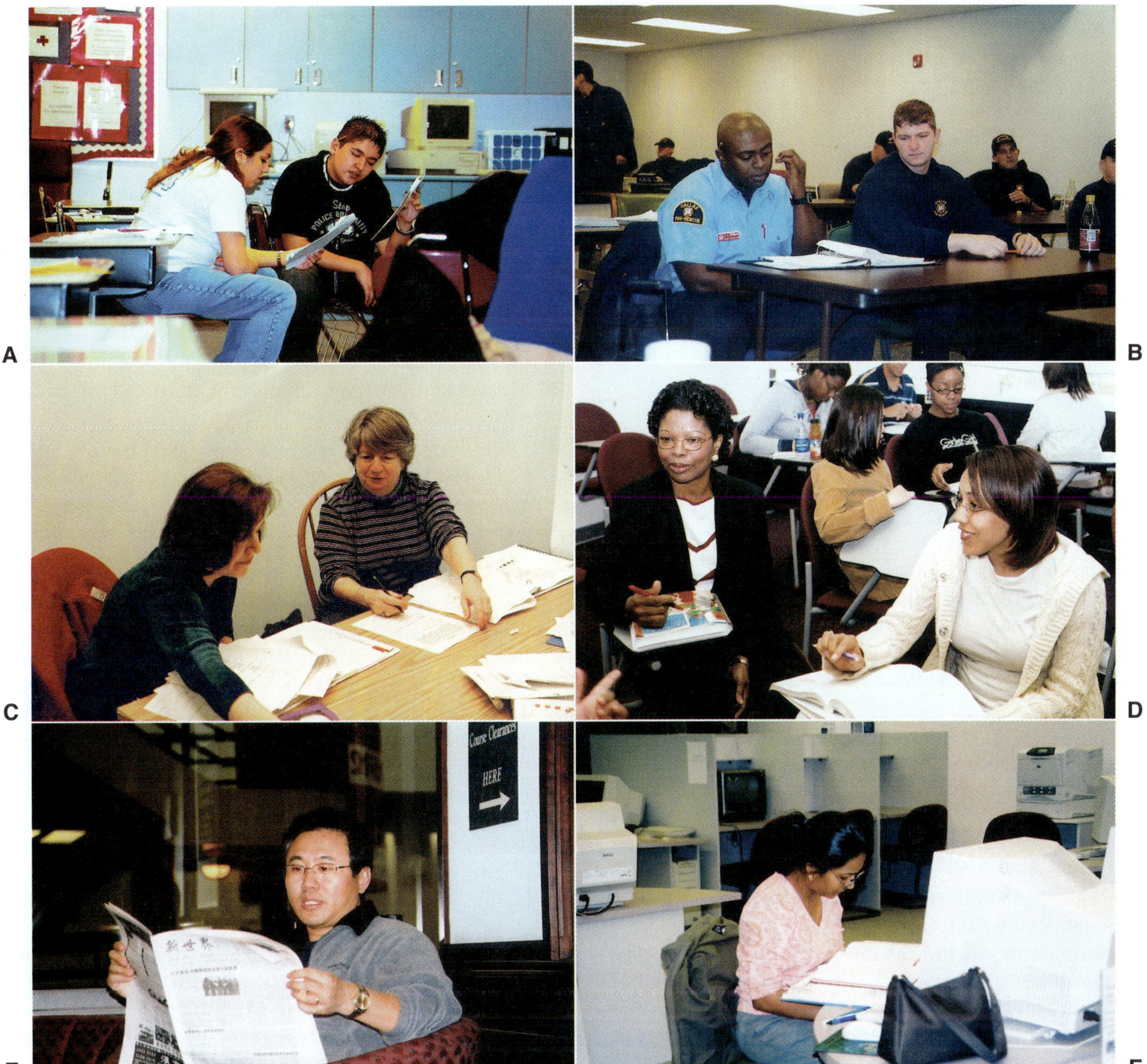

Figure 5-1 Instructors have the ability to promote understanding of diversity among students and patients.

Biases become dangerous when they are manifested as behaviors. An instructor's behavior in the classroom can and will affect the probability of success for many students. An instructor who believes students can succeed makes that prospect more likely than one who believes they will fail. Students' sense of self-efficacy (i.e., their sense of "I can do it!") is directly related to the classroom environment and the instructor's expectations of those students.[5] EMS instructors must be aware of the impact their attitudes may have on students, and they should remain diligent to prevent their own biases from negatively affecting the perceptions of those students.

To deal with or reduce bias, one first has to acknowledge its existence. Performing a critical self-reflection and recognizing one's own personal biases are ways to begin a process of self-discovery and a greater awareness of one's own potential biases. Instructors should try to see lessons and other course materials through the perceptions of others, and should consider enrolling in cultural diversity classes offered through a local college or university. For the instructor who has already critically examined and dealt with any such issues, it remains incumbent upon him or her to challenge students to do the same.

CASE IN POINT

It was the second day of the "med math" section of the pharmacology unit, and the instructor was busy working with the paramedic students, trying to convey the basic concepts of proportion and cross-multiplication to the group. The instructor noticed that a Latina woman seemed to be grasping the concepts easily, and she was using them to solve a complex dopamine drip problem. Later, he noticed her working with several other students. During a break in the session, the instructor approached the student, patted her on the shoulder, and said, "I am pleased that you were able to grasp the concepts quickly, especially considering your background. I appreciate that you are helping out the other women in the class."

The student appeared puzzled. "Why are you surprised?"

The instructor responded, "I figured that being female and *all*, that you probably were not really prepared in your high school for mathematics."

Silent for a moment, the student finally sighed and replied, "I'm not sure why you would think that. Actually, I excelled in math. Furthermore, I resent the idea that I could help only other women, especially since I helped three male students as well!"

TEACHING TIP Ask a colleague to review exams and lesson plans for cultural sensitivity.

DIVERSITY IN THE CLASSROOM

Over the past 15 years, a tremendous amount has been written about *cultural competency* within a variety of environments, including the worksite and the classroom. Earlier efforts in EMS education focused on identification of the unique traits of specific groups, based on gender, ethnic, and religious lines.[6] Although those who made these attempts meant well, the truth is that the very act of defining group characteristics can reinforce the stereotypes that such efforts are designed to minimize. Instructors who try to modify their teaching practices based on "laundry lists" of such characteristics will quickly run into issues associated with any "one-size-fits-all" approach, namely, that not all members of a specific group of individuals are completely alike. Stereotyping assumptions will likely cause discomfort for the student and the instructor. This discomfort may rise to a level of anger and open frustration that disrupts the class.

Students within the classroom may include representatives from a wide variety of groups. Alternatively, the instructor may be faced with a group of culturally similar students, and may find himself or herself in the minority. How many ways can a single group of students be dissimilar?

- Age (younger vs older, nontraditional students)
- Appearance (e.g., hair length, hygiene, tattoos, piercings)
- Disorders (e.g., physical, emotional, and psychological/psychiatric disabilities)
- Gender identification (e.g., female, male, transgender)
- Generational (e.g., Baby Boomers, Gen X-ers, Gen Y-ers, In-betweens)
- Learning ability (e.g., attention deficit disorder, dyslexia)
- Language ability (e.g., speaking non-English as first language, using poor grammar, depending heavily on slang)
- Marital status (e.g., cohabitating, divorced, married, single, widowed)
- Parenting (e.g., no children, older or younger children, stepchildren, or older parents that need to be taken care of)
- Political views (e.g., conservatism, liberalism, libertarianism)
- Race/ethnicity (alphabetical categories listed here are from the US Census Bureau and are used on most federal and state forms: American Indian/Eskimo/Aleut, Asian Pacific Islander, Black [sic], Hispanic, and White [Although the term Black is used by the Census, the term African American should be considered in accordance with current nomenclature])
- Religion (e.g., Buddhism, Christianity, Islam, Romany, Wicca)
- Sexual orientation (e.g., bisexual, heterosexual, homosexual)
- Socioeconomic status (e.g., indigent, poor, middle class, wealthy)

Careful review of this list should lead the Reader to the realization that even apparently homogeneous students may be different in many ways. This should not be surprising, as it reinforces what is commonly known: Each student is an individual and does not deserve to be limited to being seen as a "representative" of any one group. Students should be seen as complex beings with much to offer the class. Each possesses experience and knowledge that can add to the richness of the classroom experience for other students and for the instructor.

POWER IN THE TEACHING RELATIONSHIP

The relationship between student and instructor can be a powerful one, although not in the sense of *power* meaning "strength." Rather, in this case, "power" refers to the *control* that an instructor exerts upon the relationship with the student. For example, the instructor sets the teaching schedule, grades the tests, assigns the clinical rotations, and designs the curriculum, just to name a few obvious tasks. The student usually has little or no control over these areas. Another aspect of that control is the ability to decide what is taught in the classroom. The instructor may, knowingly or not, taint the material that is being taught by injecting elements of bias into lessons. Effects of bias can be seen in individual lessons and even throughout an entire curriculum. For example, although many major publishers have worked to minimize this, not all EMS textbooks equally portray individuals from ethnic minority groups and women in positions of authority.[4] The images and the *feel* of a textbook can influence an entire course. This is not to say that diversity is the only element to consider when one is choosing a text; however, it is something that should be evaluated closely.

TEACHING TIP When selecting a textbook, the instructor should be aware of the level of diversity (and equity) demonstrated in that text.

Instructors should not be afraid of embracing diversity. Some instructors may be tempted to ignore student diversity when it could in fact contribute to the learning environment not only of those individuals but of the whole group. For example, an instructor may have students from a rural, agricultural community who could directly speak to the hazards of farm machinery. Their unique cultural experiences could help to make the material more relevant for the entire class.[7] It would be tragic to ignore this wealth of information and to rely solely upon textbooks.

OPPORTUNITIES TO INTEGRATE CLASSROOM DIVERSITY

There are many ways for an educator to create an environment that takes advantage of a classroom's diversity, rather than minimizes it. Not all approaches will work with every instructor. Instructors should decide which of the following suggestions might work for them, based on their background and comfort level. Then, they should try these suggestions or develop their own ideas; they may find these efforts to be surprisingly interesting and effective.

INSTRUCTIONAL MATERIALS

Ethnicity and Gender

Spoken and written language should be ethnically/racially and gender nonspecific or used with equal frequency. Contrived or forced neutrality (e.g., using "he/she") should be avoided. The instructor can use "he" or "she" in alternating scenarios and test questions, or can use generic phrases such as "the patient" and "the doctor." Scenarios can be used to challenge misperceptions and to strengthen positive role models. For example, a scenario might be written in which the nurse is male and the EMS supervisor is female. By challenging traditional perceptions, these scenarios help to expose students to greater possibilities, so they can develop an openness to incorporating those possibilities into their practice.

Identifying the ethnicity or gender of patients in written scenarios is not always necessary. So, in general, this information can be legitimately omitted, allowing students to focus on the *real* issues at hand. However, there are times when these characteristics are significant elements of a person's medical history (e.g., when genetic disorders such as sickle cell or Tay-Sachs disease are considered). When needed, ethnic and gender identifiers should be used. Care should be taken, however, to avoid reinforcing negative—and unfounded—stereotypes. It may be helpful to discuss the contributions of different ethnic groups to the field of medicine as part of the curriculum, not as a side topic; a reference librarian can serve as an excellent resource.

Printed Material and Visual Aids

The educator should ensure that models and simulated situations reflect a wide variety of cultural backgrounds. For example, computer images of people of different genders and from various ethnic, cultural, and/or religious backgrounds may be used. Scripted scenarios should also incorporate a wide range of socioeconomic factors. Frequent reviews of textbooks by instructors for issues of equity and diversity will help to ensure not only the quality of the text but also the degree to which it encourages diversity. Feedback from students will be helpful as well.

INSTRUCTIONAL STRATEGIES

Presentation

Rather than using only one type of presentation format (e.g., lecture), the educator should use a variety of teaching strategies. The student body within any given classroom community is likely to represent a wide range of learning styles. The use of multiple methods of instruction will help to enhance the learning of the class. Examples of teaching methods include small group exercises, take-home case studies, debates, large group discussions, Internet-based lessons, and role playing.

Assessment

Instructors must be aware of their own biases when they are evaluating a student's performance. It may be helpful to have students identify all written assignments with a code name or only a portion of their social security number, so their identities are shielded during grading. Multiple instructors may grade practical scenarios and role playing to establish an "average" score. (*Note:* If these scores vary greatly, it may be appropriate to discount the highest and lowest scores, averaging the remaining middle scores.) These safeguards work in two ways: They help students by ensuring that they are not unfairly penalized, and they help instructors to avoid favoritism.

STUDENT-EDUCATOR RELATIONS

Awareness

One must recognize that students come from diverse and complex backgrounds. Nothing about them should be assumed. For example, comments about social activities that assume all students are heterosexual, middle class, or Christian should be avoided. One must not assume that the most obvious perception of a student's ethnicity (or even gender) is correct (e.g., a person who might be thought of as Hispanic American may self-identify as white American). As the nation becomes increasingly diverse, the percentage of people who identify with a multiplicity of heritages (and races) also increases. Students must be permitted to explain who and what they are and how they want to be identified.

Terminology

The educator must be sensitive to changing terminology. For example, Asian Americans may not want to be called *Oriental* (sic), Hispanic Americans may prefer to be called Chicano or Latino, and persons from diverse families may wish to be referred to as multiracial. If it is *necessary* to categorize, ask which labels are comfortable or preferable.

Spotlighting

One must not force a student to be the spokesperson for any group. For example, when describing the higher frequency of alcoholism or diabetes within a particular group, the instructor must not single out a member of that group to be its spokesperson. However, students may volunteer to share firsthand information about their community. This type of contribution should be encouraged.

Knowledge

The instructor should get to know his or her students (Figure 5-2). Office hours, class "down time," and any other lull in activity can be used to find out about personal background and learning styles. The educator can become better informed about different cultures by researching, reading, and participating in culture-specific activities. Students should be encouraged to write scenarios for the class that are based on personal experiences. This approach helps to validate students' lives for the group, and it shows that the instructor values what is shared.

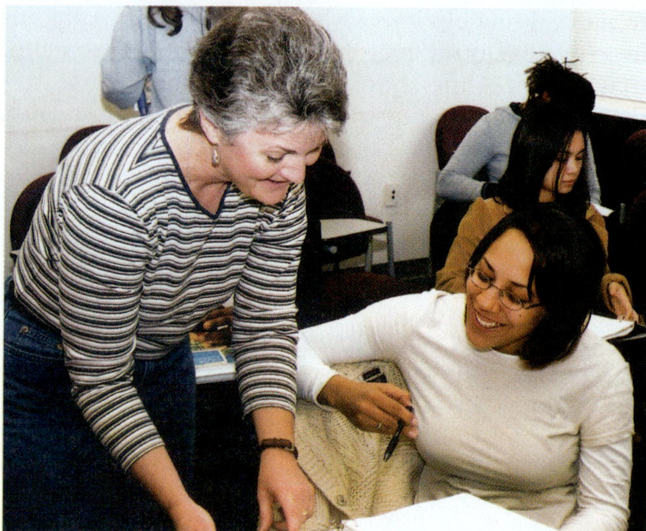

Figure 5-2 Getting to know students as individuals enables the instructor to better understand their backgrounds and values.

Behavior

One must lead by example. The instructor should exhibit the actions desired in his or her students. If comments are made in the classroom that focus on negative stereotypes, the instructor should take time to discuss and counter them with accurate information. If the instructor does not have the information available at the time, he or she should reach out to *key informants* in the community for help. Typically, these people are well-known and highly respected members of a community who are eager to help share information about their community.

Environment

The educator must create a classroom environment that is a safe haven for discussion and exploration. Distasteful or abusive remarks, even if spoken in jest, must not be tolerated. It is important to remember that what is humorous to some may be hurtful to others.

Acceptance

Many elements of everyday behaviors are influenced by cultural rules. For example, some cultures may consider eye contact between an elder (the instructor) and a child (the student, regardless of age) to be disrespectful, whereas many in our society view such contact as just the opposite. The instructor who is aware that such *cultural disconnects* exist can avoid embarrassing and even infuriating moments.

PREPARING STUDENTS TO INCORPORATE DIVERSITY AWARENESS INTO THEIR PRACTICE

Culture

When the word *culture* is mentioned, images of racially or ethnically based differences often come to mind. Many social scientists, however, define *culture* as an amalgamation of customs, experiences, languages, and beliefs common to a defined group. For example, various regions of the nation are described as having uniquely identifiable cultures with predominant characteristics for that area (e.g., Southeastern states, Appalachia, inner city urban areas). The same can be said for regions of the world (e.g., Central America, South Pacific, Middle East).

Social scientists define culture as a group of people who share experiences, language, and values that permit them to communicate knowledge not shared by those outside the culture. An example of a culture is EMS itself. How many providers have used the jargon

CASE IN POINT

It was early Monday morning, and an EMT instructor was just about to begin her class. About half of the students were in the classroom; some were reviewing their textbooks, while others were reading the newspaper. As the instructor came into the room, she noticed that a few students were congregated toward the back of the room. One animated student was relating to a group of students the details of an EMS call he had observed the previous day. The instructor overheard a few laughs but did not really pay any attention to the conversation. Soon, the class came to order, and the day's lesson on cardiac emergencies began.

During lunch, a student came to see the instructor in her office. This student was visibly angry and obviously needed to talk. Concerned, the instructor closed the office door and listened carefully to her. Apparently, the conversation that the animated student was leading earlier involved a patient who was suffering from end-stage AIDS, necessitating an urgent call for EMS. The student had described how he had been riding along as an EMT observer with the crew. The student who was currently upset had overheard the other student saying comments such as, "homosexuality is a sin," and, "AIDS is what you get when you're gay." Even though she was not part of the discussion, this student was angered by the comments, especially because her sister had died of AIDS only 6 months earlier.

The instructor asked the student if she said anything to the other student about his comments. She shook her head no; she felt very uncomfortable talking to him directly. Angrily, the student said, "I just want him to know that not all AIDS patients are gay, and even those who are do not deserve to suffer like that!"

Follow-up

After the upset student left the instructor's office, the instructor spent the remainder of her break finishing her lunch and thinking about how she could manage the situation. Despite her own discomfort and anger about what the other student had said to his classmates, she knew she had to intervene to try to turn a tense situation into a learning experience for all involved. In her conversation with the instructor, the upset student had indicated that she was not seeking an apology from the other student, nor did she want to get him "into any trouble."

The instructor decided to implement the following plan:

1. At the next break, she would pull the student who had made the negative comments aside and determine what he had actually said during the discussion. She would advise him that the comments, if stated as reported, were hurtful to another student and would not be considered professional behavior in her class. The instructor would also provide the student an opportunity to express his feelings about what was said and about how another person perceived his comments. However, she would make sure that he understood that the comments he had made were inappropriate, and that he should avoid making similar ones in the future. Later that day, she would document her conversations with both students, possibly having each student sign a copy of the respective incident reports.
2. At the next class, she would engage the class in a short discussion about verbal behavior in the classroom, as well as in the clinical setting. It is important to reinforce to the entire class how critical it is to be mindful of other people's feelings and perceptions, in case a conversation is accidentally overheard. The instructor will be careful to avoid "shutting down" the student who had made the comments and will make sure that he continues to feel valued as a member of the classroom community.
3. Later in the semester, she would provide additional information about HIV and AIDS through handouts, Internet links, and discussions in class.
4. She would schedule clinical rotations with a local AIDS hospice. Each student would be required to submit a written summary of his or her experiences and to share those experiences with the entire class in a discussion or presentation.

of the profession ("10-8," "code 3," "ALS") in a conversation with people outside the industry, only to have someone look quizzically at them? When EMS providers get together and begin talking, they should take pity on the non-EMS person who tries to keep up with the discussion. Any person who is looking from the outside in would likely be very confused about what is being said and meant. This lack of "getting it" is an example of low *cultural competency.* It is possible that students in the EMS classroom come with culturally specific elements in their communication. The EMS instructor must be aware of this potential challenge and should build tools to overcome it. One strategy would be to invite students to write down a list (with definitions) of the slang words they commonly use. Another strategy would be to simply ask students what they mean any time an unknown word is noted in the classroom.

Transcultural communication can open doors to greater understanding, but it can also lead to misunderstanding. Misunderstanding, often caused by ignorance, can make or break the medical management of an event. The following section provides some suggestions on how to reduce the occurrences of misunderstanding; ways to implement a culturally aware medical curriculum are discussed.

DEVELOPING A CULTURALLY SOUND TEACHING CURRICULUM

Needs Assessment

Not all areas of the nation are similar in terms of the cultures that exist there. For example, the incidence of homelessness may be greater in an urban, inner city area than in a sparsely populated, rural area. A needs assessment, or evaluation, should be conducted by the EMS instructor for the purpose of ascertaining which terms, customs, and other cultural elements should be introduced into the curriculum to best serve local, regional, and national needs.

Sometimes what is needed is evident. For example, the rapid influx of an ethnically based population, for whom English is not the primary language, may necessitate a specific training effort to educate the EMS system about basic practices and traditions within that population. Many texts are available to learn more about the theory of evaluation techniques. (For more information, see the works of Guskey, Tyler, and Scriven in the "Recommended Reading" section of this chapter.)

Research

This can often be the most labor-intensive step of developing a culturally sound curriculum. What information is needed during preparation of the lesson plan that will deliver the concepts? Often, the information cannot be found in traditional EMS textbooks. However, it can be found in many places, including libraries, the Internet, journals, and textbooks. (See, for example, Sue and Sue, *Counseling the Culturally Diverse,* 4th ed.) Other sources may provide more accurate and relevant information to EMS than can be found in published writings. One such source consists of those persons identified as community leaders or key informants within the population in question.

Other Resources

Local service agencies often focus on specific groups within a community and can offer a wealth of information about their clientele. Many such agencies are more than happy to share their expertise with anyone who wishes to become more enlightened. For example, a local council on aging might offer an entire presentation on the psychosocial issues the elderly face when living alone, or they might help to arrange for elderly persons to serve as patients during presentation of a unit on Geriatrics.

In addition to local resources, many helpful sources of information are available at the federal and national levels. Organizations such as the American Medical Association (AMA) and the American Association of Medical Colleges (AAMC) have released compendiums of references on the needs and resources of specific populations. The American Association of Universities and Colleges (AAUC) has compiled resource information on culturally aware teaching practices. (Some of these sources can be located in the Resources section of this chapter.)

INSTRUCTIONAL STRATEGIES

Many cultural concepts can be integrated directly into the medical curriculum that is being taught. In doing so, the instructor must take the time needed to develop and establish the "ground rules for a safe environment." These rules must include statements that assure all students that they will have the opportunity to speak and to be heard. Students must know, however, that there are limits to this free speech. This limit in the classroom, as in society, means that *one person's right to expression stops at the next person's nose.* That means students may speak, they may be honest, and they may disagree; they may not, however, attack one another. So, although *ideas* may be torn apart (i.e., with the use of reasoned arguments, or *discourse*), *people* may not be. The instructor must present these rules to the class and must ensure that all participants understand and agree to abide by them. Students should be given an opportunity to read and add to or argue against the specifics of the list of rules, but in the end, they must all sign a contract of agreement with the final document.

Instructors can incorporate diversity into a classroom community by employing a variety of educational methods, including some of those discussed in the following paragraphs.

Case Studies

These scenario-based lessons tell students about an event, the actions taken, and the outcomes. For example, students may be given a written exercise that contains a short scenario about an elderly woman who was found "down" in her apartment by neighbors. The case proceeds to detail what the responding crew found, how they treated the patient, and how the patient responded. These types of scenarios may be created to include a wide variety of diverse elements.

Guest Presentation

If the community of interest is a particular religious group, a member of the local house of faith could be invited to present a lecture to the class. This lecture might include a brief history of the group, an explanation of its core beliefs, and any special information that would be particularly useful during an emergency (e.g., perhaps members of this faith do not accept blood products or medications, or perhaps they permit female patients to be touched only by female caregivers). Students should be encouraged to ask questions, and the presenter must be made to feel welcome, even when his or her beliefs seem strange or extreme.

Community Outreach

Students often engage in community-minded projects, such as staffing first aid stations, providing blood pressure checks, and giving bicycle safety lectures (Figure 5-3). It could be helpful for the instructor (or the program) to sponsor such efforts in targeted communities. Students could set up a health education booth at a community center in an ethnic minority neighborhood, or they may provide free cardiopulmonary resuscitation (CPR) classes for a low-income, single-parents group. The communities that receive these services may, in turn, share intimate knowledge about the group. Students may be invited to attend local festivals or events, an opportunity that would further their understanding and appreciation of that culture.

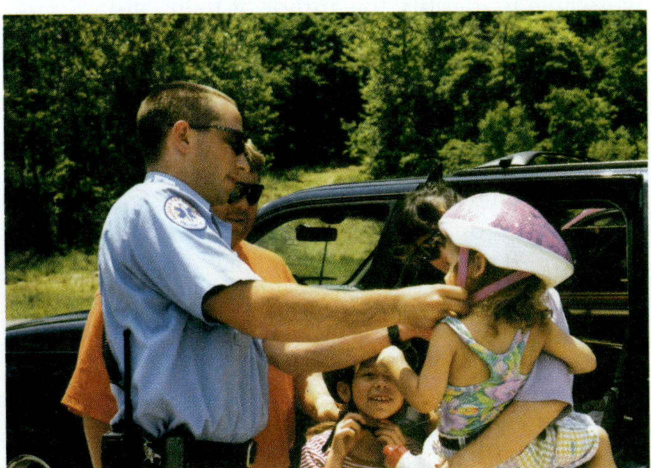

Figure 5-3 Injury prevention activities sponsored by the educational program in a minority neighborhood can be educational for the community, as well as for school-age students.

CASE IN POINT

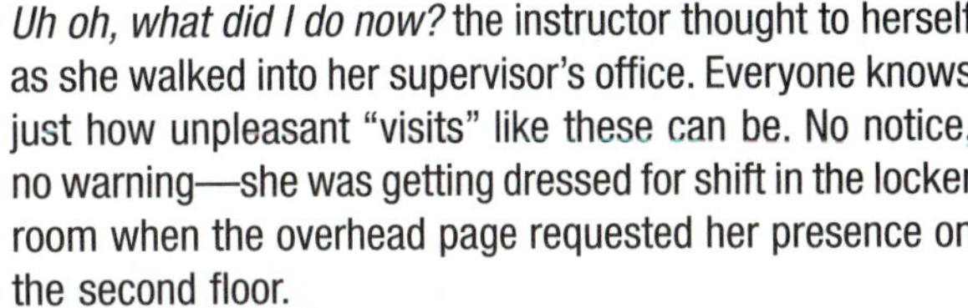

Uh oh, what did I do now? the instructor thought to herself as she walked into her supervisor's office. Everyone knows just how unpleasant "visits" like these can be. No notice, no warning—she was getting dressed for shift in the locker room when the overhead page requested her presence on the second floor.

She was a bit surprised when she entered the office. In addition to her supervisor, an elderly man was sitting in the room. Smiling, her supervisor introduced her to the director of the senior citizen assistance office of the county health department.

"Remember when you were talking about the number of hip fractures you were handling at the elder care high-rises downtown?" her supervisor asked.

"Uh huh," the instructor replied. (She was actually ranting and raving about how ambulance resources were being used to handle these cases. It seems like a city rig goes to a report of a "person found down" once or twice a week!)

"Well, by chance, I was talking to the director here about another issue, when I mentioned this might be a problem. He has offered to listen to your complaint and offer some assistance." The three began a discussion about identifying the nature of the problem.

Follow-up

First, the instructor established a common ground with all interested parties—everyone involved in this case understands the serious effects of a fractured hip for elderly patients. Next, the three discussed the possibility of performing a risk analysis to determine what factors increase or decrease the likelihood of a fall. The county's public health office probably has a tool for gathering such information. Those data could be used in the design of a safety program that eliminates hazards (e.g., loose carpeting replaced with a nonslip version, hand rails added to all rooms) and teaches residents how to monitor their personal risk index. Lastly, the instructor decided to establish a *train the trainer* model by which she would prepare her staff to go out into the community and educate the staff at the elder care centers.

From The George Washington University Emergency Health Services Program. Courtesy of A. Hsieh.

Group Discussions

An open forum is best supported by clear guidelines and goals. If some students in the class identify themselves as members of the community of interest, they should be invited (not compelled) to share their thoughts and experiences. Other sources of information are local community leaders (e.g., ministers, business owners, and instructors). The instructor must begin such discussions with a brief outline of the rules for the event. These rules must establish that ideas are welcome but attacks are not. Each student must feel safe if open and frank discussions are to occur. The instructor should function as the facilitator, guiding the discussion but not controlling it. The instructor will be *the guide on the side—not the sage on the stage.*[8]

CASE IN POINT

During a recent class discussion, the instructor presented information about initial scene assessment (the global survey). He stated that some EMS agencies provide bullet-resistant vests for their personnel. One local agency does this, and they allow the employees to wear the "over the shirt" type of vest whenever the employees believe it is justified. A student asked why most of the EMS personnel she knows wear the vests only when they get a call to go to areas of town that are primarily populated by ethnic minorities. The class immediately began a debate about the "facts" that these parts of town have more calls that are violent, and that EMS is more likely to be threatened in these areas. Some members of the class describe this as a reasonable precaution. Others describe it as racial profiling. They turn to the instructor and look for guidance. What does he do?

Follow-up

First, the instructor distills the arguments on both sides to their most salient points (e.g., crime rates, number of past EMS assaults, overall violence in the areas). Then, he gets each side to do some research to back up their beliefs. They could examine publicly available statistics and invite local community leaders to discuss the issue. He asks that each side bring their results back into class and present them to one another. This case is based on local practices, so it would be appropriate to bring in a representative of the local EMS to explain the reasoning that went into the policy's creation and implementation.

Practical Skills

Ideally, an actor is brought into the skills laboratory for each practical scenario. The actor must be prepared to play his or her role. Care should be taken to create scenarios that inform students and even challenge perceptions. For example, a scenario about a pregnant teenager should not always include a person of one particular racial/ethnic or socioeconomic group. If actors are not available, students can be coached to take on the patient roles, and to conduct the research necessary to perform the role accurately. Although they may be labor intensive, such exercises can stimulate alternative learning opportunities for all students involved.

Clinical Rotations

Clinically oriented rotations can be supplemented by limited observations in nontraditional settings. For example, if the community of interest includes severely mentally retarded patients, students may be assigned clinical rotations with a center that specializes in the care of these patients. Such rotations could provide students with expert opinions and a chance to put a face on the disorder, thereby making it more meaningful to them.

Identity

Instructors and students make assumptions about others. These assumptions include labels of ethnicity, religion, disability, and more. One strategy that is useful for challenging such potentially erroneous assumptions is known as the "identity game." During this type of exercise, students might be asked to elaborate (by writing on an index card) on how they see *themselves* (e.g., "heterosexual, Christian, male"). Each student could label his or her card using a code name known only to the instructor. These completed cards would be turned in to the instructor, who would then randomly assign the cards to other members of the class. Each student's assignment would be to try to identify the classmate whose card he or she was given. The class would be polled to see how many students were able to identify the author of their card.

Role Playing

Students are asked to identify a group (e.g., ethnic, gender, religion) that is different from their own. They are then assigned to play parts in a patient care scenario based on their new identity. For example, a Christian female student may play the part of an elderly Jehovah's Witness male patient, or an ethnic minority male student might play the part of the nonminority male firefighter. This exercise has been used in EMS classrooms with great success. However, a degree of caution must be issued here. These portrayals can be full of stereotypes and clichés. Some will break down walls and use humor to demonstrate the ridiculousness of such beliefs. Others may cause needlessly hurt feelings and have the potential to create disharmony within the classroom community. It is recommended that this exercise be used in classrooms in which there is a tradition of open dialogue, and one in which the instructor feels comfortable that a safe environment will be maintained.

Communication Games

Through games, students can learn the importance of communication and ways that it can be affected. One example of such games would be to split students into two groups. Group A would be asked to leave the classroom and go into the skills laboratory to prepare equipment for spinal immobilization. Once in the lab, this group would be told to reverse the meanings of their words (e.g., they will say "more" when they mean "less," or "right" when they mean "left"). When Group B enters the lab, they would be told to partner with those persons already there. The ensuing confusion can be humorous. It can also demonstrate how communication, although usually taken for granted, can lead to misunderstanding and can even be counterproductive.

SUMMARY

Although the United States is often referred to as a *melting pot*, perhaps a better analogy is that of a *stewpot*, in which distinct elements are blended together to make up a delicious concoction that is far greater than its parts. By supporting and celebrating diversity in the EMS classroom, students can become better prepared to deliver care with greater empathy for, and understanding of, the many cultures and groups they will encounter. These future healthcare providers may become more attuned to the diversity of the EMS profession itself and, where needed, they may even improve it.

REFERENCES

1. US Census Bureau, 2001. Available at: http://www.census.gov/prod/2002pubs/p23-211.pdf and at http://www.census.gov/pubinfo/www/hotlinks.html. Accessed December 1, 2003.
2. US Census Bureau, 2000. Available at: http://www.census.gov/prod/2001pubs/statab/sec01.pdf. Accessed November 24, 2003.
3. Brown WE, Dickison PD, Misselbeck WJA, Levine R. Longitudinal Emergency Medical Technician Attribute and Demographic Study (LEADS): an interim report. *Prehospital Care Research Forum.* 2002;6:433-439.
4. Hunter SL. Defining and valuing diversity in EMS. *Emergency Medical Services: Journal of Emergency Care and Transportation.* 2003;32:88-89.
5. Bandura A. *Self-efficacy: The Exercise of Control.* New York: W.H. Freeman and Company; 1997.
6. Honeycutt L. Cultural diversity: essential education. *Journal of Emergency Medical Services.* 1997:39.
7. Cole H. Stories to live by: a narrative approach to health behavior research and injury prevention. In: *Handbook of Health Behavior,* vol 4, Relevance for Professionals and Issues for the Future. 1997:325-349.
8. Collison G, Elbaum B, Haavind S, Tinker R. Facilitating on-line learning. Madison, Wis: Atwood Press; 2000.

RECOMMENDED READING

Sue and Sue. *Counseling the Culturally Diverse: Theory and Practice.* 4th ed. New York, NY: John Wiley & Sons; 2002.

Scriven M. The methodology of evaluation. In: Tyler RW, Gange RM, Scriven M (Eds.), *Perspectives of curriculum evaluation* (pp. 39-83). AERA Monograph Series on Curriculum Evaluation. No. 1. Chicago: Rand McNally; 1967.

Tyler RW. *Basic principles of curriculum and instruction.* Chicago: University of Chicago Press; 1949.

Guskey TR. Does It Make a Difference? *Educational Leadership.* 1998;59(6):45-51.

Guskey TR. The age of accountability. *Journal of Staff Development.* 1998;19(4):36-44.

RESOURCES

The following Internet sites focus on issues of diversity and acceptance. Many of these organizations offer free or low-cost information that can be adapted to the EMS classroom:

American Association of Medical Colleges (www.aamc.org/diversity/reading.htm)

American Association of American Universities and Colleges and Universities (www.diversityweb.org/diversity_innovations/faculty_staff_development/teaching_strategies_practices/index.cfm)

BeliefNet (www.beliefnet.com/index/index_10000.html)

Lambda Gay, Lesbian, Bi-sexual and Transexual Community Services (www.lambda.org/)

Merge Magazine (www.suzannestecker.com/pastwork/mergemag/)

Teaching Tolerance (Southern Poverty Law Center) (www.tolerance.org/teach/index.jsp)

The Multiracial Activist (www.multiracial.com/)

U.S. Department of Health and Human Services (www.hhs.gov/)

PART III

Foundations

Like a building whose integrity is only as strong as the foundation it rests upon, your teaching is strengthened and supported by a clear understanding of core concepts in education. This part of the text explains the learning domains, shows how to address them in goals and objectives, describes how to create effective lesson plans, and provides useful information about pertinent legal issues, as well as the technical tools that enhance your presentation.

Although the foundation of a building may not be as glamorous or attention getting as the architectural details found on its facade, it provides the stable platform from which those details shine. So should your teaching. Your ability to convey ideas and concepts in a brilliant way depends first on your ability to integrate the domains of learning into a comprehensive, deliberate lesson plan. Your strong implementation of that plan in a supportive learning environment is the rich architectural detail that your students will notice and appreciate.

Return to these chapters from time to time to reacquaint yourself with the material. With additional experience, you may be able to more readily apply the information and reevaluate what you are doing—and why.

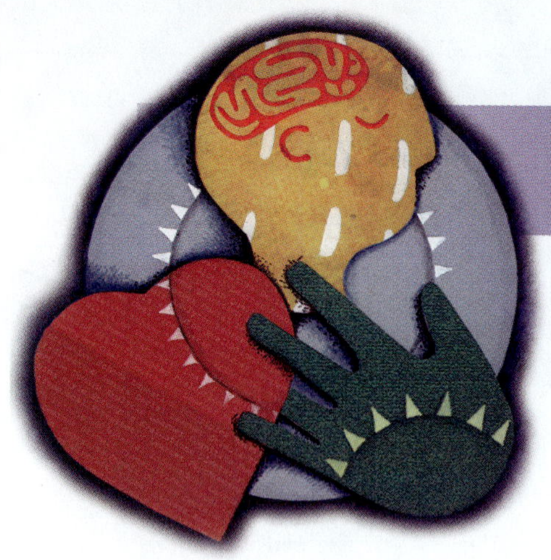

CHAPTER 6

The Learning Environment

"Teachers open the door. You enter by yourself."

—*Chinese proverb*

Being an educator involves much more than simply imparting knowledge and anecdotes. An effective educator is responsible for ensuring student success by providing an appropriate learning environment.[14] According to *The American Heritage Dictionary of the English Language,* the term *environment* is defined as, "The combination of external or extrinsic physical conditions that affect and influence the growth and development of organisms," and, "The complex of social and cultural conditions affecting the nature of an individual or community." When used to describe an educational setting, the term *environment* can be associated with positive or negative feelings of the student or the instructor. A positive learning environment is one that allows for a free exchange of ideas and information, one in which students are comfortable asking questions and the educator has or acquires the necessary tools to answer those questions. It is one in which the mood is pleasant and students are free to concentrate on academic success. Additionally, a positive learning environment is one that consistently demonstrates respect for students, as well as for the instructor. A negative environment prohibits or interferes with learning, and students may feel inadequate or may believe that their ideas don't matter or cannot be expressed.

In 1970, Malcolm Knowles reintroduced the concept that the environmental climate surrounding learning could affect learning, an idea that had been explored for many years by early educational theorists. Since that time, research has shown that a multitude of psychological, physical, and social factors can affect learning.[3,4,5,7,14,15] Psychologically, students may be intimidated by too much new information or may feel that the educator does not provide a safe environment, free from ridicule, in which they can ask questions. Physically, the environment may be extremely cold, loud, or cramped, which may divert attention from learning. Socially, teasing or hazing may occur among students, or simply, a disruptive group environment may minimize learning. This chapter explores how an educator can effectively set and maintain an appropriate learning environment for students.

THE PSYCHOLOGICAL ENVIRONMENT

The effective educator sets the psychological tone of the learning environment by establishing the psychological parameters of behavior. It is essential that the "learning rules" and the consequences for breaking those rules are established early on. The consequences must be applied equally and consistently throughout the educational experience. Moreover, the educator must create a psychologically safe environment, in which students can make and learn from their mistakes. Following are strategies that can be used to establish and maintain an effective learning climate[1,3,12,13]:

- *Mutual respect.* One should strive to establish adult-to-adult rapport with students. The educator must treat each student as an adult whose life experiences can contribute to his or her learning and the learning of the entire class. Inappropriate humor, foul language, or derogatory terms should not be used by the instructor nor permitted among students
- *Shared responsibility.* A participatory environment must be created, wherein students share responsibility for their own learning. This learning environment should encourage intellectual freedom and creativity. It should promote trial and error and should represent an interactive learning agreement between students and educators

- *Security.* In an environment laden with fear, honest assessment and learning are impossible. Typically, in a fearful environment, learners are more concerned with protecting themselves than they are with learning and improving. A positive learning environment must be safe and free of coercion by fellow students, the instructor, or the administration. In addition, the federal Safe School Act employs a zero tolerance for behaviors that threaten safety. (See Chapter 10, "Legal Issues" and more information on the Safe School Act.)

THE WELCOME

A student's introduction to the learning environment can make a lasting impression, greatly affecting the learning that takes place thereafter.[14] Sights, sounds, smells, atmosphere, and rapport with the educator established on the first day of class can potentially set the tone for the rest of the class or course. Something as simple as learning the names of students and helping them to learn one another's names can quickly break the ice, as a first step in creating a positive learning environment. Further, it reinforces that the educator values his or her students as individuals and expects that they value one another (Figure 6-1).[6,22]

TEACHING TIP: On the first day of class, an educator can play a "name game," which can take many different forms. Some suggestions include using name tags or making a class rule that a person needs to use another person's name every time he or she speaks. Another game is to start at one end of the room and have the first student say his or her name out loud. The next student has to repeat the first student's name, then add his or her name. The third student has to repeat the first and second students' names, then add his or her own, and so forth, until the last person in the classroom has to recite the entire class of names. It is important that these types of games be presented in a nonthreatening manner so that a student feels safe to "mess up" or forget a name.

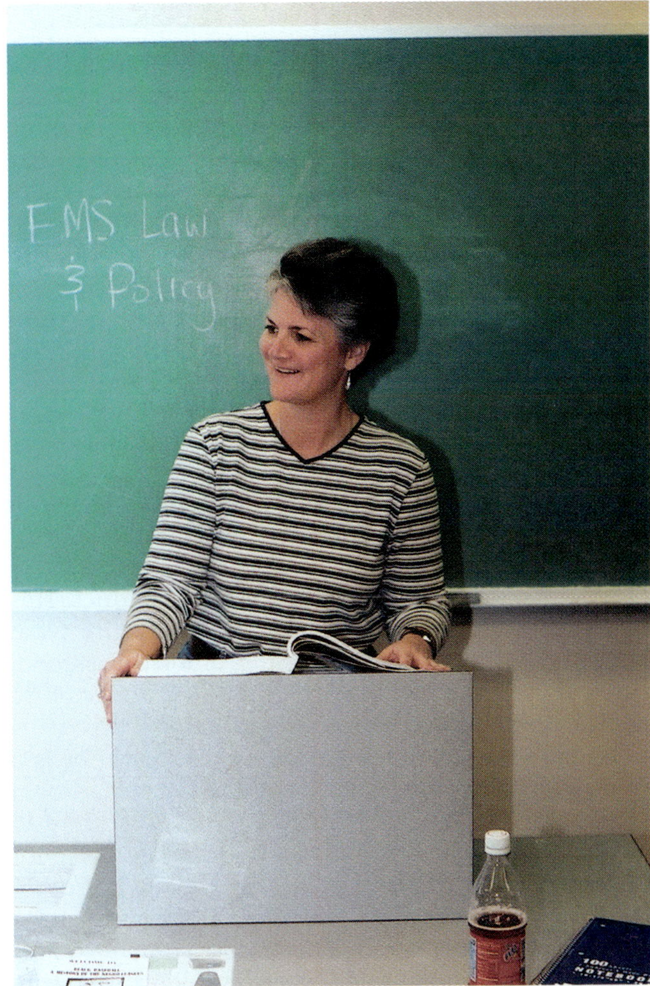

FIGURE 6-1 A warm and friendly smile from the instructor can go a long way toward setting a positive learning environment.

HOUSEKEEPING

A fundamental part of creating a comfortable learning and teaching environment is assurance that the basic needs of both the student and the educator are met. This includes giving directions about where the restrooms and refreshments can be found, and providing adequate break times so that students have time to visit the restroom or relax for a certain amount of time. A general rule of thumb is to schedule breaks approximately every 1 to 1½ hours. Breaks should be regular, so a student knows when to expect them. Most institutions use the 50-minute class hour, which consists of 50 minutes for instruction and a 10-minute break.

The class may also include handicapped students who need special consideration. Instructors must make sure that students have the opportunity to discuss their needed accommodations with a disability resource so that the instructor makes appropriate accommodations.[6] (See Chapter 10, "Legal Issues" and Americans With Disability Act, for further information.)

SETTING EXPECTATIONS

Students enter the classroom from a variety of cultures and backgrounds and with a variety of preconceptions of learning. The educator should recognize this and immediately set the standard of expected behavior and achievement. By setting a standard, the educator maximizes each student's chances for learning success.

The Syllabus

The syllabus or student handbook represents a written learning contract between the educator and the student. This contract clearly outlines the learning expectations of the course and evaluation of course work, but it should also contain information about appropriate behaviors and consequences of unacceptable behaviors. This document protects the educator and the student and provides a consistent place at which students can review class expectations. (For more information about the course syllabus, see Chapter 23, "Administrative Issues.")

Accountability

The educator plays the role of the recognized leader in the classroom. As a leader, he or she is responsible for setting and enforcing the norms of conduct, and for being the role model for those norms of conduct. This means that the instructor must clearly identify what behavior is unacceptable and must enforce classroom rules. It is important that inappropriate behavior be dealt with quickly, consistently, and fairly.[1,5,18]

Immature and sometimes disruptive behavior is a problem nationwide in the postsecondary classroom setting. Students enrolled in classes have the right to expect a safe environment and appropriate behavior on the part of fellow classmates, as well as from professional educators in the classroom setting. Immature and disruptive behavior on the part of students deters serious academic students from enrolling in future courses. Moreover, such disruptive behavior adversely affects the learning environment of all students enrolled in the course, and it distracts the educator from his or her role as instructor and facilitator.

Educators may have received little or no formal training in preparation for the major responsibility of managing the classroom environment. In addition, postsecondary educators generally do not wish to have to discipline their students as if they were in high school. Even though EMS educators are usually teaching adults in an adult setting, educators must engage in some type of discipline at some time. Educators must recognize disruptive behavior and actions that have the potential to create an unsafe environment. Moreover, they must learn techniques by which to maintain adult classrooms that are conducive to quality learning.

SOLVING BEHAVIOR PROBLEMS

When conflict erupts in the classroom between the student and the educator, tensions rise dramatically. The educator is faced with the challenge of managing the behavior appropriately. Educators should remember that violent or threatening behavior must not be tolerated under any circumstance. Unacceptable behaviors include fighting or harassing (verbal, physical, sexual), stealing, possessing illegal substances, threatening, making bomb threats, and willfully damaging school property. Occurrence of these behaviors should result in the immediate notification of law enforcement and removal of the student from the class and potentially the institution. Other behaviors such as foul language, loud voice, angry tone, and disrespect can be disruptive and should not be tolerated by the instructor. Such behaviors are stressful for the educator and can also be stressful for the class. An uncontrolled classroom limits teaching and learning time and leads to a negative, unproductive environment (Boxes 6-1 and 6-2).

BOX 6-1 Correlations Between Behavior and Cause

- If the instructor is annoyed, the student is probably seeking attention.
- If the instructor feels threatened, the student is probably seeking power.
- If the instructor feels hurt, the student is probably seeking revenge.
- If the instructor feels powerless, the student is probably seeking adequacy.

From NHTSA, Guidelines for Educating EMS Educators, Module 19 Discipline.

BOX 6-2 Examples of Behaviors

Student Seeking Attention

- Calling out
- Asking irrelevant questions
- Giving excessive examples

Student seeking power:

- Exhibiting tantrum-like behavior
- Arguing
- Lying
- Refusing to follow directions

Student Seeking Revenge

- Practicing cruelty to others
- Trying to get punished
- Carrying out pranks
- Practicing vandalism

Student Feeling Inadequate

- Passively refusing to participate
- Sitting silently
- Not answering when called on
- Asking not to be included

From NHTSA, Guidelines for Educating EMS Educators, Module 19 Discipline.

Although a caring classroom and a positive instructor foster a better learning environment and improve discipline, the fact is that there are students who will challenge the instructor. Following are a few of the trials that every instructor will face.

The Late Comer

This is the student who regularly comes to class or lab late. Fellow students watch the offending student arrive late week after week, and silent frustration begins to build in the classroom setting. If the offense is not addressed, then the instructor may find that other students may start to arrive late, or similar discipline problems can occur. Students need to know that the instructor is going to stick to the ground rules that were agreed upon at the start of class. In addition, late comers are disruptive and can interfere with the instructor's presentation style, which can slow the pace and reduce the quality of the classroom experience.

1. Pulling the student aside and counseling him or her is the first step to solving this problem. Has the student encountered any problems that have kept him or her from coming to class on time? Most EMS students are holding down a job while attending class and may have run into a particular problem. Have the student put together and sign a plan that will solve this problem, now and for the future.
2. The educator can start the class with a quiz or other classroom assignment that will encourage everyone to show up on time. A missed quiz could negatively affect the student's grade and should be a strong deterrent to coming in late. On the flip side, a group assignment can put peer pressure on the offender in that the others in the group have to pick up the slack.

The Bored One

This is the student who can bring down the instructor through body language and lack of participation. The actions of this student can be viewed by the instructor and by other students as a direct affront to the instructor's attempt to teach. The boredom can simply be related to the pace of the class, the lack of group activity, the fact that the student may be lost in the material, or the simple preoccupation of a student with work or family responsibilities.

1. This student must receive immediate counseling before the problem begins to affect the presentation. One must try to identify the problem with the student and write a corrective plan of action together with the student. The problem may be a personal issue that has nothing to do with the instructor or the material that is being presented. The pace of the class may be too slow or too fast, a fact that can be discovered in talks between the educator and the student.
2. The instructor can create an opportunity for the student to participate by allowing the student to present a portion of the material at a later date. Actively engaging students makes them stakeholders in the learning process and creates active learners. Even something as simple as operating the slide projector or laptop during a presentation can be enough to keep a student engaged and may reduce the negative effects that this type of behavior can bring to the classroom setting.

The Prisoner

Those who deal with fire agencies or corporations who require their employees to attain a mandatory EMS certification have had to deal with this group. These students shuffle into the classroom and strike an almost defiant pose for the instructor. For the new instructor, this is one of the most difficult groups to deal with and teach. Even for a seasoned instructor, a sense of dread can be noted when one has to deal with this type of student.

1. It is important that from the first day, the instructor acknowledges that this can be a difficult situation for both parties. The instructor must create a set of ground rules in light of this shared experience to involve everyone in the learning process.
2. It is imperative that these students not be allowed to interfere with an instructor's presentation. To prevent this from happening, students can be assigned to assist in classroom preparation and delivery. When these students buy into the process of helping, they become shareholders in the learning process and are more apt to maintain a positive attitude.

The Social Butterfly

These students tend to spend more time visiting with everyone as opposed to learning. They tend to hold side conversations and seem more interested in the socializing that occurs, causing problems during the instructor's presentation. A few students may even be using the classroom as a potential dating pool. Although the instructor wishes to encourage a friendly and interactive environment, clear rules and guidelines must be in place to create boundaries that both the instructors and the students have mutually agreed upon.

1. The best strategy is to pull the student aside after class and talk with him or her about concerns. Although instructors have been taught to move closer to these types of students, to increase the level and difficulty of questions directed toward them in an attempt to intimidate, or to confront

them in front of the class, such strategies are self-limiting and may lead to other problems down the road.

2. This type of student may require a job assignment in class that will allow him or her to put his or her people skills to work. The instructor can channel this type of student in a positive manner that can add rather than detract from the classroom experience.

The Elder

This is the all-knowing student who comes with or without previous EMS experience. Such a student can be a positive or a negative force in the EMS classroom. Too often, these students create frustration among fellow students and can interrupt the flow of the instructor's presentation. They have a tendency to add meaningful as well as meaningless information to the classroom discussion. They must be carefully approached so that their positive contributions to the class are not diminished.

1. Talking with students is always the first and best plan for correcting or redirecting this type of behavior. The instructor should have the student write a plan on how he or she can redirect behavior to become a more productive member of the class.
2. These students may be able to work effectively in small groups, with careful selection of students who will not be intimidated by their input. This allows the Elder to assist others in the group, giving him or her a release for some of the need to share knowledge.
3. Have the student assist the instructor before or during class. This strategy must be carefully managed as it might lead to other problems down the road with the student or with peers, if they perceive special treatment. This validation of the student's experience or knowledge must be weighed and carefully administered with the rest of the learners.

The Introvert

Every EMS classroom has a few introverts. These students are more like tourists than active participants. Like tourists, they are content to wander through the semester listening to the instructor present the material and taking snapshots of what the instructor points out to them. They remain distant and are not interested in becoming part of the tour, keeping themselves invisible in the group.

1. These students must become involved in the learning process. Traditionally, instructors were taught to bring these students out by putting them on the spot through Socratic questioning in the classroom. However, this may cause further isolation and may lead the student to drop the class, feeling that he or she is being singled out. A better strategy is to have the student lead a small group discussion or group activity. By scaling down classroom interaction to a few members and allowing the student to take a more active role, the instructor can promote a sense of belonging and ownership within the process.
2. Encouraging these students to take chances is another strategy that can work to their advantage. Small risks can lead to bigger risks that are safe and that will allow these students to pull out of their shell. The instructor must be careful not to put this type of student in a position that he or she cannot handle.

The Domineering One

This student can be extremely disruptive to the learning environment. In some cases, such students may be the ones to challenge the instructor and to face off with other students. This can lead to a hostile, or at the very least a tense, learning environment in which everyone can be the loser. The EMS profession has encouraged, to a degree, this type of aggressive student because of the nature of the business. The problem lies in the fact that the instructor's presentation can be very difficult with one or more domineering students in the room. If they go unchecked, they can have a negative effect on the class and may become the ring leaders, creating a disruptive environment.

1. This type of student must be pulled aside after or before class and spoken with about correcting this behavior. They must be made to clearly understand how their negative behavior cannot be tolerated, and a plan should be put together to ensure that the student reaches his or her full potential.
2. Small groups with other students serving as the leads can help to curb some of the negative behavior. Students in the group will, if carefully selected, be able to put enough peer pressure on this type of personality. The instructor can facilitate from a distance to make sure that this personality does not become overpowering for the group.

The Sleeper

This type of student has always been a problem for educators. Nothing drains the energy of an instructor and other students faster than looking over and seeing someone drowning in a puddle of self-produced saliva on the top of the desk.

1. At the start of the semester, set ground rules concerning sleeping. Students should understand that this type of behavior is unacceptable and can be extremely disruptive to the learning process. Should a student become sleepy, he or she may stand at the back of the room. This may be an agreed upon solution, especially for those who are coming

off a shift and who may not have been able to properly rest.

2. Ensure that students have a break every hour. Have one of the students become the official class timekeeper to ensure that breaks can be given in a timely fashion.
3. Students must be involved in activities other than the traditional lecture format. Group activities can work wonders in keeping students engaged in the learning process. Changing up the presentation style can keep students interested and is a necessary part of teaching the adult learner.

The Confused One

This is an interesting student who may have problems in grasping the material. He or she may exhibit this by not engaging the instructor or other students, or by asking a tremendous number of questions. The latter can slow down the instructor's presentation style and may lead to palpable frustration among the student's peers.

1. The instructor should assign a buddy to the student to assist him or her during and after class. Peer support can be a powerful, nonthreatening, and reassuring strategy. Tutoring can also be done by faculty at prearranged times to help clear up any confusion.
2. The educator must provide students with clear expectations and a detailed plan on how to accomplish the goals of the class. This may require the instructor to begin by outlining the classroom lecture for the day or for the week, so that the student can have a picture of how instruction will proceed.

The educator should ask himself or herself if he or she has done anything to contribute to the conflict. For example, the syllabus should be evaluated to determine if expectations are clear. If possible, one should wait until a break or until class is over to talk to the student in a private place. Comments should be focused on the breach of conduct, not on the student as a person. The instructor should ask questions such as, "What are you doing? What's going on?" This will help bring focus to the inappropriate behavior, instead of to the student. If the student does not respond to such questions, the instructor should describe what he or she is seeing that is unacceptable. One should avoid asking, "Why did you do that?" This invites the student to make excuses for the behavior and to avoid personal responsibility for the conduct. The student should be encouraged to identify the disruptive behavior, such as sleeping in class or talking disruptively during lectures; then, the student should be asked to describe what he or she can do to correct the behavior. The instructor should help the student devise a plan to correct disruptive behavior.

In any conflict between the educator and an adult student, the toughest part is staying neutral and calm. The goal of the intervention between the student and the educator is that the student will accept responsibility and ownership of the disruptive behavior. Questions such as, "What's the rule?" or "Is this helping you get what you need from this course?" can often help focus the issue.

Additionally, the educator may ask the student to formulate a plan to stop the disruptive behavior by suggesting alternatives. Students may need help in determining appropriate alternatives to disruptive behaviors. The plan for improvement should be short and concise, and should have a high probability of success. This plan can be either written or verbal, but it should be reasonable and doable. Behavioral contracts or plans should be negotiated in a neutral, nonjudgmental tone. The educator should assist the student in moving forward and in planning for a better approach to classroom citizenship that will help him or her to succeed.

It is important that all disruptions and breaches of classroom behavior be documented, so that if and when disruptions become persistent, a record of noncompliance is available to support the instructor's actions. A concise written statement of the behavior, including its impact on others and the intervention provided, is an important part of record keeping.

Although most classroom issues can be dealt with in conversations with the student, it is sometimes necessary for the instructor to deal with the issue in accordance with a formal discipline system. Instructors should check their organization's policies for the specific requirements. Formal discipline processes should be explained in the student handbook and during the first class session.

SAFETY

Learning requires an environment in which the student is at ease and is able to experiment without fear of making a mistake. Further, students should be able to develop a trusting relationship with the educator. As a general rule, in a safe and positive learning environment, the following can be expected[1,2,3,7,20,22]:

- Students are free from harm
- Students are free from discrimination
- Students are free from sexual harassment
- Students are free from teasing
- Students and educators exhibit tolerance and acceptance
- Students and educators encourage new ideas

Physical Safety

Rules for classroom safety should be explicitly stated by the educator and listed in the course syllabus.

CASE IN POINT

The Monday night section of the EMT class is one that consists mostly of law enforcement officers from the local sheriff's department. They are friends and know one another well. They tend to joke and laugh and promote a casual yet highly competitive learning environment in the classroom. The instructor has allowed the casual atmosphere and believes it can promote a positive learning environment. However, there are two students who are not doing well in class. The instructor suspects that these two students may be intimidated by the officers in class. They do not ask questions, and when they do, the instructor notices nonverbal clues that appear to be somewhat condescending from the officers in class. These two students seem reluctant to practice during skills sessions and are pushed to the back of the line by more aggressive students. The poorly performing students seem to lack confidence and are behind schedule in acquiring their skills. Instead of suggesting that the two students transfer sections, the instructor talks to the class about the class environment and the importance of respect for all students in the class. If improvement is not noted, the specific offending students should be talked to individually, and discipline procedures will be implemented, if necessary. Or, the educator might find a way to pair the two students with specific officer students in the class who have good leadership skills and will serve as mentors for these students. Whatever the best solution, the plan for improvement likely requires an improvement in the psychological environment of the class. Both individuals and groups of individuals must be held accountable for expected behavior and must be encouraged to contribute to a safe and positive learning environment for everyone involved.

TEACHING TIP: It is easier for an instructor to lighten up on class control than to start with less control and attempt to tighten up.

Students should exhibit appropriate behavior around special equipment and with other class members to prevent harm to anyone in the classroom. Examples of safety precautions include the following:

- Lifting and moving: Have additional class members act as "spotters" when students are performing lifting and moving techniques to make sure that proper procedures are followed
- IV initiation: If students are practicing IV initiation skills on one another, the instructor should be readily available for each attempt, until a certain level of competency has been established

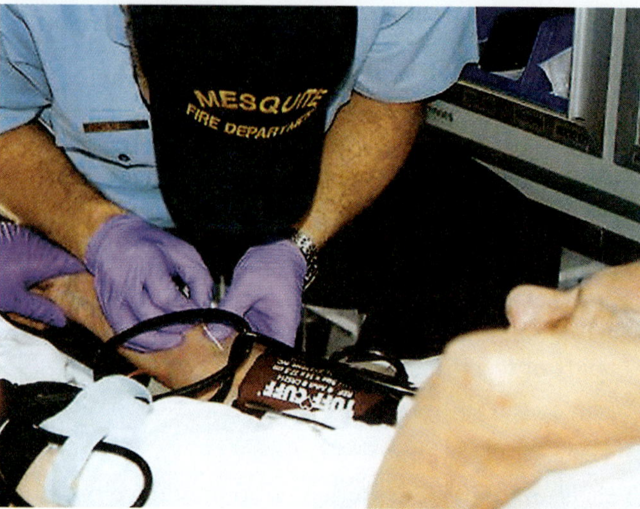

FIGURE 6-2 Safety in the clinical area is more likely if it is practiced in the classroom and skills laboratory.

- Body substance isolation (BSI): In practice, instructors should require the use of appropriate BSI precautions so that this use is reinforced and, consequently, remembered when the student is working in the clinical setting

Safety From Failure

It is important for an educator to establish from the beginning of a class that making mistakes is a normal part of learning. Trial and error should be encouraged, and students should not feel that they will be punished for making mistakes. It is important for an educator to realize that his or her response to student mistakes is critical. The instructor can acknowledge that the incorrect answer may seem plausible under the circumstances, then discuss the correct answer with an explanation as to why it is correct. The instructor should find something positive to say about the answer before explaining why it is incorrect. Every attempt should be made to have a positive reaction to mistakes. Discussion of a student's poor performance should always be conducted in private. Laughing or inappropriate tone, body language, or gestures that will potentially embarrass or ridicule are unacceptable from the instructor and from other students. Providing a safe environment for practice is essential. The student must feel comfortable enough to "get it wrong" if the student is to progress to a point where he or she can "get it right."[1,14,19]

INTELLECTUAL CHALLENGE

Research shows that there is increased interest in learning and stimulation when students are challenged to think and react just above their current threshold of learning and understanding.[3,22] Setting a challenging pace, even sometimes to the point of discomfort, is an important aspect of creating a positive learning environment. This pace must be set accurately so it does not overwhelm students and cause them to give up, but it also shouldn't be so easy that nothing is accomplished or learned by the experience.

CASE IN POINT

A college uses scenarios to introduce the real world to EMT-Basic students. Approximately halfway through each course, students are invited to a night of working through scenarios. These scenarios are carefully constructed to provide multiple stimuli and promote critical thinking, decision making, and learning. Examples include scenarios with special safety considerations or mass casualties. The purpose of the scenarios is to give students a real sense of whether or not they can handle the real world and really understand safety issues, failures, and mistakes. The stress created in this environment helps students to learn.[17]

THE PHYSICAL ENVIRONMENT

The instructor should be able to evaluate the class and answer such questions as the following[10,11,14,15,16,21,22]:

- Is there adequate space for each student to sit, take notes, and view the reference materials?
- Is there adequate space for each student to practice skills?
- Can each student see the instructor and any audiovisual presentations?
- Can each student hear the instructor and any audiovisual presentations?
- How can the lighting be changed so that there is adequate light for skills, lecture presentations, or discussion activities?
- If the classroom has windows, how can natural light be blocked or adjusted to achieve optimal lighting for audiovisual presentations?
- How can environmental controls be adjusted if it gets too hot or too cold?
- Where is the space for breaks that allow for eating and drinking?
- Where are the emergency exits?
- Where are the restrooms?
- Where is the equipment stored? Is it accessible to students?
- If a lab session must be conducted outdoors, where is easy access?
- Where will students be able to secure personal belongings during class?
- Is the classroom space accessible to students with a variety of physical abilities, such as the need to use a wheelchair?
- How can distractions from the outside environment be minimized (e.g., closing doors or windows to minimize interfering noise)?
- Are adequate electrical resources available for both instructor and student usage?
- Is lighting/security for the parking area adequate when dark?
- Is the facility clean and well maintained? Do students respect the physical facility and equipment and care for manikins properly?
- Do students pick up after themselves and properly dispose of trash?

Room Temperature

The temperature in the classroom should be at a comfortable setting for the task at hand. This may mean having the heat turned down a little for skills days when the students are actively moving around. Students should also be advised that they might wish to bring a sweater to class if they are normally cold, as the environment will be controlled to ensure the comfort of the majority.

Lighting

The lighting should be adjustable so that it can be dimmed to make best use of audiovisuals but light enough for demonstrations or taking notes, or perhaps completely off to simulate a nighttime environment for a scenario.

Distractions

Distractions such as noise, bright sunlight, and interruptions can also affect the learning environment.[11] Although some sources of distraction are out of the educator's immediate control, anything that can be done to minimize distractions will improve the learning environment. For example, the educator should ask that students shut off pagers and cell phones, or turn them to vibrate and accept only emergency calls. The instructor should set an example by putting his or her electronic devices to vibrate also. When conducting outside simulations, the instructor should hold the class in a discrete area that prevents pedestrian traffic from coming through. Shades for the windows and closed windows may further prevent distractions.

Seating Arrangements

Ideally, an educator should be able to configure and reconfigure a classroom in a variety of ways to accommodate the instructional strategy for that session.

Furniture that can be rearranged is preferable. Furniture should be comfortable and should fit students and the classroom well. Large firefighter students may require larger chairs or tables than other groups. If 8-hour class sessions are planned, padded seats are essential. If class will not last longer than 2 hours, padded seats may be optional. The physical comfort of the seats should be taken into account, as well as the arrangement of the seats in light of the focus of the instruction.

A variety of classroom setup strategies are possible, depending on the instructor's goals.

- *Traditional.* The traditional classroom setup is ideal for a large number of students. This style is not recommended, however, for small group work or for psychomotor skill development. This structure may allow students to "hide" behind others, and it can be difficult for some students to see over others. The educator at the front of the room may also have difficulty seeing all the students in the room and may focus only on the first row
- *Theater.* The theater classroom setup is optimal for a very large number of students. In this type of configuration, the seats rise from the front to the back, allowing better visibility of the educator and any instructional media or demonstrations. In addition, this arrangement allows the educator to have better eye contact with the group as a whole. This style is not recommended for small group work
- *Circle, square, and rectangle—open.* This style places the educator in the center of a U-like shape. The educator may sit with the group or may enter the center area. This can be an ideal setup when all students are expected to participate in a discussion, as it allows them to see one another. It can also work well for a psychomotor demonstration. It does not work well, though, for a lecture scenario, as someone will ultimately end up sitting with his or her back to the presenter
- *Circle, square, and rectangle—closed.* This classroom setup places the educator either sitting or standing off to the side after instructions are provided. It can be an ideal setup for a larger discussion group when all students are expected to participate, as it allows students to see one another. Similar to the open version, this type of setup is not recommended for lectures or presentations, because the focus may not be on the educator but on the person sitting across the way
- *Round table.* With this classroom setup, small groups are arranged around different round tables or workstations. The focus of instruction is within the space of each individual table or station. It is important with this style that the educator circulates around the room, or that additional educator facilitators assist in monitoring the work at the individual stations. This setup allows some privacy between workstations. Visualization of each station may not be an issue, but it can be controlled with partitions or room dividers. It is important to maintain adequate room between stations or tables to allow for movement and to reduce the noise level. Groups can be working on the same activity simultaneously (but independently), or they can be working on different activities. With this setup, the educator balances between monitoring and allowing students to direct their own learning. This setup is not as useful for lectures or presentations, as inevitably some of the students' backs will face the presenter (Figure 6-3).

Audiovisual Equipment

As part of the physical environment of the classroom, the educator must ensure that audiovisual equipment is in working order and that a backup is planned and available. (See Chapter 11 for more information on audiovisual equipment.)

THE SOCIAL ENVIRONMENT

It is important for the educator to remember that the learning environment is dynamic. As a group of individuals gets to know one another, the social interactions between them may change. This can create an evolving learning environment, which can be positive. For example, if everyone is speaking up and asking questions and learning from one another because they feel safe to do that within the group, that is obviously a positive change. However, the change can also be negative. For example, if two students have really hit it off as friends, they may spend all of their time talking and disrupting the learning environment, other students, and the educator.

At a fundamental level, the classroom experience can be thought of as a social arrangement. At the center of the social participation is the educator, who may possess a high degree of expertise in an academic discipline but may not be as skilled at promoting the effective social environment needed for effective learning.[1] It is important that the educator set the tone and keep the tone even as class dynamics change.

The instructor is the primary role model in the classroom. To act appropriately as a role model, he or she might clearly identify the behaviors that students should exhibit. The instructor has a primary role in developing the attitudes of the learner. By modeling appropriate conduct, the instructor stands the best chance of developing the desired behaviors in students.

ENCOURAGING TEAMWORK

Emergency medical services is a team activity; therefore, teamwork skills are essential. It may be difficult for an instructor to ensure that team activities

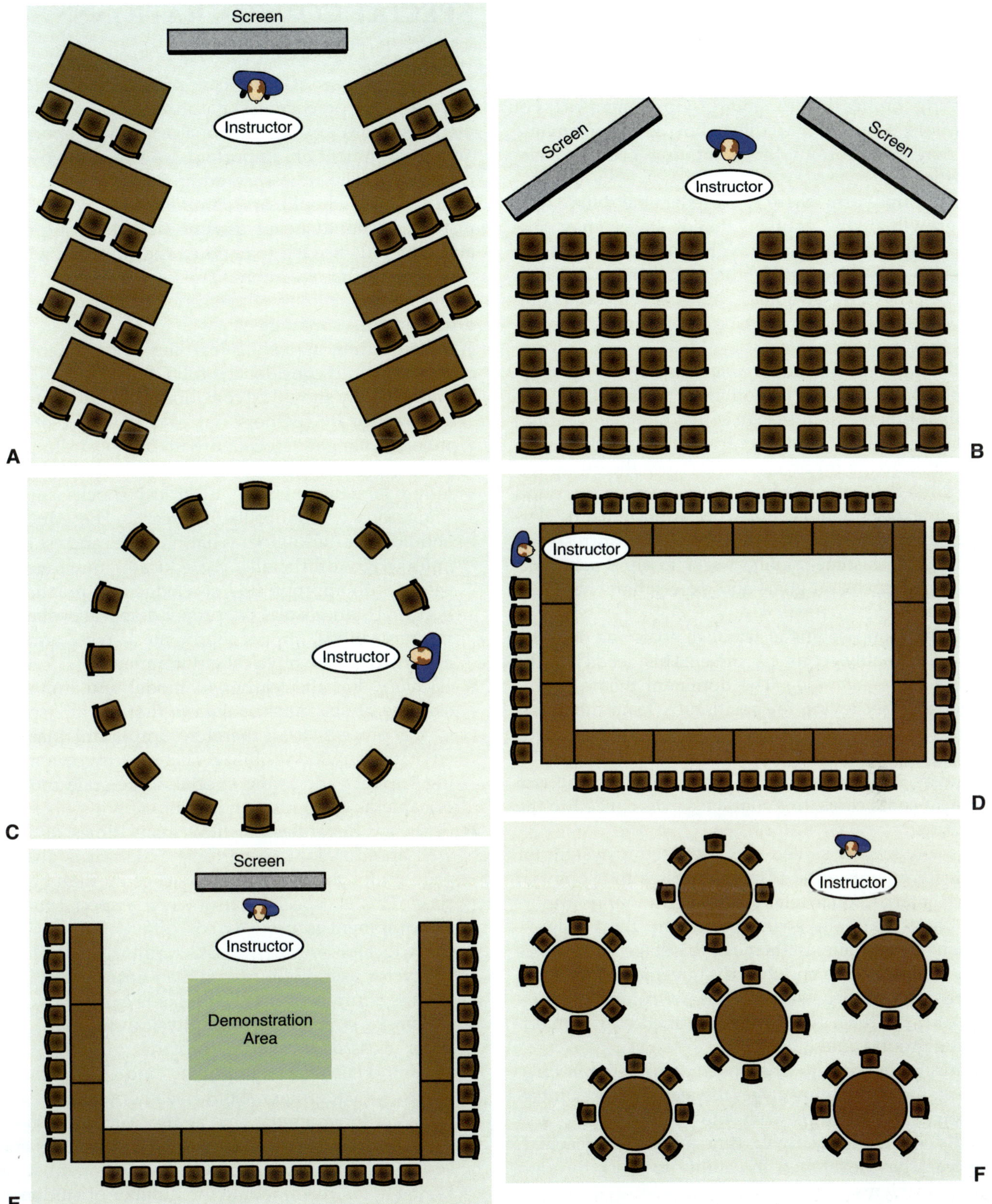

FIGURE 6-3 Types of classroom arrangements. **A,** Traditional. **B,** Theater style. **C,** Open circle. **D,** Open square. **E,** U shape. **F,** Round table.

contribute to a positive learning environment. Although the instructor may encounter students who have already developed excellent team skills, he or she is more likely to find students who need coaching on teamwork and group dynamics.[1] For educators, a basic knowledge of how groups form and function is important for promoting positive team activities.

As groups form, there is a predictable dynamic to the growth of the team. Different stages may take varying amounts of time to evolve. Awareness of team stages seems to shorten their duration, as team members have an awareness of what will occur and know the language to describe group dynamic problems that they encounter.

The first step is the *forming* stage, wherein team members encounter one another for the first time. The dominant theme of this stage is that members attempt to define the task assigned to them, and they start to determine the future course. Because the group has not worked together before, there are no set ground rules or expectations. These expectations must be clarified before the team can progress. This can result in impatience, as some members seek to jump into tasks before consensus on goals and expectations has been reached.

As the group begins to establish goals and expectations, invariably, conflicts arise. This leads to the second stage—*storming*. The dominant theme of this stage is the jockeying for position by team members, as they struggle to define the team's leadership. This struggle can cause arguing and conflicts among team members, even when there is agreement on the real issue. In some cases, this conflict is externalized to the educator.

As conflicts are settled and a leadership system for the team emerges, the team progresses to a point at which interpersonal relationships grow more important than the team goal. This is the third stage—*norming*. The dominant theme of this stage is emphasis on getting along, even when disagreements and open discussions are necessary. A sense of cohesion develops, and the team has now established and is maintaining ground rules.

This gives rise to the fourth stage—*performing*. During the performing stage, the team balances interpersonal relationships with the team's needs, and results begin to occur. By the time this stage is reached, the team has developed the ability to work through group problems.

Although it is difficult to observe teams going through this process, it is important for the educator to realize that the process itself is what allows students to learn teamwork skills. The role of the educator in team development is to guide students through these phases, pointing out landmarks and assisting them in working through obstacles.

SPECIAL CONSIDERATIONS

The Skills Environment

An essential part of healthcare provider education is learning and practicing skills in a skill lab environment. As with any instructional activity, preparation and environment are important aspects of the overall experience. The necessary equipment, supplies, and teaching aids should be identified and secured. An instructor should never assume that the equipment and materials needed to conduct the skills lab will be available in the classroom. This is especially true in multiple-use facilities, where different instructors and different classes may meet.

When setting up a skills learning environment, the educator should consider the following[6,9,22]:

- *Safety.* Safety should be considered not only in terms of practice by learners but also in terms of any inherent danger associated with demonstrating the skill. For example, caution is needed when defibrillation is demonstrated. Electrical shocks can be dangerous to nonfibrillating hearts. The educator should clearly define what is safe and should enforce it. Additionally, the educator must ensure safety with appropriate knowledge and practice of body substance isolation, proper disposal of sharps, immunizations, proper body mechanics, and all aspects of a safe physical environment.
- *Visibility.* For the learner to model and imitate a skill, he or she must be able to first see all aspects of the process. It is, therefore, important that the educator provide visibility. This may involve moving learners and using special, large-scale models or cameras and video projectors.
- *Rehearsal.* Regardless of how many times or how well an educator can perform a skill, it is always prudent for the educator to practice the skill before class. This is especially true when a special model or equipment is used that is different from what the educator routinely uses. Nothing will kill an instructor's credibility more than not being able to use the equipment that he or she is explaining.
- *Classroom preparation.* The physical setup of the skills classroom should provide visibility and accommodate the equipment and instructional props. All equipment should be checked to ensure that it is functioning. This is also a time to check such things as electrical or oxygen connections and venting. Moreover, adequate equipment must be available to accommodate the number of students.
- *Practice space.* If the learners will practice the skill, the educator must ensure that sufficient space is provided, as well as equipment, at each skill practice arena. If a classroom will be rearranged by the learners before they begin practice, the educator must ensure that this can be done and will not be overly disruptive to the learning process.

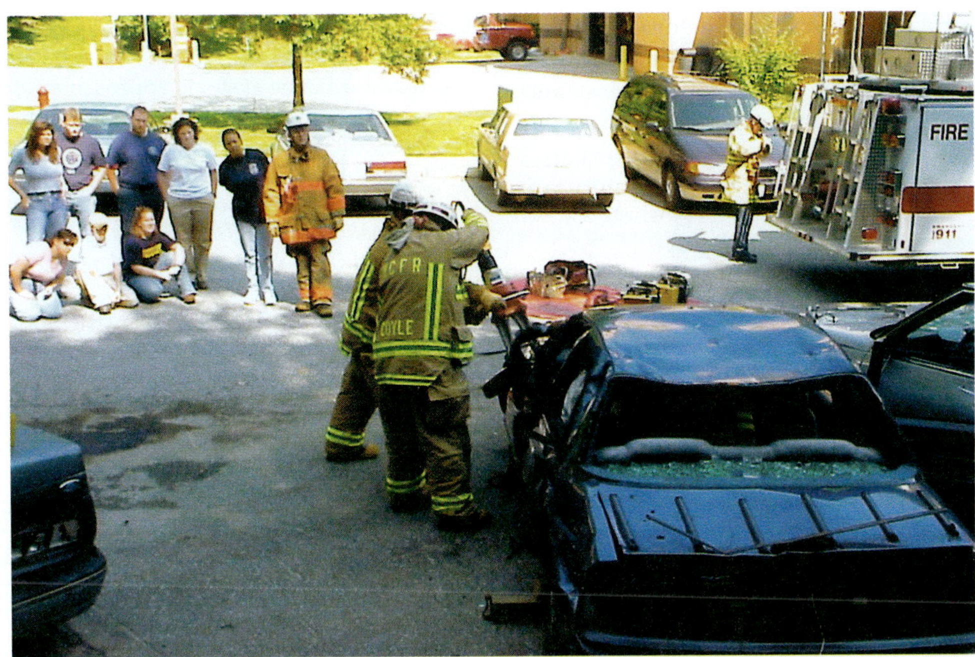

FIGURE 6-4 Special precautions may be necessary when students are introduced to extrication exercises.

- *Encourage self-learning.* Set the expectation that learning, especially skills learning, is not dependent on an educator. After an instructor demonstrates a particular skill, he or she should expect that students will watch one another, go through a skills checklist, and work through their mistakes before asking the instructor to watch them perform the skill. This type of self-learning practice encourages lifelong learning.
- *Simulate real environments.* Where possible, an educator should use "real" props in the skills lab to simulate an actual working environment. For example, moving a patient off of a sofa is different from moving someone off of a classroom chair.
- *Appropriate dress.* Students should be advised about when they will be performing psychomotor tasks so that they may wear or bring appropriate clothing—for protection and to prevent embarrassment. This applies to the instructor as well.

Nontraditional Environments

In EMS education, typical learning environments include the classroom, skills lab, hospital setting, or the field. As settings become more complex, they integrate higher levels of thinking skills and psychomotor skills. No longer is simple knowledge adequate for performing a task; the student must function at the application level or problem-solving level to perform in this different environment. (See Chapter 7, Domains of Learning.) When psychomotor skills are taught, students in clinical settings must apply these skills to a patient situation. For example, it is one thing to recite the steps for cardiopulmonary resuscitation (CPR) in class, but quite another to recognize that a patient is "down" at a scene, then manage the situation and the patient. A change in learning environments can be an effective tool for improving performance.[17,22] Increasing the complexity of the learning environment may promote critical thinking or, conversely, simplifying the environment by removing complicating factors may restore student confidence and enhance performance.

The learning environment can also be specific to location. For example, a student who has come from a rural area may be very comfortable transporting patients for 30 to 60 minutes but is failing to get all treatments done in a timely fashion in the urban setting, where transport times are less than 10 minutes. The problem in this case is likely the change in the environment, and not the student's knowledge base. Skill training around efficiency, multitasking, and delegation may provide keys to this student's success. An EMT student who has worked for a private ambulance provider for 3 years may have a level of discomfort during his internship at a large, urban fire department. His emotions and stress may be interfering with his ability to recall information and perform adequately on calls. Acclimating to the fire service will do more in this situation to improve his performance than any amount of studying; therefore, the plan for improvement should include activities to increase his comfort level at the station and with station personnel. His best option for adjusting may include additional observation time provided before patient care tasks are added to his assignment.

Students entering a clinical environment for the first time, where they are introduced to staff members and oriented to the facility, feel more comfortable and are set up for more successful learning.[19] However, as each new environmental element is introduced to a student, previous feelings of comfort and safety are challenged.[5,18]

Using New Technologies

The Internet, computer-based teaching and learning tools, and satellite education are just some examples of technologies that can be used to enhance the learning environment.[8,9,22] Use of technology to create a simulated "real environment" for students may result in successful practice and, ultimately, in learning.[8] In addition to simulations, examples of using technology in the classroom include such innovations as an online library database or computer-generated "Jeopardy-like" games. The use of different types of technology can create a dynamic and fun environment that facilitates learning. This also allows the instructor to evaluate learning and student responsiveness in a more stressful and competitive environment. Technology can be used to create a fun place for learning.

SUMMARY

The environment in which learning is expected to occur is an important aspect of education that must be taken into consideration. An effective educator makes every effort to create a psychologically, physically, and socially safe environment, where students can feel free to make mistakes and learn from one another, the educator, and different situations. It is a place that creates positive feelings, and in which the educator and students are free to focus on academic success. The tactics and resources needed to foster an environment that promotes positive learning may change with each new class of students. Instructors should continually evaluate each situation and each new group of students and should review all acquired information, then devise a plan that will promote a positive learning environment for the given situation.

REFERENCES

1. Anderson JA. Faculty responsibility for promoting conflict-free college classrooms. *New Directions for Teaching & Learning.* 1999;77(Spring).
2. Backes C. The do's and don'ts of working with adult learners. *Adult Learning.* 1997;8:January/February.
3. Billington D. Seven characteristics of highly effective adult learning programs. New Horizons for Learning 2002. Available at: http://www.newhorizons.org/lifelong/workplace/billington.htm. Accessed October 21, 2003.
4. Biswalo P. The systems approach as a catalyst for creating an effective learning environment. *Convergence.* 2001;34.
5. Cleave-Hogg D, Rothman AI. Discerning views: medical students' perceptions of their learning environment. *Evaluation & The Health Professions.* 1991;14.
6. Davis BG. *Tools for Teaching.* San Francisco, Calif: Jossey-Bass; 2001.
7. Diamantes T. Improving instruction in multicultural classes by using classroom learning environment. *Journal of Instructional Psychology.* 2002;29.
8. Dwyer CA. Using emerging technologies to construct effective learning environments. *Educational Media International.* 1999;36.
9. Ferrington G, Loge K. Virtual reality: a new learning environment. *The Computing Teacher.* 1992;9.
10. Harrison C. *Learning Management.* Retrieved from ERIC Digest No. 73. Available at: http://www.ed.gov/databases/ERIC_Digests/ed296121.html. Accessed 1988.
11. Hutchinson L, Cantillon P, Wood D. Educational environment. *BMJ.* 2003;326.
12. Imel S. *Guidelines for Working with Adult Learners.* Retrieved from ERIC Digest No. 154. Available at: http://www.ed.gov/databases/ERIC_Digests/ed377313.html. Accessed 1994.
13. Imel S. *Teaching Adults: Is It Different?* Retrieved from ERIC Digest No. 82. Available at: http://www.ed.gov/databases/ERIC_Digests/ed305495.html. Accessed 1995.
14. Imel S. Inclusive adult learning environments. Retrieved from ERIC Digest No. 162.
15. Magolda MB. Teaching to promote holistic learning and development. *New Directions for Teaching & Learning.* 2000;82.
16. Mann KV. Thinking about learning: implications for principle-based professional education. *The Journal of Continuing Education in the Health Professions.* 2002;22.
17. Moore A, et al. EMS stress training concept "Kobayashi Moru" scenarios. Domain 3. National Association of EMS Educators, Spring 2003.
18. Morris W, ed. *The American Heritage Dictionary of the English Language.* Boston: Houghton Mifflin Co; 1976:438.
19. Newble DI, Hejka EJ. Approaches to learning of medical students and practicing physicians: some empirical evidence and its implications for medical education. *Educational Psychology.* 1991;11.
20. Robins L. A predictive model of student satisfaction with the medical school learning environment. *Academic Medicine.* 1997;72.
21. Scholtes P. *The Team Handbook.* Madison, Wis: Joiner Associates; 1988.
22. Simplicio JS. Some simple and yet overlooked common sense tips for a more effective classroom environment. *Journal of Instructional Psychology.* 1999;26.
23. Villaume S, Brandt S. Extending our beliefs about effective learning environments: a tale of two learners. *Reading Teacher.* 1999;53.

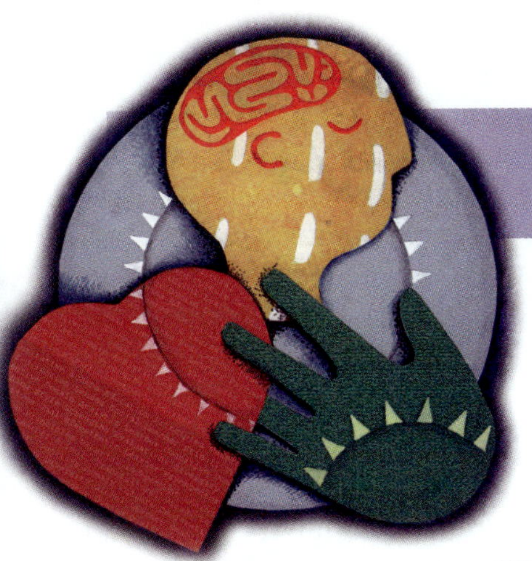

CHAPTER 7

Domains of Learning

"There are one-story intellects, two-story intellects, and three-story intellects with skylights. All fact collectors, who have no aim beyond their facts, are one-story men. Two-story men compare, reason, generalize, using the labors of the fact collectors as well as their own. Three-story men idealize, imagine, predict—their best illumination comes from above, through the skylight."

—*Oliver Wendell Holmes*

Teaching, it is often said, is both an art and a science. The science arises from the research that educators conduct into modes and methods of learning for the purpose of developing best practices and techniques for the classroom. The artistic aspect refers to the practice of teaching—those trial-and-error methods that individual educators employ to hone and master their craft.

Researchers have identified different domains, or categories, of learning that educators can use in several ways in their practice of teaching. In the instructional design process, the domains are considered when goals and objectives are established and written. Educators also identify student knowledge and behaviors that exemplify the domains of learning; for example, in the context of an emergency call, these domains are targeted in lesson plans and choices regarding teaching strategies. Finally, educators consider each domain when formulating evaluation criteria and methods. The domains of learning lie behind nearly every stage of the learning and teaching processes.

CATEGORIZING THE DOMAINS

Dr. Benjamin Bloom and a team of researchers first categorized the domains of learning in 1956.[1] Bloom and colleagues described three distinct domains of learning: cognitive, affective, and psychomotor.

Bloom chose the term *domain* to describe the major division of his concepts because *domain* means a related collection of things or items. Collectively, his work is known as *Bloom's taxonomy of the domains of learning*.

Since the time of Bloom's original work, other researchers have built upon his concepts and have developed several other strategies of classification and additional categories of learning domains. However, because Bloom's strategy is commonly used in the medical field, this is the only strategy described in this textbook.

Cognitive Domain

Simply put, the cognitive domain describes learning that takes place through the process of thinking—it deals with facts and knowledge. For example, a student who reads a textbook and learns the contraindications of administering a certain drug is operating in the cognitive domain.

Affective Domain

The affective domain describes learning in terms of feelings/emotions, attitudes, and values. For example, a student who participates in case scenarios and learns to appreciate how vulnerable patients can feel when they are sick or injured is operating in the affective domain.

Psychomotor Domain

The psychomotor domain describes learning that takes place through the attainment of skills and bodily, or kinesthetic, movements. For example, a student who practices in a skills station how to properly immobilize a cervical spine is working in the psychomotor domain.

It is important for educators to understand that, although Bloom and his colleagues described learning processes that take place within three distinct categories, learning seldom takes place solely within one category in isolation from the other two. For example, for a student to properly perform a psychomotor skill, he or she must possess cognitive, affective, and psychomotor knowledge. A Basic Emergency Medical Technician (EMT-B) who performs cardiopulmonary resuscitation (CPR) effectively must first know the correct order of the steps for CPR (cognitive domain), must make a decision regarding whether or not to begin resuscitation efforts through the application of ethical and moral values dictated by protocol or standing orders (affective domain), and, once the decision to treat has been made, must correctly and efficiently perform the skills (psychomotor domain).

DOMAIN LEVELS

Each domain is structured into distinct divisions, or levels, that reflect the increasing depth and breadth of understanding an individual achieves as he or she progresses through the domain. Several strategies or systems of categorizing these levels are applied within each domain; these are classified as formal or informal. The formal systems provide greater structure than do the informal ones, and they can lead to greater precision by the instructor in determining how much content to cover on a given topic and in identifying the appropriate depth and breadth of content for evaluation purposes.

Two formal and one informal system are described here. The two formal systems are Bloom's taxonomy and the three-level system. The informal system described in this chapter is the high- and low-level system. The reader must keep in mind that, regardless of the strategy, these systems all progress in a linear fashion, beginning with the lowest level of sophistication and progressing toward the highest level.

Bloom's Taxonomy

Bloom and associates originally identified and described five levels within each of the three domains of learning; a sixth level, which was named *evaluation*, was added to the cognitive domain after 1956 (Table 7-1). It should be noted that specific action verbs can be used to describe behavioral characteristics required within each level. A partial listing of some of the action verbs that are appropriate for each level is found in Chapter 8, Table 8-1.

Cognitive domain levels

Level 1: Knowledge focuses on memorization and recall of information.

Level 2: Comprehension focuses on interpretation and understanding of the meaning behind information.

Level 3: Application deals with relating classroom information to real life situations and experiences. At this level, students should be able to identify subtle differences between concepts and should begin to see how differences can be used in practical application. They will still, however, require assistance from instructors in thinking through these ideas.

Level 4: Analysis requires that the student should be able to separate whole concepts into individual, smaller parts to analyze their meaning and understand their importance.

Level 5: As students progress to *Synthesis,* they are able to combine pieces of information into new and different whole ideas. They are beginning the process of combining seemingly unrelated ideas together and can use logic to defend why they have made certain choices.

Level 6: In *Evaluation,* the student has attained cognitive mastery of the concepts and is able to make judgments and decisions about and with information. The evaluation level represents metacognition (thinking about thinking), in which the thought process is scrutinized as closely as is the product of the thinking process.

TABLE 7-1 Bloom's Taxonomy of the Domains of Learning

Levels	Cognitive Domain	Affective Domain	Psychomotor Domain
1	Knowledge	Receiving	Imitation
2	Comprehension	Responding	Manipulation
3	Application	Valuing	Precision
4	Analysis	Organizing	Articulation
5	Synthesis	Characterizing	Naturalization
6	Evaluation*		

*Note that the level of evaluation, the sixth level in the cognitive domain, was added a few years after Bloom's original work was completed in 1956.

CASE IN POINT

A student first learns the contraindications of administering a specific drug and is able to list them (level 1: knowledge). Next, she comprehends the adverse effects of the drug on a patient for whom it is contraindicated (level 2: comprehension). In level 3: application, she can explain the physiologic principles behind why and how the adverse effects occur. Next, given a specific patient scenario, she is able to determine whether or not the drug would be contraindicated (level 4: analysis). Moving one step farther, the student, having made the determination that the drug is contraindicated, makes a decision concerning the next appropriate treatment step (level 5: synthesis). Finally, in level 6: evaluation, the student accurately and efficiently runs through such a patient scenario in a skills practicum and performs with minimal assistance from the instructor.

CASE IN POINT

A 17-year-old student expresses a reluctance to work with elderly patients. After discussing this with him, the instructor determines that he has had limited exposure to elderly individuals and arranges for the student to spend time visiting with residents of an independent living community (level 1: receiving). The student develops a relationship with one of the residents and begins to visit him regularly (level 2: responding). The student begins to understand the importance and value (level 3: valuing) of geriatric patents. He continues to visit elderly patients. He even becomes a geriatric EMS (GEMS) course instructor so that he can teach other EMS providers about geriatric patients, and he structures his opening presentation around the value of elderly people (level 4: organizing and level 5: characterizing).

Affective domain levels

Level 1: Receiving occurs as the student acquires awareness of the value or importance of learning information and expresses a willingness to learn. At this level, students may not agree on or value the actual concepts, but they are open to listening. *Level 2: Responding* expands upon level 1 as the student actively participates in the learning process and begins to derive satisfaction from it. At *Level 3: Valuing,* the student individually perceives that the behavior has worth or value. If the concept or idea was previously a part of a student's value system, this is the level at which he or she begins within the affective domain. At *Level 4: Organizing,* students integrate new, refined, or different beliefs into their existing value system and reconcile differences between old and new beliefs. They should also begin to replace preexisting values that conflict with the newer ones that are being adopted. *Level 5: Characterizing* is the most sophisticated level in the affective domain. It requires the development of one's own value system that governs one's behavior and, like *Level 6: Evaluation* in the cognitive domain, it involves a degree of metacognition in the process as the student scrutinizes the processes used in deriving his or her values, beliefs, and opinions.

Psychomotor domain levels

Level 1: Imitation occurs as students repeat and mimic demonstrations given by an instructor. *Level 2: Manipulation* occurs as students practice the skill and begin to create their own styles of performance. Because students lack sophistication at this point, experimentation and trial and error are expected and should be encouraged by the educator. As a student reaches *Level 3: Precision,* the skill should be performed without mistakes. Students should also begin to transfer its use to other situations or circumstances. However, this will be done with a high degree of error in performance, necessitating resumption of the trial-and-error process—but with a new emphasis on exploring "what-if" concepts. *Level 4: Articulation* occurs as students become proficient and competent in the performance of the skill, adding their own style or flair. At this level, students should be able to modify the performance of the skill in appropriate ways and defend their choices and decisions. *Level 5: Naturalization* is the mastery level of skill performance. In contrast to the cognitive and affective domains, this level is attained when the student performs the skill seemingly without any cognition required. This level is sometimes referred to as "muscle memory," or automatic. True naturalization occurs when skill performance is correct *despite* the environment or circumstance in which the skill is performed.

CASE IN POINT

When a student begins the megacode skill for cardiac arrest resuscitation, he or she must integrate the application of many skills, including those of team leader. The first time these concepts are presented, the instructor role-plays a megacode scenario in which he or she acts out each of the roles. The student is then encouraged to function as the team leader (level 1: imitation). The student practices the role of team leader, directing classmates through a programmed megacode scenario, while the instructor observes and provides feedback (level 2: manipulation). As the student gains confidence in performing a megacode, the instructor begins to introduce "what if" scenarios into the simulations, causing the student to react and adjust his or her treatment plan (level 3: precision). The student reacts appropriately in most scenarios and, when questioned, can defend his or her treatment choices with logical reasoning (level 4: articulation). When the student attends an advanced cardiac life support (ACLS) class, he or she correctly performs the megacode skill and can carry on a conversation on an unrelated topic during the drill (level 5: naturalization).

THE THREE-LEVEL SYSTEM

When the distinct levels within each of the domains in Bloom's taxonomy are analyzed, it is clear that movement from one level to the next can occur in a nearly seamless fashion between certain levels. For example, imitation (level 1) and manipulation (level 2) are strongly interlinked in the psychomotor domain. Analysis (level 5) and synthesis (level 6) are closely related in the cognitive domain as well. Over time, educators began to see distinct points of separation in the increasing sophistication within the levels of each domain. They also noted that these points seemed to fall in similar places. These natural breakpoints led to the development of a three-level system.

In the three-level system, the descriptive terminology is consistent for each domain: Level 1 is knowledge, level 2 is application, and level 3 is problem solving. This three-level strategy of classification is common to fire service instruction, as well as EMS. Table 7-2 shows the application of the three-level classification strategy to Bloom's taxonomy.

TABLE 7-2 Bloom's Taxonomy Sorted According to the Three-Level System

Levels	Cognitive Domain	Affective Domain	Psychomotor Domain
1: Knowledge	Knowledge Comprehension	Receiving Responding	Imitation Manipulation
2: Application	Application	Valuing	Precision
3: Problem solving	Analysis Synthesis Evaluation	Organizing Characterizing	Articulation Naturalization

Level 1: Knowledge

Level 1: Knowledge is the least sophisticated of the three levels, requiring only a rudimentary understanding of concepts, feelings, and skills performance. Students who master this level comprehend basic facts, feelings, and procedural steps. It includes such behaviors as imitation, recall, defining of terms, or receiving and responding to new information. A student who is functioning at this level cannot yet extrapolate this information to other concepts. An example of a student who is functioning at this level is one who can define the terminology for the *ABCs of CPR* and perform the simple steps of airway opening. At this level, the student lacks the sophistication to know when to use the jaw-thrust method instead of the head-tilt chin-lift. When students have a firm grasp of knowledge at this first level, they are ready to progress to *Level 2: Application.*

TEACHING TIP: If a firm foundation of knowledge is not achieved in level 1, a student may require remediation before he or she can truly master the concepts within levels 2 and 3. The student will demonstrate this lack of foundational knowledge in poor performance during both formal and informal evaluation processes.

Level 2: Application

Level 2: Application builds upon the concepts learned in level 1. It involves the integration and execution of principles, procedures, and values in specific situations. Students are now capable of precision in skill execution, application of principles, and valuing of feelings and beliefs. Students can transfer learning that has occurred in level 1 to new situations. They can form new meanings with and from the deconstruction and reconstruction of concepts from level 1. For example, as the CPR student continues in the program, he or she learns all the skills and can perform standardized patient care scenarios. As students master this level, they should progress to level 3.

Level 3: Problem Solving

Level 3: Problem solving builds upon the concepts from the previous two levels. Success in level 3 indicates that true mastery of the concepts has been achieved. It involves thoughtful analysis of information, procedures, and feelings. Students can successfully modify and adapt specific tasks depending upon situations. Metacognitive processing is the hallmark of this level for the cognitive and affective domains, along with automation (or naturalization) of skills in the psychomotor domain. Continuing with the previous example, as the CPR student progresses to this level, he or she will correctly alter his or her treatment plan, depending upon the environment or circumstance, in such a manner that the correct solution will result a high percentage of the time.

The High- and Low-Level System

The informal system of categorizing domain levels, called *the high- and low-level system,* sorts the existing levels within Bloom's taxonomy into one of two categories: high level or low level (Table 7-3). This strategy is presented because it was used in the past to develop EMS and fire science curricula. Now, this strategy is used less frequently, as the three-level system has gained popularity.

Although the high- and low-level system may appear to be the easiest strategy for an educator to use because it comprises only two categories, the system is problematic. There is no clear consensus as to whether the elements that fall within the middle ground of the taxonomy (i.e., level 2 of the three-level strategy and level 3 of Bloom's original description) belong to the "low" level or the "high" level; some instructional designers and educators consider them to be high-level concepts, whereas others consider them low-level concepts. The only clear consensus is that level 1 of the three-level system is "low," and level 3 of the same system is "high." The real problem with this informal strategy emerges when instructors attempt to guess where the middle ground lies as they plan instruction and evaluation. For this reason, it is not recommended that an informal strategy be used in the design or development of instruction or teaching.

TABLE 7-3 Bloom's Taxonomy Sorted According to the High- and Low-Level System

Levels	Cognitive Domain	Affective Domain	Psychomotor Domain
1. High	Knowledge	Receiving	Imitation
	Comprehension	Responding	Manipulation
	Application	Valuing	Precision
	Analysis	Organizing	Articulation
2. Low	Synthesis	Characterizing	Naturalization
	Evaluation		

*Color in the second row indicates ambiguity regarding which midlevels fall within the high and low categories.

ADDRESSING THE DOMAINS IN GOALS AND OBJECTIVES

The domains of learning are used in the instructional design process for writing goals and objectives. Educators must understand the language of an objective or goal and must discern specific meaning from the verbs used to write them. (See Chapter 8, Goals and Objectives.) This enables the educator to plan instructional and evaluative processes that assist students in meeting the objectives and provide a means of measuring their achievement.

In the knowledge level of cognition, the following terms are useful: *arrange, define, describe, identify, label, list, name, match, memorize, order, recall, recite,* and *repeat.* The analysis level of the cognitive domain uses such action verbs as *analyze, calculate, compare and contrast, differentiate, and examine.* In the psychomotor domain, level 1: imitation employs terms such as *repeat, mimic,* and *follow,* whereas level 4: articulation uses *demonstrate proficiency* and *perform without assistance.* In the affective domain, terms such as *accept, attempt,* and *willing* are appropriate for level 1: receiving, and *join* and *participate* are found in level 5: characterizing. Goals and objectives are more explicitly addressed in Chapter 8.

ADDRESSING THE DOMAINS IN TEACHING STRATEGIES

Learning within one domain is often interdependent on learning in another domain. For example, psychomotor skill development requires cognitive knowledge and concepts for hands-on practice to be most effective. A student will achieve mastery of endotracheal intubation more quickly if he or she can identify the necessary equipment, understand the indications for the skill, and recite the sequence of events required for completion of the skill before he or she ever attempts to perform it.

At the same time, mastery of knowledge in one domain does not imply mastery in the other domains. For example, a student who can answer multiple-choice exam questions about the procedure for spinal immobilization is not necessarily able to fully immobilize a patient without compromising the spine.

As educators plan learning, they should consider the level of learning that has taken place within each domain and how it relates to their instructional objectives. The process of building new learning upon previous learning is called *scaffolding.* In the building trade, scaffolds allow an individual to move from one floor, or level, to another. They are often fragile structures that depend on firm attachment to multiple points below them. Learning scaffolds are also highly dependent upon successful performance at lower levels (Figure 7-1).

To properly scaffold, teaching strategies and evaluation methods must target the top of the level in which students are learning. To do this, the instructor should review objectives from the course, unit, or lesson to determine the appropriate depth and breadth at which to teach the material. To determine depth and breadth, one of the two formal strategies should be used to identify the level of the objective.

Depth and breadth examples:

- Objective A states that the student should take a supplied list of names of seven organs and label those organs on a manikin
- Objective B states that the student should draw a human skeleton and label all the major bones from memory. Objective A deals with cognitive knowledge (level 1), whereas objective B deals with synthesis (level 3)
- Objective C states that the student should be able to take an empty oxygen cylinder and switch the regulator to a full tank. If the instructor demonstrates the skill, then some—but not all—of the students mimic him or her, it is unlikely that the students will be successful in an evaluation of this skill. Skill demonstration and practice are level 1 activities, whereas performance of a skill for testing purposes with confidence and proficiency is a level 3 activity

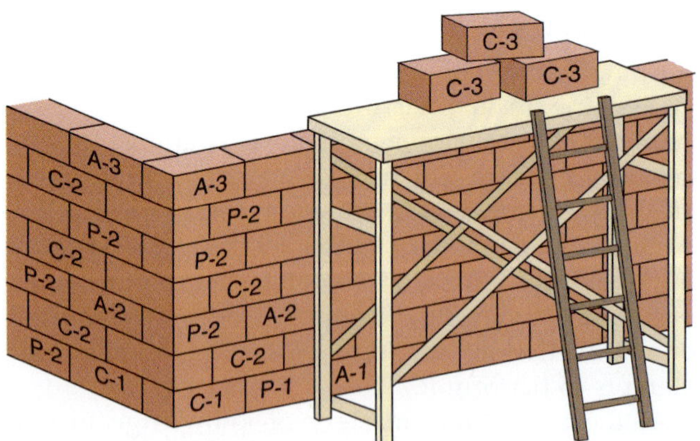

FIGURE 7-1 The process of building new learning upon previous learning is called *scaffolding.* In the building trade, scaffolds allow an individual to move from one floor, or level, to another. They are often fragile structures that depend on firm attachment to multiple points below them. Learning scaffolds are also highly dependent upon successful performance at lower levels. To properly scaffold, teaching strategies and evaluation methods should target the top of the level at which students are learning.

- Objective D states that the student should be able to list the "five patient medication rights." In reviewing what an instructor taught in class, the instructor realizes that he or she stressed only four of them. It is unlikely that students will be able to successfully test on this objective unless they are highly self-motivated and learned it on their own through reading or participating in a study group or tutoring session

Clever educators can devise methods for integrating learning across several domains to enhance both depth and breadth of knowledge. This is accomplished by engaging as many senses as possible to enhance retention, for example, use of multimedia, class discussion, and role playing. Studies on retention suggest that, as more senses are engaged in the learning process, more learning takes place. Additional studies show that greater retention occurs as concepts are revisited and reviewed.[2,3]

TEACHING TIP: A common strategy used to assist students in attaining mastery of depth and breadth is to teach one level beyond that required by the objective to account for memory degradation. If time is at a premium, which it often is, this may not be possible.

Individual student learning styles and preferences magnify the interdependence of the different learning domains. (Also see Chapter 4, Learning Styles.) Students who are strongly kinesthetic (hands-on) in their learning preference may have difficulty understanding cognitive concepts until they are able to experience their psychomotor application. On the other hand, students who identify most strongly with "global" tendencies may be more attuned to feelings than are analytic individuals and may, therefore, require more (or less) attention to the affective domain.

TEACHING TIP: Chapter 4 contains information on learning styles and preferences. An instructor should, while reading that chapter, consider how this information influences the domains of learning.

The application of learning domains to teaching strategies is more explicitly discussed in Chapters 12 to 18 of this text.

ADDRESSING THE DOMAINS IN EVALUATION METHODS

Educators must devise evaluation strategies that determine the mastery of each level of each domain as it is reached. Educators who assume competency and fail to evaluate students quickly learn the importance of doing so. In addition, evaluation should occur to ensure that students retain concepts from the previous level(s).

Current Department of Transportation (DOT) National Standard Curricula guidelines for each level of EMS training recommend that equal consideration be placed on the evaluation of each of the three domains of learning, with one-third emphasis on cognitive, one-third on affective, and one-third on psychomotor. This represents a paradigm shift for many EMS educators, who may have placed little emphasis on evaluating the affective domain.

TEACHING TIP: An instructor can take a quick look at the course grading policy to determine whether a program places equal emphasis on each domain of learning.

Even veteran educators may find it difficult to target evaluation methods to the specific domains of learning. Written and oral exams are useful for evaluating the cognitive domain. Class participation, demonstrated leadership, and peer supervision are useful for evaluating the affective domain. Skill competency exams and evaluation within the clinical setting are useful for evaluating the psychomotor domain. The application of learning domains to evaluation methods is more explicitly covered in Chapters 19 to 21 of this text.

SUMMARY

Ultimately, students must achieve proficiency in all three domains of learning if they are to be competent EMS providers. The domains of learning levels are a scientific tool that instructional designers and educators should use to craft objectives, identify the appropriate depth and breadth of content to plan lessons and teaching strategies, and effectively evaluate learning and retention. Savvy educators recognize their importance and know how to use them in practicing and honing the art of teaching.

REFERENCES

1. Bloom BS, et al. *Taxonomy of Educational Objectives, Cognitive Domain.* New York: Longman; 1956.
2. Cicchetti G. *Cognitive Modeling and Reciprocal Teaching of Reading and Study Strategies.* Watertown, Conn; 1990.
3. Mayer RE. (1998) Cognitive, metacognitive and motivational aspects of problem solving. *Instructional Science.* 1998;26:49-63.

WORKS CONSULTED

Hardt UH. *Determining Goals, Objectives and Strategies for the Domains of Learning and Instructional Intents. A Guide to Lesson and Unit Planning.* 1977.

Hodell C. *Basics of Instructional Systems Development.* ASTD Info-line, Issue 9706, 1997.

Learning to Learn. ARIS Information Sheet, 2000.

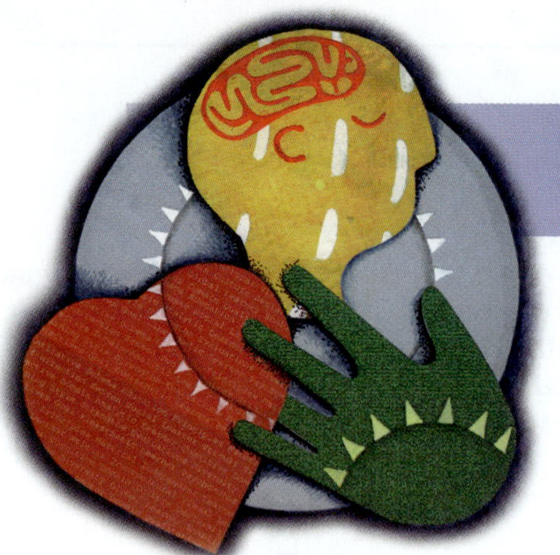

CHAPTER 8

Goals and Objectives

"'Would you tell me please, which way I ought to go from here?'
'That depends a good deal on where you want to get to,'
said the Cat.
'I don't much care where—' said Alice.
'Then it doesn't matter which way you go,' said the Cat.
'—so long as I get somewhere,' Alice added as an explanation.
'Oh, you're sure to do that,' said the Cat, 'if you only walk
long enough.'"

—From Alice's Adventures in Wonderland by Lewis Carroll

Goals and objectives are the backbone of the instructional process. They provide meaning for instruction by identifying what educators should teach and what students are expected to learn. This chapter discusses how the taxonomy of the domains of learning categorize learning into discrete levels. This chapter then builds on that concept by using those levels in the process of writing goals and objectives.

During instructional planning, educators use goals and objectives to determine the appropriate depth and breadth of content required to teach a given topic, including differentiating between necessary and unnecessary content. This planning helps to ensure that instruction is targeted to specific goals. Goals and objectives are also used in the test item writing and evaluation processes to effectively evaluate student learning. Finally, these tools are useful for measuring the effectiveness of the educator's teaching activities.

Through goals and objectives, students focus their learning and begin to differentiate important content from unimportant content. Students should be able to track their individual progress in the course by evaluating their ability to perform (or answer questions regarding) class objectives and meet course goals. Instructors should ensure that students have course goals and objectives and that they use them to focus their studying.

Although several strategies for writing goals and objectives may be applied, this chapter focuses on a single, generic technique for writing both that uses two tiers: goals followed by objectives. Although this technique is common to emergency medical services (EMS), educators should determine whether their specific agency or department uses a different strategy; if that is the case, this chapter will still be helpful, as the concepts explained here are similar to those associated with other objective and goal writing methods.

TEACHING TIP: Although an entry level educator may not be required to write objectives, it is important that the educator understand how goals and objectives relate to the planning and evaluation of instruction.

WHAT ARE GOALS AND OBJECTIVES?

Educators can make the best use of goals and objectives when they have acquired a keen understanding of exactly what these instructional tools are—and can identify the differences between them. The words *goal* and *objective* are often used interchangeably or without regard for their actual meaning, which can lead to confusion. In this textbook, a two-tiered system is described wherein the term *goal* is used only to describe the uppermost level of instruction and the term *objective* is used to describe the subordinate level.

A great deal of support is available for use of this method. In many instructional materials, goals and objectives are presented in two distinct levels, with objectives being subordinate to goals. The first level (which is generally the goal) identifies the overall goal of instruction for the course or specific instructional event. Confusion arises when this tier is called a *terminal objective* instead of the *primary goal of instruction.*[1]

Objectives are always subordinate to the goal. In completing each objective, a student makes progress toward meeting the overall goal. Sometimes, objectives are called *enabling objectives.* This terminology is common when goal statements are named *terminal objectives.* Every goal statement should have at least one objective that relates to it, and every objective should relate to at least one goal. The content of the lesson (sometimes called the *declarative* material) should relate to the goals and objectives, and should not contain information that does not relate to the goals and objectives. (See "Performance Agreement" for further details.)

TEACHING TIP: Another strategy for writing goals and objectives applies three tiers, or levels, of distinct goals and objectives. In this strategy, the goal is the upper level, or tier. The second tier is often called the terminal objective, and the last tier is called the enabling objective. In this strategy, various enabling objectives are grouped together under a single terminal objective that directly relates to the goal. Completion of the enabling objectives leads to completion of the terminal objective. Completion of several terminal objectives leads to completion of the goal. This strategy of classification is useful when one is describing a program with multiple class sessions that is offered over a certain length of time. It can also be used to break down each block of instruction for a semester-long course.

Goals

Goals are philosophical statements about what learning is intended to produce. They are often broad, generalized, and overarching with no specific information on *how* learning is to be accomplished or measured. Goals are similar in nature to mission or vision statements. An educator may establish goals, for example, for an entire course, a learning module, a 1-hour skills practice, or a single case scenario.

Examples of goal statements include the following:

- The goal of this chapter is to explain the concepts of basic airway management
- Students who attend this cardiopulmonary resuscitation (CPR) course will perform all required CPR techniques correctly on a manikin
- At the completion of English 203, the student will be able to compose essays using a technical writing style

Objectives

For a goal to be accomplished, specific and measurable objectives must be identified. The word *objective* literally means *observable.* Objectives are expressed statements of expected learning outcomes, which include products or behaviors that students are required to exhibit. As with goals, an educator may establish objectives, for example, for a course, a particular lesson, a skills practice, or a single classroom exercise.

An objective should be detailed enough to encompass the *who, what, when, where,* and *how* of behaviors that are appropriate for accomplishing that goal. To provide this information, an objective should clearly identify four distinct items:

1. Target audience
2. Expected behavior
3. Condition under which that behavior will be performed
4. Measurement tool or strategy used to evaluate the objective for successful completion (or outcome)

Each of these elements must be expressed in such a manner that anyone who reads the objective will clearly understand the pass/fail point for each objective and will know exactly what behavior is expected.

This format describes the *ABCD model* (Audience, Behavior, Condition, and Degree) for writing objectives. This generic strategy is basic to most behavior-based goal and objective models. Examples of complete objectives include the following:

- The Basic Emergency Medical Technician (EMT-B) student will use his or her own words to correctly define at least five of the following six terms pertaining to respiratory emergencies: dyspnea, apnea, eupnea, hyperpnea, tachypnea, and bradypnea
- At the completion of this module, students in Advanced Chef Techniques will be able to bake basic soufflés and crème brûlé without assistance from recipes provided by the instructor
- Given an assortment of paintings of various styles, the Art History 101 student will be able to identify without error all paintings classified as "Impressionist"

PERFORMANCE AGREEMENT

The linkage of goals and objectives is established through an evaluation process called a *performance agreement*. Performance agreement is the process of critically evaluating the goals, objectives, and declarative content for the purpose of validating their logical relationships to one another, and to ensure that they adequately support one another. For performance agreement to exist within a body of planned instruction, each goal statement must be supported by one or more objectives that link (or relate) directly to it. At the same time, each objective should link to at least one goal. The declarative content should provide the depth and breadth described by the verbs written in the objectives. Refer to the previous chapter for a discussion of the levels of sophistication for each domain of learning.

Any goal or objective within the block of instruction that does not have a clear link should be evaluated further for appropriateness. These "unlinked" goals or objectives may represent omissions in the content required for the lesson. Or, they may highlight unnecessary material that should be deleted from the section altogether or perhaps moved into another lesson. (See Figure 8-1 for an example of performance agreement and an example without performance agreement.)

CASE IN POINT

A paramedic educator is reviewing his lesson plan for his next presentation, which is about how to interpret 12-lead electrocardiograms (ECGs). He begins by reviewing the goals and objectives for the session. He notes that all four of the goals listed are covered by at least one of the objectives, and each objective is linked to at least one goal. He then reviews the content for the presentation and discovers two places that lack performance agreement because there is a disconnection between the goals, objectives, and declarative content. The first error he discovers is that two of the objectives listed do not seem to be covered in the declarative section of the lesson plan. He adds the necessary material to make certain that he has covered all objectives. The second problem he notes is that a section of the material is not described in either the goals or the objectives for the lesson plan. As he reviews this material, he decides that it is not really appropriate for this lesson but should be covered in the next lesson. He moves this information to the next lesson after discussing his findings with his mentor. He updates this lesson plan with these changes so that the next time this plan is used, it will be more complete. His mentor compliments him on his plan and on finding the problems before attempting to teach the material.

<table>
<tr><th>Performance Agreement</th><th>No Performance Agreement</th></tr>
<tr><td>Topic: Cake Baking

Objectives:
1. Assemble and identify ingredients
2. Mix and measure ingredients
3. Bake as directed

Presentation Content:
A. Ingredients
1. Quality of ingredients
2. Acceptable substitutions
B. Mixing and combining
1. Measuring accurately
2. Ordering of steps
C. Baking as directed
1. Using an oven safely

Performance agreement is attained. Every objective is covered in the presentation and there is not anything additional in the presentation that does not relate to an objective. NOTE: The discussion of ingredient substitutions MAY be beyond the requirements for this presentation. This should highlight some of the difficulty with vaguely worded objectives.</td><td>Topic: Cake Baking

Objectives:
1. Assemble and identify ingredients
2. Mix and measure ingredients
3. Bake as directed

Presentation Content:
A. Mixing and combining
1. Measuring accurately
2. Ordering of steps
B. Baking as directed
1. Using an oven safely
C. Frosting and decoration

Performance agreement is NOT attained. The first objective is not covered in the presentation and the presentation included additional material that was not listed under the objectives (frosting and decorating). The possible impact of this is that the students may not be able to complete objective 1 on a test or may be able to work their way through it on their own, but clearly they did not receive any sort of instruction on it.</td></tr>
</table>

FIGURE 8-1 Performance agreement.

For the educator, the exercise of looking for and validating performance agreement is useful for identifying unnecessary instruction or any holes in a lesson plan. It helps to ensure that the content found within the lesson plan (which may or may not have been developed by the same educator) and the content presented in the classroom match the goals stated for the lesson in the curricula. In general, educators can focus on teaching only the necessary and appropriate content when they evaluate performance agreement.

TEACHING TIP: When performance agreement is assessed before instruction is provided, adjustments can be made before mistakes are made in the classroom. When performance agreement is assessed after instruction has been provided, content omissions or areas requiring remediation or reteaching can be identified.

Whenever possible, an educator should conduct a postpresentation evaluation for performance agreement. This should occur immediately after instruction has been provided for the purpose of reviewing what was taught and identifying whether any omissions, sidetracks (superfluous content), or other deviations from the lesson plan occurred. One method for conducting this type of performance agreement is to ask students to summarize the lesson or to provide their impressions of the key points covered. Another method of conducting this assessment is through the use of posttests. Omissions that are identified during this performance agreement assessment can be made up during future teaching sessions or through alternative learning opportunities outside of the face-to-face meeting.

TEACHING TIP: The postpresentation evaluation for performance agreement provides an excellent time for the educator to draft exam questions or select questions from a test item bank. Once an instructor has determined that performance agreement exists and this review is fresh in his or her mind, then he or she can select test items that most closely reflect the content delivered.

PARTS OF AN OBJECTIVE

Many methods, models, and templates are available for teaching an educator how to write objectives. The generic ABCD model, which is commonly used in EMS, lists the parts of a behavioral objective, where ABCD indicates the required elements of information. In this model, A = Audience, B = Behavior, C = Condition, and D = Degree.[2] Objectives need not be written in the ABCD order but should contain each of these four elements. (See Box 8-1 for a checklist for writing complete objectives.)

BOX 8-1 Checklist for Writing Objectives

- All four parts of the ABCD behavioral objective are present
  - Audience
  - Behavior
  - Condition
  - Degree
- Accurate terminology is used to reflect the domain of learning level
- Expected outcome is clearly articulated and measurable
- Expected outcome is written in terms of behaviors to perform or observe
- The point (score) for pass/fail is clearly articulated
- A measurement tool is discussed or described
- Objective supports overarching goal (performance agreement)

Two simple models to follow in constructing the order for an objective include:

1. The (Audience) will (Behavior) under (Condition) to (Degree).
2. Given (Condition), the (Audience) will (Behavior) to (Degree).

Audience

The *audience* describes the receiver (student) of the instructional activity (Figure 8-2). When reviewing objectives before providing instruction, the educator should ensure that the intended audience matches the actual audience for the instruction. If, for example, the intended audience for the lesson is identified in the objective as an advanced life support (ALS) provider, but the educator is using it for basic life support (BLS) providers, he or she will need to compensate for the disparity. In this case, the educator could supplement the lesson with additional material or stretch the presentation over a longer time period to account for deficits in the BLS provider's depth of knowledge.

In another example, the audience identified in the objective may have significantly different prerequisites from the audience that the instructor is about to teach or may be at a different intellectual level. In this situation, the educator could plan additional learning opportunities, make adjustments in timing, or rearrange the lesson entirely to suit the new target audience.

Because the audience remains constant throughout a series of objectives in, for example, the same lesson

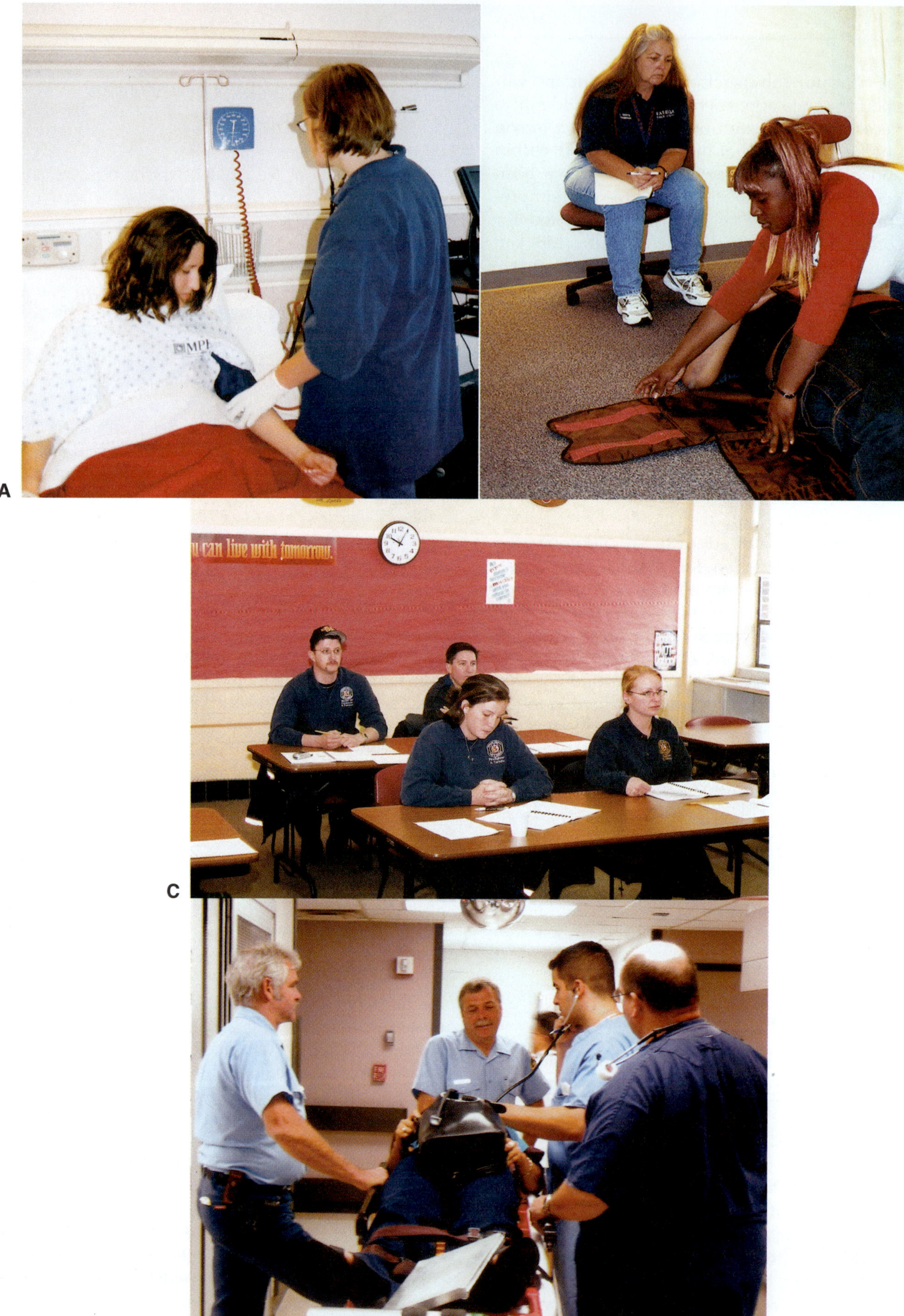

FIGURE 8-2 The audience (students) may be in the hospital **(A),** the skills lab **(B),** the classroom **(C),** or the field **(D).**

plan, textbook chapter, or block of instruction, the audience statement is often limited to the goal or first objective found in that series. In this case, the educator can assume that the stated audience carries through for the remainder of the objectives in that section.

Examples of audience statements include:

- The Columbia Community College freshman student . . .
- The EMT-Intermediate refresher course participant . . .
- The firefighter cadet attending this seminar . . .

TEACHING TIP: In light of this discussion, it may become clear that the Department of Transportation (DOT) objectives found in the National Standard Curricula (NSC) for each provider level appear to be written without the benefit of measurement information. Rest assured that this was deliberate. Bodies of work like the DOT NSC curricula serve as guidelines and are not meant to provide measurement criteria. It is the responsibility of training programs, regulatory bodies, and testing and certification agencies to establish these criteria.

Behavior

The *behavior* statement describes the expected outcome or capability that the learner should exhibit after the instructional event has occurred. Robert Mager, a behavioral theorist, is credited with the concept that goals and objectives should be tied to measurable outcomes.[3] The term that he used to describe this relationship was *concrete.* That is, any statement, or objective, tied to measurable behavioral outcomes is concrete; those that are not tied to measurable behavioral outcomes are called *fuzzy,* meaning that they are immeasurable statements. Mager believed that objectives should always be written in terms of performance so that learning can be measured. This concept is the foundation for the EMS process of writing objectives. If an objective is written so that it can be measured or observed, it becomes concrete enough to form the basis of evaluation. The relationship between goals and objectives and evaluation is explored at the end of this chapter.

Review the following two objectives. According to the criteria established by Mager, objective number one is not measurable, and number two is measurable.

- Objective 1: The EMT-B student will identify equipment used to immobilize a patient to a long backboard
- Objective 2: Given a BLS ambulance stocked with all the equipment and supplies identified by Maryland protocol, the EMT-B student will identify every piece of equipment used to immobilize a patient to a long backboard.

Objective number one states the audience and behavior but does not articulate any conditions or degree. It does not state how or what equipment will be used in the test, nor does it state the required score for successfully satisfying this objective. Thus, it would be difficult for an instructor to perform an evaluation of this objective. Objective number two tells both the instructor and the student that he or she will be required to identify all required equipment and supplies, and that he or she will be working with an ambulance stocked according to an established standard. This objective leaves little room for subjectivity in interpretation.

If objectives are observable and measurable, a tangible product or outcome that can be scrutinized and evaluated should be the result. This product or outcome can take the form of demonstrated knowledge, performance of a skill, or expressed or modeled feeling or emotion. It can come from any of the domains of learning (cognitive, affective, or psychomotor) and can be written to correspond to any of the levels of sophistication within a domain. It should be a realistic behavior that is related to the real life scope of practice for the student.

Examples of behavior statements include:

- . . . should be able to describe the steps used to initiate a peripheral IV . . .
- . . . should demonstrate how to put on sterile gloves . . .
- . . . will be able to challenge statements that do not support professional behavior and conduct . . .

Verbs such as "understand," "know," and "think" are not measurable and should be avoided in writing objectives.

In some educational settings, the terminology used to construct the behavioral statement carries legal connotations. In this case, there is a significant difference between phases such as *should be able to* and *will be able to.* It is important for the instructor to determine whether such a circumstance exists, and if it does, to follow the requirements accordingly when developing goals and objectives.

Condition

The *condition* portion of the ABCD objective describes any circumstance that influences the performance of behavior. It may include a list of tools or equipment that may or may not be used in completion of the behavior; it may describe environmental or weather conditions or identify specific locations or situations, such as time of day or season of the year. Time limits may also be imposed as a condition of the performance of a skill.

Examples of condition statements include:

- . . . in swift running river water with class II rapids . . .

- Given a table of assorted EMS equipment, . . .
- . . . within 1 minute . . .

Take this example of a measurable objective for a trauma lesson: The BLS student will perform a trauma patient assessment on a simulated patient placed in a difficult-to-access place, without committing any critical errors. The conditions that affect the performance (in this case, the skill of trauma patient assessment) of this objective are the use of a simulated patient (necessitating the finding of predetermined signs or symptoms) and a challenging environment. Because the condition is well articulated, both the instructor and the student can determine what behavior is expected and how it should be tested. This leaves little room for surprises during testing and helps create realistic expectations for both students and instructors.

Degree

The *degree* portion of the objective provides the standard of accuracy required for acceptable performance. It describes the actual measurement tool used to assess the student's performance and clearly identifies the point at which the student will be successful in his or her performance. Objectives can be measurable by both quantitative and qualitative criteria. Quantitative (quantity) criteria identify behaviors through conditions that impose or describe limitations (e.g., the lowest acceptable passing score, time limits, or limits on number of attempts) and provide this information as a percentage or point value. Qualitative (quality) criteria include nonnumerical observations that show underlying dimensions or patterns of relationships (e.g., expressing the value or acceptance of a concept or idea, defending a decision or action, or adopting a new behavior pattern). Quality standards are often more difficult to attach numeric scores to, but they can be observed for performance. The use of rubrics as evaluation tools can be helpful in qualitative measurements (Box 8-2).

Here are several qualitative examples of degree:

- . . . using therapeutic communication strategies throughout the simulation . . .
- . . . by using all of the 11 affective domain characteristics described in the EMT-B National Standard Curricula that apply to this scenario . . .
- . . . without committing any critical fail point errors . . .

Additional factors to consider in measuring performance according to an objective are whether steps required to perform a skill are ordered (and if this order is important), and whether any factors or steps are critical to the performance. Examples of critical factors include the wearing of gloves when one approaches a patient and the performing of an assessment before one begins CPR. Such factors are often labeled *critical criteria* or *critical fail points*, and failure to satisfy or perform them may result in immediate failure in the performance of an objective. Critical fail points are generally absolute, which means that failure is imposed despite an otherwise acceptable performance. For this reason, critical fail status should be reserved for extremely important steps or considerations. The psychomotor examination check-off sheets of the National Registry of EMTs include at the bottom of each skill sheet critical criteria, called *critical fail points*.

Some additional examples of degree statements include:

- . . . seven out of ten times . . .
- . . . to 80% accuracy . . .
- . . . for every patient care encounter . . .

It is important that the performance level be specifically stated; otherwise, an educator may assume that 100% accuracy is required. Note that a performance level of 100% accuracy for quantitative or qualitative measures is not required for every objective. Educators should scrutinize objectives carefully to determine the acceptable level of performance and should plan instructional time and emphasis accordingly.

BOX 8-2 What Are Rubrics?

A rubric is an evaluation tool that uses scales with examples to provide a framework for evaluation. Rubrics have many applications for both qualitative and quantitative evaluations. Rubrics work well with qualitative criteria because they provide concrete examples of the expected behavior, along with the scores or grades that will be awarded for each category. Rubrics can also be useful for evaluations that are more subjective than objective because they quantify the process. Essay questions are generally considered selective but are less so when graded with rubric tools. In this case, a group of instructors has determined ahead of time the criteria required for each level of grade or points assigned for each level. For example, the rubric may state that the student will receive 5 points for each key concept that he or she explains in his or her essay, up to a total of 50 points. It may also include a deduction of 5 points for every unrelated concept or incorrect item that he or she includes in the answer. Another rubric may score the essay by creating a scale for punctuation and spelling errors, awarding up to 10 points for 0 to 5 errors, 9 points for 6 to 10 errors, 8 points for 11 to 15 errors, and so forth. Scoring within the rubric should allow for evaluation of each of the dimensions of the project. Students can even be provided examples of answers for each grade range. Tools for developing rubrics can be found on various Web sites on the Internet, along with the spectrum of topics from K-12 to adult education. A rubric for evaluation of the affective domain is provided in the Appendix of the DOT EMS Instructor Guidelines.

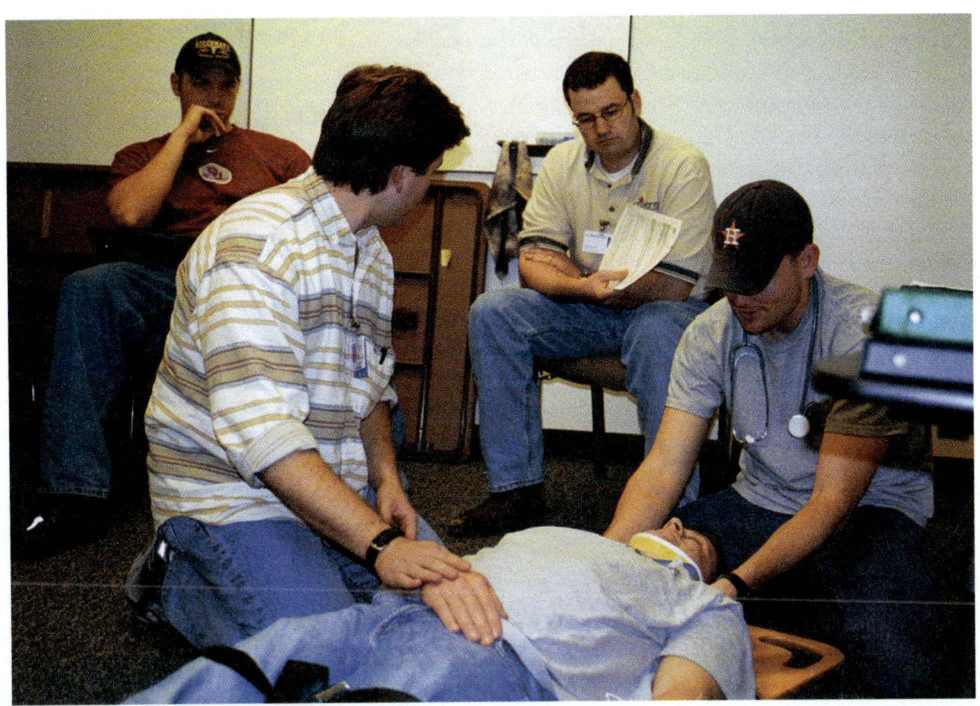

FIGURE 8-3 Skill performance criteria should include critical fail points that must be completed properly if the student is to successfully perform the skill.

Sometimes, it is difficult to distinguish between some of the ABCD parts of an objective, as there seems to be crossover between them. Take, for example, the following objective: *At the completion of this lesson on trauma, the Howard County Fire and Rescue Training Academy Firefighter Cadet will be able to correctly demonstrate the application of a rigid splint to a simulated open fracture of the upper extremity within 7 minutes, without committing any critical errors.* Instructors may debate whether the statement *within 7 minutes* represents a condition or a degree. They may also debate whether the words *correctly demonstrate* indicate that a score of 100% accuracy is required to satisfy this objective. This objective leaves little doubt about what behavior is expected of the student (apply a rigid splint to an open upper extremity fracture) and about how the student will be evaluated (it must be done correctly within 7 minutes, and the student cannot commit any critical fail errors). The word *correctly* may cause minor confusion, but most instructors would overlook this wording because the phrase about committing critical errors sets a clear boundary.

This example draws attention to the fact that the writing of objectives is not a simple task. In this case, it is important for the educator to identify the behavior portion of the objective and to place that behavior in the proper context within the domains of learning. In so doing, the instructor can identify the depth and breadth required to teach the content so that the objective is satisfied. This objective requires problem-solving behavior via cognitive level 3: application, level 4: analysis, and level 5: synthesize, as well as psychomotor performance at least at level 3: precision.

TEACHING TIP: When working from goals and objectives that have been supplied to him or her, it is critical that the educator review the objectives to ensure completeness and relevance to the audience and situation.

CASE IN POINT

An instructor is reviewing lesson plans for the next several class sessions. He compares what students have already learned with what is coming next. He notes that so far, students have not spent a lot of time practicing psychomotor skills, but they have a practical skills test coming up in 2 weeks. He is concerned because students are performing on level 1 (through imitation of the instructor's performance and practicing with assistance), and they will be tested at level 2: precision. The instructor decides to alter the schedule so that students will have an extra practical session. During the session, the instructor makes certain that he verbally quizzes the students on cognitive content, in addition to monitoring their psychomotor skill development.

TERMINOLOGY AND PRECISION

Objectives must be written with clear, unambiguous terminology that is free of jargon. All acronyms and potentially confusing terms should be clearly defined. Statements must be written in observable and measurable terms, with careful attention to ensure that action verbs used to describe the required behavior/expected outcome reflect the desired level. Table 8-1 provides a listing of appropriate verbs that correspond to the various levels within Bloom's taxonomy.[4]

Objectives are always results-oriented. Unlike broader goal statements, objectives describe specific expectations. When they read an objective, there should be no doubt in the student's and instructor's minds about exactly what behavior is expected. Returning to a previous example *(The BLS student will perform a trauma patient assessment on a simulated patient placed in a difficult to access place, without committing any critical errors),* imagine the difficulty that this student would face if, every time he or she practiced a trauma patient assessment, it was on a manikin lying supine on a blanket in the middle of the classroom floor; yet, on the night of the test, the simulated patient was placed head-down on the side of a hill outdoors in the dark.

CASE IN POINT

A paramedic student meets with the primary course instructor with the intent of informing her that he intends to drop out of the program. The student tells the instructor that he is having trouble with medical terminology and feels that he cannot possibly memorize all the terms that the instructor went over in class in preparation for the upcoming test in 3 weeks; he feels that he will be unable to keep up in the program because of this. The course is 18 months long, and this lesson occurred during the second week of the program. This student successfully passed two semesters of anatomy and physiology at the community college and has 1 year of experience as an EMT-B. He is becoming a paramedic because of his desire to help others, and he left a successful career in banking. He is in his late thirties and has a bachelor's degree in finance. Using the objectives in the course syllabus, the instructor works with the student until he understands that he is not required to memorize all the terms covered in the lesson for the test in 3 weeks, but that by the end of the course, he will be required to know all these terms. She emphasizes that for this test, the student needs to understand how to break down a medical term into its component parts (word root, suffix, and prefix) in order to properly define a term. She also suggests that he begin to memorize commonly used terms, and she recommends that he create flashcards to help him study. She also agrees to provide the student with a list of required medical terms for each section of the course to assist him with studying.

TABLE 8-1 Action Verbs Corresponding to Bloom's Taxonomy

Domain	Levels	Appropriate Verbs
Cognitive	1 Knowledge	Arrange, Define, Describe, Identify, Label, List, Name, Identify, Match, Memorize, Order, Recognize, Recall, Recite, Repeat
	2 Comprehension	Classify, Discuss, Distinguish, Explain, Identify, Indicate, Locate, Review, Rewrite, Summarize, Tell, Translate
	3 Application	Apply, Choose, Compute, Demonstrate, Operate, Practice, Prepare, Solve
	4 Analysis	Analyze, Calculate, Compare, Contrast, Criticize, Diagram, Differentiate, Distinguish, Examine, Experiment, Evaluate, Relate, Separate, Select
	5 Synthesis	Assemble, Compose, Construct, Create, Combine, Design, Formulate, Organize, Prepare, Set up, Summarize, Tell, Write
	6 Evaluate	Appraise, Evaluate, Judge, Score
Affective	1 Receiving	Accept, Attempt, Willing
	2 Responding	Challenge, Select, Support, Visit
	3 Valuing	Defend, Display, Offer, Choose
	4 Organization	Judge, Volunteer, Share, Dispute
	5 Characterization	Consistently, Join, Participate
Psychomotor	1 Imitation	Repeat, Mimic, Follow
	2 Manipulation	Practice with minimal assistance, Create, Modify
	3 Precision	Perform without error, Perform without assistance
	4 Articulation	Demonstrate proficiency, Perform with confidence, Perform with style or flair
	5 Naturalization	Perform automatically

THE RELATIONSHIP BETWEEN THE DOMAINS OF LEARNING AND OBJECTIVES

There is a strong link between objectives and the domains of learning, a fact that is thoroughly explained in Chapter 7. As a simple review, Benjamin Bloom grouped learning into three distinct domains, or categories of related elements: cognitive, psychomotor, and affective domains.[4] These domains reflect the fact that learning can take place in a variety of ways, depending on how we feel emotionally about an issue, how we perform skills and procedures, and how we think about concepts and ideas.

Each domain is subdivided into five or six distinct sections. These sections are arranged into levels. As an individual's learning progresses within a domain, increasing sophistication (more internal processing with less reliance upon the instructor's input or guidance) is required, and greater mastery is attained. In the three-level system, level 1 is the knowledge level, level 2 is application, and level 3 is problem solving. The degrees of sophistication that require less depth of knowledge (e.g., when a student defines words or matches terms with meaning) are referred to as the *lower level* or *level 1* objectives. Level 2 (application) objectives are at an intermediate level between levels 1 and 3. Level 3 (problem solving) represents the *highest level* of learning and requires that students think critically about a topic, debate it, and understand it in depth.

GOALS AND OBJECTIVES AND THE EVALUATION PROCESS

Once the level has been identified for the goal or objective, the instructor can determine which level the evaluation tool should address. Formative evaluation tools can target any level: knowledge, application, or problem solving. Generally, evaluation tools are summative in nature and focus on the higher levels of application and problem solving. Summative tools should include some assessment of verification of competency in the knowledge level, as well as at higher levels. This condition will be important in the event that the student does poorly on the evaluation, as this information can help focus the remediation process by identifying where the deficit occurred. (Chapter 19, Principles of Evaluation of Student Performance, takes an in-depth look at formative and summative evaluation tools.)

Use each of the following objectives (presented earlier in this chapter) to determine at what depth the instructor should evaluate, and to stimulate discussion of possible evaluation tools:

1. The EMT-B student will use his or her own words to correctly define at least five of the following six terms pertaining to respiratory emergencies: dyspnea, apnea, eupnea, hyperpnea, tachypnea, and bradypnea.
2. At the completion of this module, students in Advanced Chef Techniques will be able to bake basic soufflés and crème brûlé without assistance from recipes provided by the instructor.
3. Given an assortment of paintings of various styles, the Art History 101 student will be able to identify without error all paintings classified as "Impressionist."

Objective 1 asks the student to provide definitions. Bloom's taxonomy places this type of cognition in level 1: knowledge. Thus, a fill-in-the-blank question format would be an appropriate evaluation tool.

Objective 2 asks the student to apply his or her baking skills, so he or she must possess knowledge (level 1) but must also apply techniques of baking and cooking (level 2). The student also may encounter problems that would require him or her to troubleshoot and use critical thinking skills (level 3). The student in this situation would need to operate on all three levels to satisfy this objective, but the objective concentrates on level 2. The objective states that the student must perform baking skills (a psychomotor activity), so a demonstration of those skills is the appropriate requirement for evaluation. The evaluator should also ask knowledge questions to ensure that level 1 has been mastered. It would not be appropriate for the evaluator to introduce problems deliberately into the examination, as the objective does not state that such a high level of performance is expected. Also, in the event of a problem, it may be appropriate for the evaluator to assist the student. Even though this is an "advanced" chef course, the objective speaks of performing basic skills. It would be helpful to place this objective within the context of the overall program. If this happens early in the course, the student may not possess many problem-solving skills. However, because this is an advanced course, the student may be expected to have already mastered a certain number of problem-solving skills.

Objective 3 may appear to be of a higher level upon first glance, but it is operating primarily at level 2: application. In this objective, the student will be shown a group of paintings, and he or she must apply the rules and knowledge obtained in level 1 to make some decisions about paintings that don't meet the criteria. The student is not asked to defend his or her choices or to determine whether the artwork presented is even considered a painting or not. Because the objective states that students will be given a finite grouping of paintings to look at, all they will really be doing is sorting the paintings into one of two categories: those paintings that meet the criteria and those that do not. This involves mainly knowledge level 1 activities, along with some level 2 skills, in that they are applying their knowledge of the rules. An evaluation approach that would be appropriate for this situation would be showing students a series of slides and asking them to write "yes" or "no" on an answer sheet. Another way to evaluate this objective would be to give students a pile of cards with the images on them, and asking them to sort the cards into two piles: one with Impressionist paintings and one with images that are not.

SUMMARY

As the backbone of instructional planning, goals and objectives clarify for the educator and for the student precisely what learning should take place and how learning will be evaluated. Educators can use the ABCD method to write complete and accurate measurable objectives that address the three domains of learning: cognitive, affective, and psychomotor. By evaluating for performance agreement, the educator can determine the appropriate depth and breadth of content that should be taught on a given topic and can determine whether lesson plan content is complete. Goals and objectives are also used in decisions about appropriate evaluation tools.

REFERENCES

1. Hardt UH. Determining goals, objectives and strategies for the domains of learning and instructional intents. In: *A Guide to Lesson and Unit Planning*. 1977.
2. Hodell C. Basics of Instructional Systems Development. ASTD Info-line, Issue 9706, 1997.
3. Mager RF. *Goal Analysis*. Belmont, Calif: Fearon Publishers; 1972.
4. Bloom BS, et al. *Taxonomy of Educational Objectives. Book I: Cognitive Domain*. New York: Longman; 1956.

WORKS CONSULTED

Nooman ZM, Schmidt HG, Ezzat ES, eds. *Innovation in Medical Education*. New York: Springer Publishing Company.

Novak JD. *A Theory of Education*. Ithaca Cornell University Press; 1977.

Smilkstein R. Acquiring knowledge and using it. *Gamut*. 1993;16:41-43.

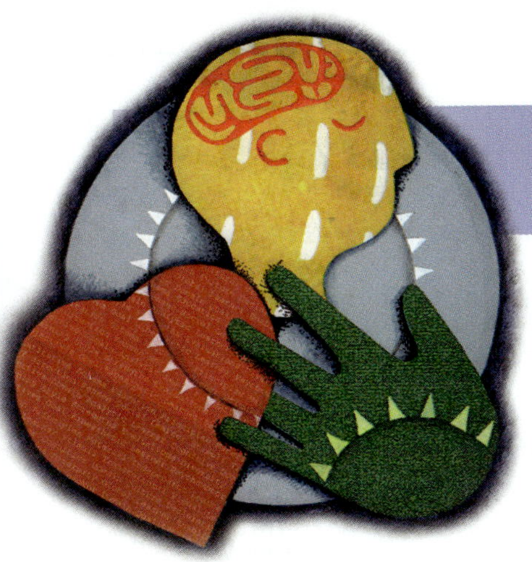

CHAPTER 9

Lesson Plans

"The whole art of teaching is only the art of awakening the natural curiosity of young minds for the purpose of satisfying it afterwards."

—*Anatole France*

The process of education can be described as a journey. As with any journey, the traveler or student has to know where he or she is going and the path he or she will take. Along the way, various waypoints will indicate the progress that is being made. In an educational journey, the final destination is indicated by the course or terminal objective. Waypoints along the way correspond to the student performance objective, and the map that keeps the learner on track and heading toward the final destination is the lesson plan. Thus, it can be seen that the lesson plan plays a key role in the educational process.

OVERVIEW OF LESSON PLANS

The lesson plan is a valuable teaching tool on many levels. In addition to keeping the instructional process on track, it serves a variety of other important functions. For the instructor, it provides the basic information needed to teach as well as to prepare the lesson. A properly formatted lesson plan includes not only the materials needed to meet the lesson objectives, but also the introductory material needed to prepare the lesson. It provides information and guidance on the development and use of instructional aids. And, because it is tied to the lesson objectives, it serves as a basis for, and even provides, student evaluation.

Lesson plans assist the instructional process and directly help the instructor. Lesson plans explain the depth and breadth of the lesson and tie together the student objectives. And, perhaps as important as the assistance they lend to the instructor, lesson plans ensure continuity and consistency in instruction. So, even if multiple instructors are involved in an educational program, the lesson plan serves as the "common map" that guides the course instruction.

For the new instructor or even the seasoned instructor who is moving into a new content area, the lesson plan takes on increased importance. In such cases, the instructor will most likely not be the one developing the lesson plan. Standardized courses such as Emergency Medical Technician-Basic (EMT-B) and Advanced Cardiac Life Support (ACLS) typically use lesson plans provided either by the sponsoring agency or by the institution for which the instructor is teaching. The availability of prepared lesson plans frees the new instructor to concentrate on the instructional process and not on course and lesson development. Although advanced instructor training programs teach ways to develop lesson plans, the knowledge and process awareness needed to develop plans may be beyond the scope of the typical Emergency Medical Services (EMS) instructor. However, even the rookie instructor should be familiar with the required components of a lesson plan and should be able to evaluate a plan for completeness and appropriateness.

PURPOSE OF A LESSON PLAN

The lesson plan is truly a multipurpose tool. It serves a number of functions in the educational process, including the following:

- Ties all lesson objectives into a coherent plan of instruction
- Provides a structure or framework from which the lesson is presented
- Ensures that important material is covered and learning objectives are met
- Helps the instructor prepare to teach the lesson
- Matches declarative material with each objective
- Provides a basis for the development of student evaluative activities

- Serves as a means by which instructor performance can be evaluated
- Helps to keep the instruction on track and on schedule
- Assists substitute or secondary instructors and instructional assistants

SOURCES OF LESSON PLANS

Lesson plans are available from a variety of sources, ranging from the course instructor to outside agencies to textbook publishers. Some common sources of lesson plans include the following:

- State EMS agencies—A state EMS agency may develop lesson plans for courses specific to a particular state or region, or it may modify curricula such as the National Standard Curriculum (NSC) to meet the needs of a particular state. This is especially true if the curriculum content conflicts with local scope of practice or protocols
- Primary or senior instructors—Instructors who have been teaching a course for some time most likely will have modified existing lesson plans or developed their own. These instructors may be adept at writing lesson plans, thus serving as a lesson development mentor for new instructors. However, instructor-modified lesson plans can be very personal and may be tailored to a particular instructor's style and preferences in teaching. Therefore, they should be carefully reviewed before they are used
- Lesson plans for nationally recognized courses are frequently obtained from publishers. Publishers of textbooks often provide not only lesson plans, but also complete instructional support packages to supplement their texts. One must remember that these lesson plans and accompanying materials are designed for a wide audience and may be biased toward a particular product or approach. They often need modification and must frequently be tailored if they are to address local system issues. Instructors should avoid relying totally on these instructional packages; they must be sure to invest sufficient time in their own lesson preparation and delivery
- Several national organizations and groups produce specialty courses that cover a specific topic in detail. Examples of these "alphabet soup" or "boutique" courses include ACLS, Pediatric Advanced Life Support (PALS), and Basic Trauma Life Support (BTLS). Lesson plans provided for these courses vary in complexity. However, most are very basic and are designed to follow closely an accompanying slide or PowerPoint presentation. Lessons are planned around a specific time frame and evaluation process. Because of the administrative control associated with many of these courses, instructor variation through tailoring of lesson plans is limited. Instructors must follow the lesson plans and schedule closely because they are often one of a cadre of instructors who have been assembled to teach such courses
- One of the missions of the National Association of EMS Educators (NAEMSE) is to prepare and disseminate model curricula on various topics. Produced as packages for the instructor, these curricula contain lesson plans designed to be modified and customized by the EMS instructor
- Perhaps one of the most maligned sources of lesson plans is the NSC developed for each national level of EMS provider. Early versions of the NSC were produced by the US Department of Transportation as complete instructional packages. Not only was a lesson plan provided, but the 1983 version also included a student manual. Over the years, the complexity and philosophy of the NSC have changed. The 1996-1998 editions greatly reduced the amount of declarative material provided, thus precluding use of the curriculum as a stand-alone lesson plan. However, these versions of the NSC do provide a comprehensive and organized skeleton for the development of lesson plans. As EMS education moves toward embracing the *EMS Education Agenda for the Future,* the NSC as it is known will change and will be replaced by a model scope of practice and educational standards
- Institutions and agencies such as fire departments and ambulance services may produce their own lesson plans to ensure consistency and uniformity in instruction. This is usually the case with recruit and procedural training courses, especially when instruction is scheduled to occur at various geographically separated locations. A training officer or central office staff may prepare lesson plans for distribution to instructors at various locations.

TEACHING TIP: An instructor who is selecting lesson plans must make sure that the source is appropriate for the students. An instructor wouldn't want to use a lesson plan on the cardiovascular system at the paramedic level to teach a citizen CPR course. Note that some commercial lesson plans have costs or restrictions associated with them. Proper permission to use a lesson plan must be obtained.

PARTS OF THE LESSON PLAN

As has been stated, lesson plans can come from numerous sources and may be written in a variety of formats. The instructor may have little control over how a lesson plan is constructed. However, for the sake of this textbook, a standard lesson plan format will be used.

The standard lesson plan consists of the following:

- Audience description
- Lesson goal(s)
- Cognitive objectives
- Psychomotor objectives
- Affective objectives
- Recommended list of equipment and supplies
- Recommended schedule
- Suggested motivational activity
- Content outline and instructor notes
- Summary
- Evaluation
- Next assignment/lesson
- References

The format of lesson plans varies greatly according to the source. However, as a rule, most lesson plans include these listed parts in some form. If the lesson plan an instructor has selected does not comprise all of these parts, he or she should add missing sections. If he or she is inexperienced with curriculum development, the instructor should seek help in preparing more complicated parts of the lesson plan.

Front End

The first few parts of the lesson plan comprise what can be called the "front end," which contains administrative details and information. This section should contain a title for the lesson or some other scheme by which the lesson can be identified and sequenced. Specific parts of the front end are as follows.

Audience description

The audience description is just what the name implies. It is a statement describing who the intended audience is for the lesson. In a certification course, this description may be the same for all lesson plans. An example would be "Entry level EMT-B students." For a more advanced course, the description might be "Senior paramedic with command responsibility."

Lesson goal

Course designers develop an instructional goal for the entire course, as well as a goal or goals for each particular lesson. This is presented as a broad statement of what will be accomplished during the lesson. For example, "At the conclusion of this lesson, the student will be able to identify and describe the functions of the endocrine system." The lesson objective is supported by the listed affective, cognitive, and psychomotor objectives that follow. The action verb used in the lesson goal determines, to a large extent, the instructional approach. A goal that uses verbs such as "identify," "describe," and "discuss" will most likely be pursued through a lecture or presentation format. A goal that identifies "demonstrate" as the desired outcome behavior will be addressed as a practical session. The same applies to design of the evaluation method. Lesson goals that are predominantly cognitive will be assessed through paper tests, such as multiple choice and short answer. Psychomotor goals will be evaluated by methods such as observation or a skills check sheet.

Lesson objectives

The lesson objectives portion of the lesson plan is a listing of student performance objectives that support the lesson goal. Objectives are categorized according to the three domains of learning: affective, cognitive, and psychomotor. Depending on the lesson plan format or the institutional preference, objectives may be assigned a numeric sequencing. This allows the objective to be referenced on tests and other course materials without the need for the instructor to write out the entire objective. Similar to the lesson goal, lesson objectives should be reviewed with students, so they know in greater detail what will be covered in the lesson. This is especially important for concrete and field-dependent learners.

TEACHING TIP: Students should be given a complete list of objectives for each lesson of a course. That way, they know what material will be covered. Objectives also make a good study guide.

Recommended list of equipment and supplies

Classroom success for the instructor is most often ensured by careful preparation. This preparation process includes reviewing the material, refreshing knowledge and skills, preparing the learning environment, and preparing instructional materials. The lesson plan contains a list of equipment and supplies needed for the lesson to be taught effectively. This list may include such items as instructional models, audiovisual materials and equipment, handouts, student practice materials, and practical training equipment. This list is also useful at the completion of the lesson as a checklist to ensure that materials are accounted for and returned to their proper storage locations.

TEACHING TIP: Instructors should not forget to prepare the basic "tools of instruction," such as chalk, whiteboard markers, erasers, a laser pointer, and a podium.

If any part of a lesson is going to fail, it most likely will be the part that is related to or dependent on equipment or technology. For this reason, the instructor should begin by familiarizing himself or herself with all material and aids to be used. Instructors should not assume that they know how something works. Instruction manuals are an excellent source of information and usually contain additional facts worth presenting to learners. Because of this, instructors should arrive well in advance of the class start time and should check and review all equipment. The instructor should not assume that because a particular audiovisual device or piece of equipment was in the classroom during the last session, it still is available. Also, instructors should know whom to contact if assistance is needed with equipment. The complexity and costs of current educational technology preclude replacement or repair by the average instructor.

The instructor must have a backup plan in the event of equipment failure or other such problems that can occur with technology-dependent lessons. A common example of this is failure of an in-service ambulance to show up. An instructor who is planning to conduct a lesson on ambulance operations should definitely have a backup plan if he or she is relying on an in-service unit. The backup plan may involve alternative aids to accomplish the lesson, material to be presented until the unit can arrive, or an entirely different lesson to replace the intended one. The good instructor always has one or two lessons "in the can" in the event of an unforeseen problem.

TEACHING TIP: If a planned lesson cannot be presented and no backup lesson is available, the instructor can always do skills practice. Even at the beginning of a course, the instructor can review prerequisite skills. He or she should never waste a lesson by canceling class. Practice and review are always needed.

An area of concern in EMS education is the quality and amount of equipment available for training. Too often, outdated or broken equipment is relegated to training, or the amount of equipment is insufficient for active student participation. This sends a negative message about the service and its appreciation of training for the learner. It also violates basic educational principles in that learners are not receiving the most realistic experience during the learning process. Behavioral modeling may have as great an impact on learner development as what students are taught by the instructor. The lack of equipment identical to that used in the field also requires that the provider must be trained again before he or she can begin functioning in the field. If he or she is participating in a field internship, the provider may become confused and frustrated because of differences in equipment and procedures between the classroom and the field.

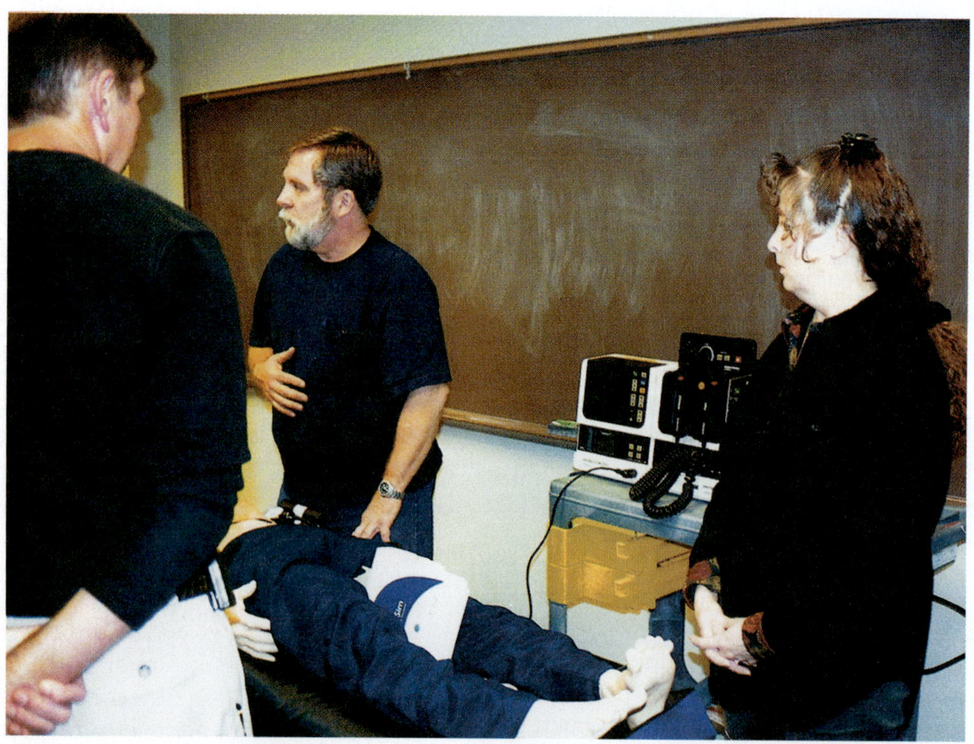

FIGURE 9-1 An equipment list is an important part of the lesson plan that should not be overlooked. Equipment should be kept updated and in working order.

TEACHING TIP: A lesson plan may be designed to "teach" a particular model or type of equipment. This is especially true of lesson plans provided by equipment manufacturers. The instructor must make sure that what he or she is teaching matches the equipment the students will be using for practice.

If the instructor is teaching students who provide a mixture of services, he or she can ask students to provide an inventory of equipment carried on their units. In this way, the instructor can determine whether students will be using different or unusual equipment in the field. If the instructor does not have a specific piece of equipment in his or her training cache but students may benefit from instruction on it, he or she can make arrangements to borrow equipment from the service for a single class session.

Recommended schedule

This is the estimated time needed for the instructor to teach the lesson. For a practical session, it may include a schedule for practice activities. If the number of learners in a class is variable, this section may list time frames in terms of a set number of participants. For example, each group of five students will require 20 minutes to cycle through the skills stations. The recommended schedule may include information on planned breaks.

TEACHING TIP: As a rule of thumb, an instructor should plan 3 hours of preparation time for each hour of instruction.

Suggested motivational activity

Learner motivation can vary greatly over the duration of a course. In the beginning, learners are often highly motivated in anticipation of the course. This is especially true for courses leading to a certification level. However, as the course progresses, motivation may wane. Even the most dynamic instructor would find it hard to keep paramedic students motivated after 3 weeks of cardiology. Thus, instructors must continually motivate learners at the beginning of each class session. Lesson motivation also serves to increase learner interest in the material of each individual lesson. Most importantly, it establishes the environment, or what is also called the "set," in which learning occurs.

The suggested motivational activity should be designed to appeal to as many learner motivational needs as possible. It should serve to move the learner mentally from the external environment to the lesson. It should both peak and focus the learner's attention. Some motivational activities include the following:

- Show a picture and pause for reflection. The instructor may show a picture or a video clip related to the lesson topic and follow up by asking the learners how this picture affected them
- Play a dispatch tape of an actual 911 call. The instructor may ask the learners whether they feel ready to respond to such a call
- Tell a "war story" about a personal experience
- Invite a survivor or former patient to address the class. Depending on the topic and the class length, this may not be practical for short lessons
- Engage the students in an "icebreaker" activity that relates to the class topic
- Invite a provider to tell about a significant experience that would be motivational to the learners

Regardless of the technique used, instructors must be cautious of two things: patient confidentiality as required by the Health Insurance Portability and Accountability Act (HIPAA) guidelines, and overstimulation of learners to the point that a negative emotional response may be created. An example of the latter would be use of an event that may have emotional and personal ties to the learners, such as a call in which members of their rescue squad were killed or injured.

Body of the Lesson Plan

Content outline

The sections covered thus far form the front end of the lesson plan. Once the instructor and learners are prepared and motivated, it is time for the instructor to present the actual material that will allow learners to meet the lesson goal and objectives. To do this, the instructor must have a complete understanding of the lesson objectives and of the depth and breadth of material to be presented. Is material being presented for awareness or for mastery? This can be determined by the action verbs used in the course goal and objectives. Each domain of learning has a hierarchy that determines the required level of learning or mastery. The cognitive domain, for example, comprises six levels of mastery: knowledge, comprehension, application, analysis, synthesis, and evaluation. These six levels can be grouped into the following three levels of understanding:

1. *Basic.* The learner acquires new information or develops a new skill with instructor feedback. Includes objectives that demonstrate knowledge and comprehension (Level One)
2. *Intermediate.* Learners connect the knowledge learned in the basic level with knowledge gained through experience. Includes objectives that demonstrate application (Level Two)

3. *Advanced.* Learners move toward learning why events occur as opposed to how to perform a skill. The instructor serves as a facilitator in a coaching or mentoring role. Includes objectives that require analysis, synthesis, and evaluation (Level Three)

Often, instructors or institutions assign a level code, similar to these for the cognitive domain, to each objective. This helps the instructor know which level of mastery is required for each objective. This approach has been used with some versions of the EMT National Standard Curriculum.

TEACHING TIP: The instructor should teach Level One material before Level Two information is presented, and Level Two before Level Three. Students should be evaluated for mastery before they are permitted to move on to the next level.

Once the level of instruction is known for each lesson objective, an actual teaching outline is developed. Objectives are arranged and grouped in the order in which they will be taught. This teaching cycle is used to integrate affective, cognitive, and psychomotor objectives. The actual ordering of objectives can be based on a number of different schemes that will determine the order in which declarative material is presented. This will be the actual order of instruction during the class. It is important that the declarative material be presented in a coherent fashion that supports learner understanding and retention. Some examples of schemes include the following:

- Whole-part-whole
- Procedurally from beginning of a procedure to end
- Chronologically
- As specified in protocol
- Body or organ system based
- Simple to complex
- Small to large
- Algorithm based
- ABCs
- Head to toe
- Dispatch to return to service
- Known to unknown
- Following textbook content

However, in another way, a simple plan is to "tell 'em what you are going to teach 'em, teach 'em, and then tell 'em what you taught 'em." More specifically, explain the importance of the lesson, deliver the content, allow students to apply or practice the material, gather feedback, provide remediation, and evaluate performance. An easy way to do this is to open with a quick overview of lesson material and close with the same overview used as a summary.

The lesson plan developer has chosen a level of specificity for the content portion of the lesson plan. The specificity of the outline, that is, the number of levels used in the outline, varies according to the complexity of the material being presented and the instructor's teaching ability and familiarity with content. A primary instructor may simply need "B. Start IV" and be able to teach the entire process. A new instructor, however, will want the lesson broken down to list the various knowledge points and skills necessary to start an IV. The extent of the outline is really a matter of personal preference. However, a lesson plan that is developed for use by various instructors must be adaptable to various levels of instructor expertise; toward that goal, sufficient declarative material must be included. When one is teaching skills, it is especially important to provide sufficient detail to the learner. An experienced practitioner may be so comfortable doing a procedure that he or she may not realize the many small steps and nuances important to its successful completion; thus, he or she may not emphasize or share these with new learners. It is also good practice to include in the lesson outline formulas and drug names to ensure that they are properly presented to the new learner.

As shown in Figure 9-2, a good format for a lesson plan is the use of two facing pages with the right page divided into two sections. The left page contains the declarative material in outline form. The first column of the right page includes notes for the instructor. This format allows lesson plans to be easily personalized by different instructors. In the notes space, the instructor can include notes and comments that he or she wants to cover in class, additional information that may be needed to answer student questions, drawings to be written on the board, and questions and answers. If teaching formulas or problems, the instructor should include the solving methods and correct answers in this area. This format is especially helpful for new instructors who might become flustered or confused during a lecture. The far right column is used to list audiovisual aids, handouts, or activities that support the declarative material. Again, it is easy for even the experienced instructor to get off track and forget to use a teaching aid. This format also provides a complete and integrated lesson plan that can be used easily by substitute instructors.

TEACHING TIP: An instructor can place the pages of his or her lesson plan in clear sheet protectors. This not only protects the pages, but it allows the instructor to write class-specific notes and comments on the page protectors with a transparency-marking pen. Notes can be wiped clear for use with another class. Additionally, other material such as instructions or protocols can be tucked between the sheets for easy access if needed during class.

Lesson Plan Title	Instructor Notes	References and Aids
Audience: Lesson Goal: *After completing this lesson, the student will be able to...* Objectives: *Affective* *Cognitive* *Psychomotor* Equipment & Supplies: Schedule: Motivational Activity:		
Lesson Content Overview Outline Summary		
Evaluation Assignment Next Session		

FIGURE 9-2 Sample lesson plan format.

Back End

The remaining parts of the lesson plan constitute the back end, which contains sections that pull the lesson together, check student understanding, and prepare learners for the next lesson.

Summary

Regardless of the format used or the complexity of the material presented, the instructor must provide closure to the lesson. Just as the motivational activity sets the stage for the lesson, the summary brings it together for closure. A simple summary involves using the overview that began the presentation of the declarative material. It is even possible for the motivational activity to be used again, if it is a simple one such as a picture or video clip; this allows students to appreciate the importance of the lesson material and relate it to reality.

Evaluation of learning

To ensure that learning has taken place during a lesson, the instructor must evaluate learner mastery of the material. Various approaches may be used to conduct such an evaluation, and discussion of each is beyond the scope of this chapter. More information on this can be found in Part V, Evaluation. However, the instructor should specify in the lesson plan an evaluation method that will be used to determine learner mastery of the material presented. This may be as simple as a few overhead questions asked at the conclusion of the lesson to gauge learner understanding or student self-assessment undertaken to determine whether a particular objective has been mastered. Or, it may take the form of an announcement that a 20-question, multiple-choice quiz on the material will be given at the beginning of the next session.

The evaluation section concludes the formal parts of a lesson plan. However, a few additions to the end of the lesson plan that may be helpful to the instructor

---

TEACHING TIP: An instructor should number the pages of a lesson plan. If the instructor removes a page to take with him or her while writing on the board or doing a demo, he or she might forget where it goes. Then there is the risk of dropping the whole lesson plan during a class presentation and not knowing how to quickly get it in order.

CASE IN POINT

THE LAST-MINUTE LESSON PLAN

An instructor has just finished teaching a session of EMT-B to new hires at a commercial ambulance company. As she is walking back to her office, the director of training comes rushing up to her. She informs her that another instructor who teaches the company's paramedic course is tied up on a long critical care transport and will be at least an hour late for his class that starts in an hour. She asks the instructor to fill in for the absent instructor until he gets back. The instructor hesitates, then says okay. The instructor asks the director if she has a copy of the class lesson plan. The director says that she doesn't, but she is sure the other instructor has all his lesson plans in his office. The two walk to the instructor's office, and the director lets both of them in. To put it mildly, the other instructor is not the most organized person! Papers, books, teaching materials—everything is strewn about the office. The two can't even find a place to begin looking for lesson plans. After a quick search, the instructor realizes it is hopeless and that time is getting short before class begins. She knows the lesson topic—obstructive pulmonary disease. At least that is the topic listed on the schedule the director had on file. What should she do to prepare for the lesson?

At this point, the fill-in instructor has two major problems. First, she doesn't know the instructor's plan for that night's class. Are the students expecting a quiz or another activity? She also doesn't know the level of the students or which topic is scheduled to be covered. Are the students ahead of schedule? Or, are they behind schedule and not ready for this lecture? Her second concern is that her paramedic course lesson plans are at her home because she has been teaching only EMT-B classes.

What should the instructor do? To help her plan a class that is on schedule, the instructor can

- Try to reach the absent instructor
- Check to see if the training director's office or human resources department keeps copies of attendance rosters. These rosters may list the topics covered in each class session. Or, the training director may be able to provide a list of students and their contact information. Someone can call students to find out what was planned
- Go to the classroom or another nearby area early to try to intercept a student who is arriving early
- Begin class by explaining the situation and finding out what was planned. Work with the students to conduct a meaningful lesson, even if it is a review session of knowledge and skills taught previously
- Give the students a brief assignment that they can complete on their own, and leave the classroom for 15 minutes to prepare a quick teaching outline

Now that the instructor knows the content scheduled for the class, how can she teach without a lesson plan? She can do the following:

- Ask students if they have an outline for each course lesson. If not, do they have a list of objectives? Any handout materials?
- Use the textbook to create a "down and dirty" lesson plan. Use the chapter heading as the main point, subheadings as secondary points, and so forth. For each heading of the "outline," she can try to think of important facts or ideas to convey. She can jot down these ideas as they come to mind, then skim the text for key points. This approach usually works best if the instructor is familiar with the material and has taught it before. The "lesson plan" won't be extensive or eloquent, but it will provide a rough organizational framework
- Use the same approach for class objectives. This is more difficult without textual material for elaboration. The same holds true if the instructor has access to a PowerPoint presentation on the lesson topic
- Use the National Highway Traffic Safety Administration (NHTSA) Web site (www.nhtsa.dot.gov) to download appropriate parts of the online copy of the *EMT-Paramedic National Standard Curriculum.* Some sections include declarative material sufficient for use as a basic lesson plan. This curriculum will provide the instructor with an organized presentation that covers all the key points
- Check the *Trading Post* on the NAEMSE Web site to see if a lesson plan or visuals aids for the lesson topic are available (www.naemse.org)
- Depending on the topic, the instructor can use his or her EMT-B lesson plan as a basis for instruction

The take-home message from this case study is that many options are available by which instructors can quickly produce a basic lesson plan for an instructional crisis. The instructor must be creative and should be sure to be honest with students about "winging it" and needing their cooperation. Who knows? This lesson may turn out to be better than one that was developed with proper preparation time.

and to the learners include assignments, the topic for the next session, related readings, and additional references. If the instructor has planned any "homework" for the learners, this can be assigned or distributed at this time. The next lesson topic serves as a reminder to the learners to prepare for the next session and reinforces any required readings or preparative assignments. The end of the lesson is also an opportunity for the instructor to announce any schedule changes and to remind students to bring special equipment, such as turnout gear, to the next session. Finally, the instructor can come to class prepared with a list of references, Web sites, or other sources that may be of interest to learners or that may provide greater detail or explanation of the material already presented. If learners have questions or concerns, they can be referred to this reference list.

Lesson plan evaluation

Once the institution or instructor has developed a lesson plan, the development process does not stop there. In addition to initial evaluation of its effectiveness, the lesson plan must be reviewed again periodically for timeliness, correctness, and applicability to the overall curriculum and learner needs.

If an instructor is teaching a new course with newly developed lesson plans, he or she may be involved more closely in the evaluation process. The initial evaluation process involves a formative evaluation that is ongoing and begins while the lesson plan is being constructed. The instructor should constantly compare the overall goals of instruction, lesson objectives, and content to determine whether performance is in agreement. Tests, audiovisual materials, student materials, and reference materials should be evaluated as well for relevance to the instructional goal.

TEACHING TIP: It is handy for an instructor to have a pad of "sticky notes" while teaching. If an instructor finds a problem with a lesson plan or class, he or she can jot down a quick note and stick it on the lesson plan. This is also helpful if he or she needs to find additional material to answer a student's question, or for noting areas that need remediation.

Even established and published lesson plans should be periodically evaluated throughout their life span. Often, lesson plans are produced according to a certain standard or medical protocol that may change over time. This can be seen in lesson plans that accompany ACLS, which change according to changes in American Heart Association (AHA) Guidelines. A summative evaluation of lesson plans is used to determine the effectiveness of the teaching strategy and to provide information on ways that future performance of the same strategy and related material can be improved. Again, tests, audiovisual materials, student materials, and reference materials should be evaluated as well.

LESSON PLAN TROUBLESHOOTING

Regardless of who creates a lesson plan, or where it comes from, the potential for problems always exists. Problems usually fall into two broad categories: structural and factual.

Structural problems have to do with the delivery of the lesson material. When structural problems occur, the material to be presented in the lesson plan is correct and up-to-date, but something is wrong with the delivery of the material. Examples include using in a 3-hour session a lesson plan designed for a 2-hour block of instruction, or working alone to teach a skills lesson designed for a four-instructor team. In most cases, the instructor can remedy the problem by keeping the lesson material but rewriting the lesson plan into a more usable format. However, the instructor must be aware of how this lesson fits into the overall scope of the course so as not to disrupt future lessons. Shrinking a 4-hour lesson into a 2-hour session may be possible, but what are the consequences? If enrolled in a certification course, students may be required to have a minimum number of instructional hours in a topic, and this change could affect their eligibility for certification.

Structural problems can often be easily corrected if they are detected in advance of the lesson. However, factual and timeliness issues are more complex. First, the problem has to be discovered. Then, the instructor has to research to find the correct information and make changes as needed. This may seem straightforward, but a problem may arise with making changes. If a standardized curriculum is being used, the instructor may not be authorized to make changes. If the program is being taught with other instructors, or if the course is being taught in multiple sections, the lesson plan will have to be changed for *all* instructors. In addition, many programs require that the medical director approve all lesson plans—a requirement that adds another level to the process. To make matters more complex, some medical practices and procedures are not embraced by all medical professionals or groups. A good example of this is the emerging research on cardiopulmonary resuscitation (CPR) that is challenging the traditional CPR method. Such research must be verified and studied in greater detail. However, the instructor may find himself or herself standing in front of a class teaching the basics of "traditional" CPR to a class that has just read in the local newspaper about a study advocating that mouth-to-mouth does not need to be performed.

CASE IN POINT

LESSON PLAN DISCONNECT

An instructor has been assigned to teach a paramedic refresher course at the local municipal fire department training academy. The class is made up of department career paramedics. The instructor is teaching the course because he must obtain instructor certification as a requirement for promotion to lieutenant. For maintenance of standardization throughout the department, he is required to teach from a lesson plan that has been developed and approved by the EMS training officer.

While preparing to teach the unit on cardiac emergencies, he finds that the lesson plan contradicts current ACLS guidelines. He also notes that although a protocol is in place for handling cardiac patients, he and most other paramedics in the department use a slightly "modified approach" rather than strictly adhering to the protocol. Because he knows his audience so well, he knows that they will give him a hard time if he tries to teach the material as outlined in the lesson plan. However, he doesn't want to "make waves" with the training officer because he is coming up for promotional review. What should he do?

This is a situation that involves dynamics beyond the scope of educational instruction. It is also a management issue. For the purposes of this chapter, the alternatives must be examined from an educational delivery perspective. In other words, how should the instructor handle this disconnect in the classroom? Possible approaches include the following:

- Teach the lesson directly as outlined in the lesson plan, and ignore any questions or criticism from the class. Such an approach would ruin credibility and could lead to loss of class control. This outcome would not make the instructor look like officer material
- Present the material in the lesson plan and state that this is department policy. Then, ask the class if they have any other approaches to handling such situations. This should lead to discussion about how things are actually done in the field
- Take a reverse approach to presenting the material. Give the class a scenario in which the responders treat the patient as is really done in the field, then ask them to contrast this with the department protocol

An instructor can use these and similar strategies to handle disconnects between the lesson plan and textbooks, protocols, guest lecturers, or other instructors. Regardless of an instructor's approach, he or she should not use the instructor's podium as a "bully pulpit" to complain or attack others. If an instructor must address a controversy, he or she should present both sides of the argument impartially so that students can analyze the situation and come to their own conclusions.

SUMMARY

The lesson plan is a valuable and essential tool of effective and successful EMS education. It provides the map that guides the learner through the educational journey. It also serves to tie together the instructional goal, the course objectives, and the teaching strategy. Moreover, it is a helpful tool that allows the instructor to present the course material in an organized and confident manner, thus ensuring learner success.

SUGGESTED READING

Gagné RM. *Essentials of Learning for Instruction.* Hinsdale, Ill: The Dryden Press; 1974.

Gagné RM, Briggs LJ. *Principles of Instructional Design.* 2nd ed. New York: Holt, Rinehart and Winston; 1979.

Mager RF. *Preparing Instructional Objectives.* 2nd ed. Belmont, Calif: Fearon Publishers; 1975.

Mager RF, Beach KM Jr. *Developing Vocational Instruction.* Belmont, Calif: Fearon-Pitman Publishers; 1967.

Tyler RW. *Basic Principles of Curriculum and Instruction.* Chicago, Ill: University of Chicago Press; 1949.

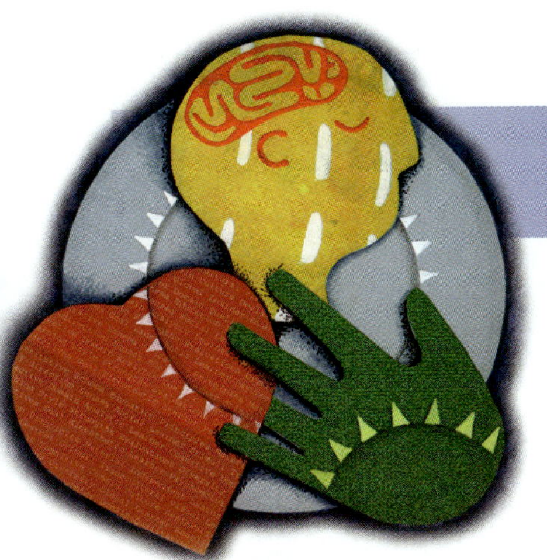

CHAPTER 10

Legal Issues for the Educator

"No man is above the law and no man is below it; nor do we ask any man's permission when we require him to obey it."

—*Theodore Roosevelt*

OVERVIEW OF THE AMERICAN LEGAL SYSTEM

America is a litigious society. Regardless of circumstances, all citizens have the right to file lawsuits. Despite the fact that no one has the right to file a *frivolous* lawsuit and attorneys are legally and ethically responsible for screening suits to make sure they have merit, Emergency Medical Services (EMS) instructors may not be able to prevent all lawsuits. The best way to avoid being placed in the position of potential litigation is to have a basic understanding of legal concepts and terminology. Such an understanding begins with an overview of America's legal system. In-depth presentations of legal issues facing educational institutions are found in *Legal Issues in Career and Technical Education,*[1] *The Academic Administrator and the Law: What Every Dean and Department Chair Needs to Know,*[2] and *Teachers and the Law.*[3]

This chapter is intended to present EMS faculty and administrators with accurate information on legal issues in education. Local, state, and federal laws and regulations, as well as appropriate jurisdictional courts, are to be considered the final authority. This chapter is provided as a supplement to legal advice. If such advice or expertise is required, EMS educators should seek the service of competent legal professionals.

Hierarchy of Laws

In the American legal system, laws are established by the three branches of government at federal, state, and local levels. These three branches of government are the legislative, executive, and judicial branches. Laws at the federal level are generated by the legislative branch (Congress). The states also have legislative branches, which are active sources of laws. Both state and federal level legislative branches enact statutes such as the Americans With Disabilities Act or state EMS statutes. The executive branches at both state and federal levels promulgate regulations that affect EMS and education. The Occupational Safety and Health Administration (OSHA) is an example of a federal agency with regulations that affect EMS. State EMS agencies generate regulations particular to each state. At all levels, the judicial branch interprets statutes and regulations and makes case law binding.

These branches comprise four sources of law:

1. Constitutions (federal and state governments)
2. Statutes (federal and state governments), Ordinances (city government), or Resolutions (county governments)
3. Regulations (agencies created by states)
4. Common law (norms of society decided by judges).

Constitutional law is based on the US Constitution. Although subject to the US Constitution, each state also has a constitution. The constitution is the highest legal standard in America, the "supreme law of the land." State and local governments may establish constitutions at their own levels that represent the highest legal standard, other than the US constitution. This means that no rule, regulation, or constitution may supersede or contradict the US Constitution.

Statutes, also known as laws, may likewise be established at local, state, or federal levels. Rules and regulations, again developed at any level, further expand and define specific statutes or constitutions. Although rules, regulations, and statutes at the local and state levels may be more restrictive than constitutions, they must not be in conflict. The judicial arm of the government, from local courts through the US Supreme Court, is responsible for assuring that all laws are compliant with the US Constitution.

Areas of Law

The American legal system is composed of two types of law: criminal and civil. Criminal law refers to "public wrongs," or crimes that violate legislative codes in statutes at the state or federal level. Criminal cases are prosecuted by an attorney for the government on behalf of the citizens, such as one in a district attorney's office. Violation of these laws can result in fines, imprisonment, or both.

Civil law involves private matters (e.g., contracts, domestic relations) between persons or legal entities such as corporations. In civil cases, a plaintiff, or individual, seeks recovery of money or other forms of relief for a breach of contract or a similar personal wrong. This claim is made against another private person or entity, known as the defendant. A tort is a "private or civil wrong or injury."[4] A tort is an act by a private person, in a careless or reckless manner, against another person or his property that causes injury or damage. A claim of medical negligence or malpractice is a tort action, as are defamation, assault, and battery.

Tort Law

The instructor must be aware of actions that can result in a tort claim and must be proactive to prevent such claims.

Assault and battery

Although these two terms are frequently used in combination, they actually are separate charges. Assault is the condition in which one person places another person in reasonable fear of harm. Verbal assault occurs when a person states the intent to harm another person. Nonverbal assault occurs when a person creates an atmosphere of intimidation, such as when brandishing a weapon. Battery is the physical, unlawful touching of another person.

CASE IN POINT

Two students in the classroom begin having an argument about sports. The argument begins as simple joking but escalates to a heated interaction. One student says, "You had better look over your shoulder when you leave class today. I'll be there to knock some sense into your thick skull." (This is an example of assault. An atmosphere of fear of physical harm has been established.)

After class, the first student physically attacks the second student. (This is a case of battery because actual physical, unlawful touching is involved.)

Defamation

Defamation is "the area of tort law which seeks to protect the interest one has in his or her reputation."[5] Libel is the written or printed form of defamation. Slander is the spoken or oral form of defamation.

Misrepresentation

In education, misrepresentation most commonly occurs when a program indicates that it is something other than what it really is. Further information on misrepresentation can be found on page 113.

Negligence

Negligence is "[t]he failure to exercise the standard of care that a reasonably prudent person would have exercised in a similar situation; any conduct that falls below the legal standard established to protect others against unreasonable risk or harm except for conduct that is intentionally, wantonly, or willfully disregardful of others' rights."[6] Negligence claims require four basic elements. These "are (1) a duty; (2) breach of the duty; (3) injury in fact which is (4) proximately caused by the breach of duty."[7]

A negligent claim against a technical institution was dismissed when the court determined that there was a lack of duty on behalf of the student. In *Judson v. Essex Agricultural and Technical Institute*, 635 N.E.2d 1172 (Mass. 1994), a student was participating in a paid activity related to her program when she fell from a barn loft. The accident occurred on the employer's farm (not the institution's facility). An agreement signed before the paid activity occurred indicated that the employer agreed to be responsible for workers' compensation insurance. In fact, the employer did not even carry such insurance. The student sued the institution, but the court dismissed the case because no duty on the part of the institution was found to exist. Although this case resulted favorably for the educational institution, courts generally do recognize a duty to protect students from unreasonable risk of harm in the classroom setting (Figure 10-1).

Delbridge v. Maricopa Community College, 893 P.2d 55 (Ct.App.Div.1 Ariz. 1994) illustrates the court's belief that educational institutions do have a duty to protect students from harm. In this case, the student (Delbridge) was injured during a training activity in a facility rented by the institution (MCC). As the result of a 30-foot fall, Delbridge was rendered a paraplegic. It was decided that MCC did have a duty to protect the student from harm.

Cases such as *Delbridge* reinforce the courts' distinction that a duty was owed to students for classroom activities. See *LaVoie v. New York*, 458 N.Y.S.2d

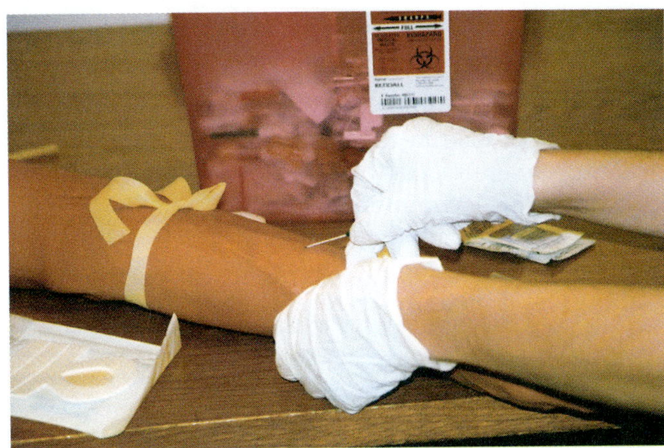

FIGURE 10-1 Teaching, modeling, and requiring appropriate body substance isolation are important methods of preventing harm to a student.

277 (1988) (university was responsible when a student was injured in a chemistry lab) and *Amon v. New York*, 414 N.Y.S.2d 68 (1979) (student was injured by a saw while working in the university shop). However, duty was not found when students were injured off-campus while performing activities not related to the curriculum. See, *e.g., University of Denver v. Whitlock*, 744 P.2d 54 (Colo. 1987); *Hartman v. Bethany College*, 778 F.Supp. 286 (N.D.W.Va. 1991); and *Beach v. University of Utah*, 726 P.2d 413 (Utah 1986).

TEACHING TIP: When students are placed in hazardous circumstances, as may readily happen in any EMS clinical situation, care must be taken by the faculty. Students are owed "a duty" or protection from dangers known to exist outside their routine assignments. However, if students are injured while involved in noncurricular activities, no "duty" is required on behalf of the educational institution.

The case of *Leal v. Hobbs*, 2000 WL 1056340 (Ga.App. Aug. 2, 2000) involves a paramedic student intern (Leal). The widow of a man brought a wrongful death case against multiple persons when her husband died of cardiac arrest in the ambulance. Leal was a paramedic student in Idaho who was completing his internship training in Georgia. He had not obtained a Georgia Emergency Medical Technician (EMT) license and was to provide medical treatment only under the supervision of a licensed paramedic preceptor. Leal was found to have acted appropriately and followed the paramedic's directions precisely. The courts found that because Leal had made no independent decisions, he was not guilty of negligence. The EMS faculty and preceptors acted wisely in making certain that Leal understood his limited scope of practice. Failure to assure that Leal was aware of this could have resulted in negligence on the part of the student, faculty, and clinical preceptors.

In loco parentis

The doctrine of *in loco parentis* means "in place of the parent." Court systems have traditionally differentiated between the duty of care afforded K-12 students and those attending schools in postsecondary systems. At the secondary level, schools are perceived to stand "in place of the parent." The student-institution relationship at the postsecondary level is generally considered contractual and the doctrine of *in loco parentis* does not stand.

Risk management

Risk management fits into the category of tort law and is "the process of preventing, or at least minimizing, harm or loss to a school, program, instructor, or student."[8] This loss may be measured in terms of physical damages or injuries. An EMS student who is infected by a contaminated needle would fit into this category. Risk management may also be measured in terms of material loss, as in the case of stolen property. When injury, either physical or material, has occurred, a person may attempt to place blame and seek compensation. Three basic defenses to negligence claims include assumption of risk, release of risk, and contributory negligence.

Assumption of risk

The assumption of risk doctrine indicates that a person who willingly participates in an activity known to involve risk cannot recover damages from another party. This is because the injured person is assumed to have accepted the inherent risk involved. Frequently, this doctrine is applied in cases of sports. (See, *e.g., Scott v. Pacific West Mountain Resort*, 834 P.2d 6 [Wa. 1992].)

Release of risk

Educational institutions frequently encourage students (or guardians) to sign release or waiver of risk forms. This is done to establish the assumption of risk doctrine. With a signed release form, it is apparent that the party involved was aware of, and assumed, the risk involved with the activity. In the cases of *Boyce v. West*, 862 P.2d (Wa.App. 1993) (student died in university scuba diving course) and *Wagonblast v. Odessa School Dist.*, 758 P.2d 968 (1988), courts upheld the release of risk and assumption of risk doctrines.

EMS educators should be cautious in the creation of release of risk waivers. These forms must be clearly written and in compliance with state and federal laws.

Minors are considered by the courts to be owed greater duty than are adults.

Contributory negligence

Contributory negligence refers to "conduct on the part of the plaintiff which falls below the standard to which he should conform for his own protection, and which is a legally contributing cause co-operating with the negligence of the defendant in bringing about the plaintiff's harm." (*Restatement [Second] of Torts,* Sec. 463.) This law varies according to state. In some areas, the amount of recovery is decided on the basis of the degree to which each party contributed to the injury. Other areas permit recovery to a plaintiff, providing the person's "negligence or comparative responsibility was not as great as the negligence, gross negligence, or comparative responsibility of the person against whom recovery is sought." (Idaho Code § 6-801.) EMS educators should be familiar with the laws within their own states.

Methods of risk management

EMS educators should adhere to two primary methods of risk management. The first method, risk control, is the process of reducing the rate and intensity of potential harm. This is a preventive process in which safety methods are employed to modify potential activities or equipment that could lead to institutional or personal liability. The second method of risk management is risk transfer. Waivers, releases, and insurance policies are all forms of risk transfer.

EMS faculty members should be actively involved in risk management in their classrooms, labs, and other educational facilities. Based on the very nature of the EMS profession itself, safety is of critical importance. Safety education should be an initial component of any EMS curriculum. Safety tests should be given to students, and a high level of success required to continue in the course. The exam results should remain on file with the institution.

Record keeping is critical for establishing a strong defense against risk management litigation. The case of *Miles v. School District No. 138 of Cheyenne County,* 281 N.W.2d 396 (Neb. 1979) involved a student who was operating machinery in a high school wood shop. She attempted to remove the wood in a manner that was contrary to the way she had been safely instructed to do so. In the process, she lost two fingers. The instructor was able to document that safety handbooks had been provided, safety tests were administered, and safety demonstrations had been completed. The court found that the student was negligent "in failing to use the ordinary care that a student of her age and maturity 'would have used under like circumstances'."[9]

Student supervision

No federal statutes require that students should be supervised at all times while performing hazardous activities. Because negligence claims may be filed if students are injured in the classroom, the EMS educator should use common sense and adhere to any appropriate institutional or state policies. Instructors should consider students' level of maturity, safety training, and activity before leaving a laboratory unsupervised.

Emergency protocol procedures

It is doubtful that anyone is more familiar with emergency protocol procedures than EMS instructors. In cases of emergency in the classroom, laboratory, or clinical setting, students and instructors alike must be familiar with emergency protocol procedures and must be able to implement them appropriately. Failure to respond appropriately increases potential success for litigation.

Site selection

EMS faculty must be cognizant of inherent dangers when selecting sites for clinical affiliations. Although no guarantee may be made to ensure students' safety as they complete clinical rotations, faculty must be aware of potential litigation based on inappropriate site selection. Specifically, *Cross v. Family Services Agency, Inc.,* 716 So.2d 337 (Fla.App. 4 Dist. 1998) involved a student placed on practicum in what may have been considered a dangerous area. The student was robbed and sexually assaulted in the parking area near the site. This lengthy case continued into *Nova Southeastern University, Inc. v. Gross,* 758 So.2d 86 (Fla. 2000). It is obvious that the legal battle took a great deal of time and money on everyone's part. Ultimately, the Florida Supreme Court decided that universities may indeed be liable for injuries sustained by students placed in externship sites located in areas previously known to be high-risk locations.

Affiliation agreements

Institutions should establish affiliation agreements with cooperating agencies involved in student activities. A standard affiliation agreement must be clearly written and approved by legal counsel. Cooperating agencies may also require that documents be reviewed by their legal counsel. Once a standard agreement has been approved, it may be used as a template for various clinical sites.

Affiliation agreements establish guidelines that are mutually acceptable to both educational and clinical facilities. A well-written affiliation agreement identifies obligations required by the educational institution, by the student, and by the clinical facility. This document should clearly define procedures to be followed. In the event that policies between the two institutions conflict, the affiliation agreement should indicate which of the regulations should be followed. Stating this information in the affiliation agreement before students are assigned to a facility is useful in addressing potential conflicts before they arise.

To minimize litigation potential, all affiliation agreements should contain basic components[10] that are deemed necessary for affiliation agreements.

Headings

Each affiliation agreement should clearly identify in the heading the parties involved. At the least, this would include the educational facility and the cooperating agency.

Dates

The agreement must identify the starting and terminating dates of the contract. Multiple-year contracts are generally adventitious in that they eliminate the need for annual renegotiations. Institutional administrators and legal counsel will determine if the affiliation agreement should be developed on a case-by-case basis or as a multiple-year contract.

Objectives

Affiliation agreements must provide the objectives required for maximal student learning. In this way, each party will be aware of their duties in the learning processes of students.

Student-employee relationship

Each affiliation agreement must define the student-employee relationship. Frequently, health education students may not receive remuneration for their clinical experiences. EMS faculty must be aware of institutional, state, and accreditation policies and must clearly identify these in the affiliation agreement.

Liability expectations

This section of the agreement is designed to define responsibilities and expectations of each party. Indemnification information must also be included. According to *Black's Law Dictionary* (1999, p 772), the word *indemnify* means "to reimburse (another) for a loss suffered because of a third party's act or default." This issue is further discussed under the section on liability insurance.

Mutual obligations

This part contains three sections:

1. The institution's obligations to the student and to the cooperating agency
2. The cooperating agency's obligations to students and to the institution
3. The obligations mutually agreed upon by the institution and by the agency

Key contacts

Names, titles, and telephone numbers for both the educational institution and the clinical site must be included in the affiliation agreement. Both parties to the contract must have immediate access to their counterparts.

Signatures

Signatures are required on the affiliation agreement. Because these agreements are considered legal documents, only authorized persons should affix their signatures. Each institutional administration must determine who this individual is and must notify faculty. Frequently, the chief executive officer is the only person who is allowed to legally sign documents on behalf of the institution.

Federal Nondiscrimination Statutes

Federal statutes are laws that are enforceable throughout the entire nation. Among the most common federal statutes that affect all components of American society are those dealing with discrimination. Although not restricted to these, three federal antidiscrimination statutes that are having a great impact on educational programs are the Americans With Disabilities Act (ADA) of 1990 (42 U.S.C. § 12101 *et seq.*), the Equal Employment Opportunity Act of 1972, and Title IX of the Education Amendments Act of 1972. These complex laws are briefly highlighted here. EMS educators and administrators should become familiar with all nondiscrimination laws and specific applications of these to their educational institutions and programs. Institutional legal counsel may be a valuable resource for providing in-depth instruction on nondiscrimination laws.

Americans With Disabilities Act

The Americans With Disabilities Act (ADA) was enacted in 1990. Before that time, the key piece of legislation addressing persons with disabilities was Section 504 of the Rehabilitation Act of 1973 (29 U.S.C. § 794). Both Section 504 and the ADA are currently in effect.

Most of the disability issues and terminology addressed in Title I of the ADA relate to both employment and postsecondary education. Title I of the ADA states, "[n]o covered entity shall discriminate against a qualified individual with a disability in regard to job application procedures, the hiring, advancement, or discharge of employees, employee compensation, job training and other terms, conditions, and privileges of employment." (42 U.S.C. § 12112.) Several terms with which the EMS educator should be familiar are clearly defined in the ADA (Table 10-1). Individuals with alcohol and illegal drug abuse problems are not considered qualified individuals under the ADA.

A *prima facie* case is one in which evidence is strong enough in favor of the plaintiff that a defendant may be required to respond to charges. To establish a *prima facie* ADA case, a plaintiff must be able to demonstrate "(1) that he or she is a disabled person within the meaning of the Act, (2) that he or she is otherwise qualified to perform the essential functions of the job with or without reasonable accommodations, and (3) that he or she suffered an adverse employment decision due to the disability."[11] In *Sullivan v. River Valley School District*, 197 F.3d 804 (6th Cir. 1999) and *Menes v. CUNY University of New York*, 92 F.Supp 2.d 294, 301 (S.D.N.Y. 2000), the plaintiffs (employees) were unable to establish *prima facie* cases of disability because they could not demonstrate the three basic requirements. As such, the educational institutions were not required to provide accommodations for those employees.

The National Registry of EMTs (NREMT) offers reasonable and appropriate accommodations for the written component of the registration examination for persons with documented disabilities. Persons who present documentation of learning disability in reading decoding and/or reading comprehension and/or written expression are permitted to take the standard format of the examination but receive an extended time in which to complete the exam, typically 3.75 hours rather than the standard 2.5 hours.[12]

Equal Employment Opportunity Act of 1972

Title VII of the Civil Rights Act of 1964 was amended by the Equal Employment Opportunity Act of 1972 (42 U.S.C. § 2000 [e] *et seq.*). According to this law, it is illegal for employers to discriminate in the hiring or terminating of individuals, or in any other act of

TABLE 10-1 Americans With Disabilities Act (42 U.S.C. §§ 12101-12213) Terminology

Term	Definition	Comments
Qualified individual with a disability	Any individual with a disability who, with or without reasonable accommodation, can perform the essential functions of the employment position that he or she holds or desires . . .	The term *handicapped* has been replaced by *disability*, which is the politically correct term to use. Alcohol and illegal drug abuse do not qualify.
Reasonable accommodation	Making existing facilities used by employees readily accessible to and usable by individuals with disabilities; and job restructuring, part-time/modified work schedules; acquisition or modification of equipment or devices; appropriate adjustment or modifications of examinations, training materials, or policies; provision of qualified readers or interpreters, and other similar accommodations . . .	An interactive process involving the EMS educational institution representatives and the disabled student determines student accommodations to be provided.
Undue hardship	Nature and cost of accommodations; overall financial resources of the facility, etc.	Financial burden may be respected in light of establishing undue hardship for the educational facility.
Major life activities	Functions such as caring for oneself, performing manual tasks, walking, seeing, hearing, speaking, breathing, learning, and working . . .	To qualify for disabilities, individuals must have substantially limited activity or activities.
Substantially limited	Unable to perform a major life activity that the average person in the general population can perform . . .	Factors to consider in determining whether an individual is substantially limited include nature and severity of impairment, duration of impairment, and permanent or long-term impact of impairment.

employment, based upon age, race, color, religion, sex, or national origin. Applicants and students in EMS programs are afforded these same rights. Related nondiscrimination laws include the Pregnancy Discrimination Act of 1978 (42 U.S.C. § 2000e[k]), the Immigration and Nationality Act of 1986 (8 U.S.C. § 1101 *et seq.*), and the Older Workers' Benefit Protection Act of 1990 (29 U.S.C. § 623 *et seq.*).

EMS educators must be familiar with medical practice acts and scope of practice laws within their own states. Tort cases may be filed against the instructor, the educational institution, and the student, in the event the EMS curriculum expands beyond the scope of practice laws held within any given state.

Title IX of the Education Amendments Act of 1972

Title IX of the Education Amendments Act of 1972 provides that "[n]o person in the United States shall, on the basis of sex, be excluded from participation in, be denied the benefits of, or be subjected to discrimination under any educational program or activity receiving Federal financial assistance" (20 U.S.C. § 1681[a]). Sexual discrimination cases are frequently filed under Title IX, Title VII (*supra*), or a combination of these two laws. The case of *Dunlop v. Colgan*, 687 F.Supp. 406 (N.D.Ill. 1988) involves a career and technical education instructor who had allegedly been dismissed on the basis of her gender. Educational programs that receive federal funds may not discriminate in admission, dismissal, or any other way based upon a student's gender. Even though not required by law, educational programs that are not federally funded would be wise to follow the same nondiscriminatory practices.

EMS EDUCATIONAL STANDARDS

Educational standards for EMS programs vary by state and by institution. EMS educators should be familiar with all accreditation, licensure, certification, and instructional regulations accordingly. State EMS offices are an important source of regulatory and administrative rules for EMS education. Refer to Chapter 23 for additional information.

TEACHING TIP: When relocating between states, EMS educators should contact the appropriate regulatory offices so they can become familiar with the laws governing their profession. One must not assume that laws are the same in every state across the nation.

EMS programs accredited by the Committee on Accreditation of Educational Programs for Emergency Medical Services Professions (CoAEMSP) reflect a high integrity of educational standards. The CoAEMSP Web site (www.coaemsp.org) provides accreditation data relevant to EMS educational standards. See Chapter 23 for additional information on program accreditation.

In following state guidelines, educational institutions may establish standards of instruction required of all instructors, including EMS faculty. Frequently, EMS faculty are required to hold some form of state teaching certification or credential. It is critical that EMS educators meet or exceed the minimum standards for both the EMS and teaching professions established by the accrediting body, institution, and state.

CURRICULUM ISSUES

EMS educators must establish a curriculum that is in compliance with state and federal laws and that adheres to accreditation standards. Beyond that, educators have traditionally believed that they have the right to control curriculum within their programs. However, in *Urofsky v. Gilmore*, 216 F.3d 401 (4th Cir. 2000. cert. Denied, 5531 U.S. 1070) (2001), the court stated that

> Significantly, the [United States Supreme] Court had never recognized that professors possess a First Amendment right of academic freedom to determine for themselves the content of their courses and scholarship, despite opportunities to do so (*Id.* at 414).
>
> In deciding the *Urofsky* case, the Fourth Circuit Court relied upon the 1998 decision of *Boring v. Buncombe County Board of Education*, 136 F.3d 364 (4th Cir. 1998), cert. Denied, 525 U.S. 813 (1998). In the *Boring* case, the Fourth Circuit Court of Appeals determined that school systems have full authority to determine instructional curriculum. Furthermore, courts in the case of *Edwards v. California State University of Pennsylvania*, 156 F.3d 488 (3rd Cir. 11998), cert. Denied, 525 U.S. 1143 (1999), determined that college professors did not have control over curriculum. In this case, a tenured professor who taught instructional media classes decided to focus the curriculum on humanism, censorship, and religion. The federal appeals court decided that Edwards must keep his personal religious beliefs out of the classroom and must adhere to curriculum determined by the university (*Id.* at 491).

No decisions contrary to the *Urofsky*, *Boring*, and *Edwards* cases have been made by the US Supreme Court. As such, both secondary and postsecondary educators must uphold curricular decisions made by the institutional or system administration.

STUDENT ISSUES

Student issues in EMS programs are similar to those of most educational programs. Common student issues include, among others, institutional relationships, handbook policies, enrollment and dismissal, health policies, and academic integrity.

Institutional Relationship

The institutional relationship with students is the basis for all EMS educational programs. Establishing a positive student-institution relationship is critical to the success of the program and its graduates. Documents, including but not restricted to catalogs, handbooks, course syllabi, and advertising materials, play an important role in promoting a positive relationship between the institution and students. All information must be correct, detailed, and readily available to the public.

Catalogs

Catalogs are perhaps the most enduring document of the student's relationship with the institution. Information generally provided in catalogs includes institutional data, academic requirements, enrollment and dismissal rules and regulations, and student support practices. Nondiscrimination policies should be printed near the front of the catalog; for example, the following statement is printed on the first page of the *Idaho State University Undergraduate Catalog (2003-2004)*:

> Idaho State University subscribes to the principles and laws of the State of Idaho and federal government, including applicable executive orders pertaining to civil rights, and all rights, privileges, and activities in the institution are made available without regard to race, creed, color, sex, age, disability, or national origin. The university is an Equal Opportunity and Affirmative Action employer. Evidences of practices which are not consistent with such a policy should be reported to the Office of the President of the University.

Student Handbooks

Depending on the size and type of institutional facility, students may receive a variety of handbooks that provide rules, regulations, and information pertinent to their educational endeavors. Some institutions combine general student handbooks with institutional handbooks or catalogs. Traditionally, student handbooks are broad in scope and include information pertinent to the entire program. Syllabi generally provide information specific to a given course within the program. For additional information on course syllabi, refer to Chapter 23.

EMS educators may develop handbooks specifically for students in their programs. This program handbook provides information on curricula, attendance guidelines, uniform or dress codes, and other specifics. EMS educators may also create clinical or field experience handbooks that provide rules, expectations, and guidelines relevant to practical learning activities.

CASE IN POINT

Two EMS students preparing for Clinical Rotation I went shopping for uniforms. One found a pale blue scrub suit on sale. She also found a pair of nonuniform clogs, which she considered the perfect match for her outfit. When she showed her planned purchase to the second student, a discussion ensued as to the appropriateness of the uniform. The second student had his *EMS Student Handbook* in the car. Before making their purchases, the students reviewed uniform guidelines in the handbook. The well-written *EMS Student Handbook* clearly stated that all uniforms must be navy blue and that only closed shoes would be acceptable. Thanks to the foresight of the EMS educator, a problem was prevented, and the students learned exactly what was expected of them.

When developing program policies, EMS educators may establish standards that are stricter than those of the general institution. No policies should be established that are less stringent or that conflict with institutional or governmental policy. EMS educators should have their suggested policies approved by appropriate institutional personnel before printing them. Legal counsel should approve all policies before the time of publication.

Related Printed Documents

EMS educators may use printed documents for recruitment or related activities. All published documents may provide information that, when interpreted by the reader, may potentially lead to litigation and should first be approved by institutional representatives and legal counsel. The 1965 Higher Education Resources and Student Assistance Act, as amended by Congress in 1976, requires that all institutions that participate in federal financial aid programs must provide key information to all prospective and current students. Such information must include financial assistance opportunities, programmatic costs, refund policies, program descriptions, ADA support, veterans' benefits, confidentiality of records, and nondiscrimination policies.

Challenges to Printed Documents

In today's educational system, catalogs and handbooks may be perceived by students as legal documents. Many institutions include disclaimer statements to protect themselves from potential litigation. The *Idaho State University Undergraduate Catalog (2003-2004)* states:

> Catalogs, bulletins, course and fee schedules, etc., are not to be considered as binding contracts between

> Idaho State University and students. The university and its divisions reserve the right at any time, without advance notice, to: (a) withdraw or cancel classes, courses, and programs; (b) change fee schedules; (c) change the academic calendar; (d) change admissions and registration requirements; (e) change regulations and requirements governing instruction in, and graduation from, the university and its various divisions; and (f) change any other regulations affecting students. Changes shall go into force whenever the proper authorities so determine, and shall apply not only to prospective students but also to those who are matriculated at the time in the university. When economic and other conditions permit, the university tries to provide advance notice of such changes. In particular, when an instructional program is to be withdrawn, the university will make every reasonable effort to ensure that students who are within two years of completing the graduation requirements, and who are making normal progress toward the completion of those requirements, will have the opportunity to complete the program which is to be withdrawn (p 1).

In *The Contract to Educate: Toward a More Workable Theory of the Student University Relationship,*[13] evidence was provided that courts sometimes decide on behalf of students who have been terminated. Courts have established "that students are citizens and do not shed their basic constitutional freedoms when they enter [education]."[14] EMS administrators and faculty must be careful not to violate students' constitutional rights when making programmatic changes. Students' constitutional rights might include freedom of speech, freedom of assembly, and freedom from discrimination.

Enrollment and Dismissal

The enrollment process in any EMS program begins with recruitment. All applicants and students must be treated equitably and according to published guidelines. The ultimate goal is to see students successfully complete the program and become employed. However, on some occasions, students must be dismissed from the program. When it occurs, this must be handled in a fair and equitable manner so that potential litigation can be avoided.

Recruitment

When recruiting students for the EMS program, institutional representatives must be certain that no discrimination occurs. Printing a nondiscrimination statement on all recruiting documents is a good way to start. However, policies must go beyond written statements and must be strictly enforced. The two most common areas of litigation involving recruitment are breach of contract and misrepresentation or fraud.

When an EMS program or institution does not perform any action or duty required by written or implied expectations, it is considered to be a breach of contract. In the case of *Wickstrom v. North Idaho College,* 725 P.2d 155 (Idaho 1986), four students filed legal action indicating that the college failed to comply with statements made in the college's catalog. The court stated that "[i]t is by now well-settled that the principal relationship between a college and its student is contractual," and that "[s]ince a formal contract is rarely prepared, the general nature and terms of the agreement are usually implied, with specific terms to be found in the university bulletin and other publications." (*Id.* at 157.) The court found that "a valid cause of action in contract could exist if the terms of the implied contract between appellants and North Idaho College were not complied with." (*Id.*)

Misrepresentation occurs when an EMS program provides photos or text that inappropriately represents the program. In cases of misrepresentation, the plaintiff (accuser) must provide the proof.

> "A common law action for misrepresentation requires a plaintiff to plead and prove (1) a false statement of material fact; (2) known by the defendant to be false, or uttered with reckless disregard for the truth or falsity of the statement; (3) upon which the plaintiff reasonably relies; (4) resulting in damages to the plaintiff."[15]

In the *Wickstrom* case (*supra*) and in *Dizick v. Umpqua Community College,* 599 P.2d 444 (Oregon, 1979), both colleges were alleged to have enhanced program outcomes. In *Wagonblast*, college documents indicated that, upon successful program completion, graduates would be employable as entry level journeymen. In fact, graduates were not so qualified. In the *Dizick* case, similar misrepresentations were made by Umpqua Community College in Oregon, which were subjected to legal action. *Andre v. Pace University,* 655 N.Y.S.2d 777 (Sup.Ct. 1996) is another case of alleged misrepresentation. Although the decision was ultimately in favor of Pace University, a great deal of time and expense was expended in responding to the charges. It is for these reasons that EMS educators should be extremely careful in determining the factuality of all printed material that will be used for recruitment and enrollment of students.

Acceptance

Once accepted, students must know what is expected of them, not only in the general EMS program but also in specific courses. Student handbooks may provide most of this information. During the first session of each class, EMS educators should provide students with course syllabi. Each syllabus must (1) be clearly written; (2) adhere to state, institutional, and federal guidelines; and (3) spell out all expectations and grading criteria. Well-written syllabi limit students' ability to pursue potential litigation.

Dismissal

Educators like to see their students succeed. Occasionally, however, students fail to meet the published educational standards or for other reasons must be dismissed from the program. This is a difficult situation that must be handled carefully for the protection of the faculty, program, and institution from student lawsuits. Just as with other aspects of student-institution relationships, fair treatment is critical. According to Toma and Palm, "if academic administrators follow their own rules, the courts are likely to uphold their academic judgments."[16]

Student dismissal is similar to employee dismissal. Common problems that may occur in the dismissal process can be avoided. Hall and Marsh (2003) identified "problems that make it more difficult to prevail in internal grievance and/or administrative proceedings and in litigation" (p 405). In terms of student issues, litigation may result if the educator fails to

- Regularly and objectively document student behaviors with examples of expected performance
- Provide educational experiences, both academic and practical, directed toward success
- Keep evidence of both positive and negative completed student work
- Maintain fair and objective student evaluations
- Communicate as though every word, written or spoken, would be broadcast in public
- Treat all students the same and objectively
- Maintain students' confidentiality before, during, and after the educational experience[17]

Because of their training, EMS professionals are experienced in the process of careful documentation. As educators, EMS professionals must adapt this ability to document to classroom and clinical activities. Again, it is critical that all students are treated equitably.

Discipline in the Classroom

One of the most common problems faced by educators is discipline in the classroom. In the case of EMS educators, this problem extends to the clinical setting. The court system has traditionally supported educational institutions in dealing with discipline problems, either academic or behavioral, provided that students' rights are not violated.

Cornett v. Miami University, 728 N.E.2d 471 (Ohio Ct.App. 2000), is a case that illustrates this point. The Ohio Court of Appeals decided in favor of the university in this case that dealt with alleged sexual misconduct. Another student discipline case is *C.B. By and Through Breeding v. Driscoll,* 82 F.3d 383 (11th Cir. 1996). This case involved two students (minors) who alleged that their rights had been violated. One student (T.P.) was suspended from school for fighting. The second student (C.B.) was suspended on the suspicion of illegal drug activity. The court system decided in favor of the school principal (Driscoll). It was found that the school's handbook and policies were appropriately followed and that students were afforded their due process rights.

Appearance

Healthcare workers, including EMS students, are traditionally held to a high standard of professional appearance. The appearance of healthcare workers not only establishes a level of professionalism, it also is a matter of hygiene and safety. Faculty should expect students to adhere to dress codes as approved and provided by the institution. Dress code policies may address personal hygiene, uniforms, hairstyles, jewelry, fingernails, and other related issues.

Policies regarding student uniforms should be established in accordance with institutional guidelines and input from advisory committees, and they should be written in compliance with regional clinical expectations. If hospitals or EMS service field agencies have dress codes that are stricter than those of the educational institution, instructors may enforce such guidelines, provided that such requirements are reasonable and constitutional.

Institutional policies must be clearly presented to students in their handbooks and/or syllabi. Instructors should not assume that students know what is acceptable appearance. If students are required to wear identification badges or name tags, it is the instructor's responsibility to notify students of this. If stethoscopes and bandage scissors are part of the uniform, students must know this in advance.

Depending on the program and the institutional policies, students may be required to be in uniform at all times. It is also possible that they may be assigned to wear uniforms only during time spent in clinical settings. Again, it is important that students are provided this information as early in the educational process as possible. By informing students, the instructor has clearly identified the standards and has established a basis for expectations.

Although students' appearances may be perceived as problematic, EMS educators must use caution in dealing with issues such as clothing and hairstyles. Courts have allowed educational institutions to establish dress codes to restrict clothing deemed to be unsafe, offensive, or unsanitary. In *Gano v. School District 411 of Twin Falls County, Idaho,* 672 F.Supp. 796 (D. Idaho 1987), the student (Gano) alleged that his right to free speech had been violated when he was suspended from school for wearing an "inappropriate"

T-shirt. Gano had designed the shirt with caricatures of school administrators appearing intoxicated on school property. "The court found that the T-shirt falsely represented the administrators in a condition of alcoholic stupor and was in violation of Idaho Code § 33-1605. It was decided that since the administrators were role models and had no history of drinking alcohol on school property, they were due protection by the court."[18]

Not all dress codes are considered constitutional. In 1970, school administrators in a New Hampshire school believed that jeans had a negative influence on student behavior. The district court found against the dress code and decided in favor of the students. (See *Bannister v. Paradis*, 316 F.Supp. 185 [S.N.H. 1970].)

While observing health and safety practices regarding hairstyles, EMS educators also must be cognizant of prohibitions that may be deemed unconstitutional. In the early 1970s, several court cases were decided that recognized students' right to freedom of speech expressed by how they wore their hair. Ethnic hairstyles have been protected by the courts, even when they violated institutional dress codes. (See *Alabama and Coushatta Tribes v. Big Sandy Independent School District*, 817 F.Supp. 1319 [E.D.Tex. 1993].)

Academic Dishonesty

Academic dishonesty in the classroom is not a new concept. It is, however, on the increase with the advent of technology, such as copy and fax machines, computers, and the Internet.

> "Internet plagiarism is a growing concern on all campuses as students struggle to understand what constitutes acceptable use of the Internet. In the absence of clear direction from faculty, most students have concluded that 'cut & paste' plagiarism—using a sentence or two (or more) from different sources on the Internet and weaving this information together into a paper without appropriate citation—is not a serious issue. While 10% of students admitted to engaging in such behavior in 1999, this rose to 41% in a 2001 survey, with the majority of students (68%) suggesting this was not a serious issue." (Center for Academic Integrity Research[19])

The Center for Academic Integrity (CAI) at Duke University was established in 1990 as the result of a national research presentation. CAI is a consortium of more than 320 institutions dedicated to researching and relating information on academic integrity. The EMS educator may find the CAI Web site a useful tool in dealing with academic integrity (http://www.academicintegrity.org). For more information, see Chapter 23 on academic dishonesty.

Printed information in institutional catalogs, handbooks, and syllabi should contain clearly established policies on academic dishonesty. Such policies must be made available to students upon enrollment and must be reinforced at the beginning of each course. In the event that academic dishonesty does occur, students will have already received the institutional policy and will know the related penalty. See Box 10-1 for a sample academic dishonesty policy.

The court system has generally supported educational institutions in matters of academic dishonesty. The most common current form of academic dishonesty is plagiarism. (See, *e.g.*, *Easley v. University of Michigan Board of Regents*, 906 F.2d 1143 [6th Cir. 1990]; *Hand v. Matchett*, 957 F.2d 791 [10th Cir. 1992]; and *Childress v. Clement*, 5 F.Supp.2d 384 [E.D.Va. 1998].)

Student-institution relationships are among the most critical and most challenging components of any educational system. Those issues identified herein provide merely a brief overview. The EMS educator should become familiar with all institutional, local, state, and federal regulations under which the program operates. It is vital that the educator have access to appropriate support by administrators and/or legal counsel to avoid being placed in positions of potential liability.

GRIEVANCE POLICIES

Every educational institution must have defined and published grievance policies for both the employees and the students. Although policies may differ

BOX 10-1 Idaho State University Academic Dishonesty Policy

Dishonest conduct is unacceptable. In cases of academic dishonesty, such as cheating or plagiarism, students will be dismissed from class, given failing grades, or otherwise disciplined by the faculty member. Before students are allowed to repeat the course, they must submit a petition and must obtain approval from the Scholarship Requirements Committee, or the designated official of the college who has jurisdiction over the course. Faculty members are responsible for deciding academic dishonesty cases that occur in their classes, except when a case involves additional violation of University policies. Such other violations may be resolved under the Student Code of Conduct, Rights, Responsibilities and Judicial Structure, or other applicable procedures. (See the complete policy in the *Idaho State University Faculty and Staff Handbook*, Part 6, Section IX, page 6.9.1, for definitions of cheating and plagiarism from the Web site http://www.isu.edu/references/fs.handbook/.)

From *Idaho State University Faculty and Staff Handbook;* http://www.isu.edu/references/sthandbook, retrieved March 3, 2004.

according to the nature of the institutional relationship, the concepts are the same. Accredited CoAEMSP programs are required to "have a defined and published policy and procedure for processing student and faculty grievances."[20]

Students

Grievance policies should be made readily available to all students upon enrollment in the EMS program. Many institutions elect to publish the grievance procedure in the institutional catalog or program handbook. When disciplining students, the EMS educator should attempt to resolve the issue at the lowest possible level. If unable to resolve the student issue at this level, the educator should be certain that the steps in the institutional student grievance policy are carefully followed and documented. Failure of educators to adhere to published policies may enhance students' opportunities for successful litigation.

CASE IN POINT

A student was dismissed from the EMS program. She sought the advice of her family's attorney, and a Notice of Tort claim was filed. As the legal action proceeded, the judge dismissed the issue, finding that the student had not followed the institution's grievance policy, which had been published before the time of the student's enrollment. Even though the case was dismissed, a great deal of time and energy had been spent on it by EMS faculty members and administrators. When handling dismissals, faculty members should remind students of the grievance policy and should encourage them to work within the system. Frequently, issues may be resolved at this level.

Faculty

EMS faculty members should also have a published grievance policy relative to their employment. This policy is frequently published in faculty or staff handbooks.

Just as students do not sacrifice their constitutional rights when they enroll in programs, educators also maintain their constitutional rights and must be afforded the opportunity to respond when those rights appear to have been violated.

SAFE EDUCATIONAL ENVIRONMENTS

Safe educational environments are established on the basis of laws and common sense. Safe learning facilities are strong defenses against potential litigation. Schools and colleges were once considered secure. However, events such as the 1966 University of Texas bell tower massacre and the 1999 shooting at Columbine High School (Colorado) are evidence that educational institutions are not free of violence.

EMS faculty, along with administrators and others, must strive to provide safe educational environments for their students. Among the federal statutes requiring safe educational environments with which the EMS educator should be familiar are the Safe and Drug-Free Schools and Communities Act (1994), the Gun-Free Schools Act (1994), the Jeanne Clery Disclosure of Campus Security and Campus Crime Statistics Act (1990), and the Occupational Safety and Health Act (1970).

School Violence

The 2001 attacks on the World Trade Center and the Pentagon aroused a somewhat complacent American society to acknowledge real and perceived terrorist threats. Educational statistics, such as those listed here, are overwhelming:

- More than 6250 teachers are threatened with violence on a daily basis
- More than 260 teachers are physically attacked each day
- An estimated 4% of American high school students carry guns to school at least on occasion
- Every day, more than 150,000 students stay home from school for fear of physical harm
- Nearly 4000 are assaulted daily[21]

With statistics like these, it is obvious that EMS educators work in situations of potential harm to themselves and their students.

Administrators must be cognizant of potential litigation involving negligent hiring practices. In *Harrington v. Louisiana State Board of Elementary and Secondary Education*, 714 So.2d 845 (La.App.4 Cir. 1998), the student (Harrington) brought charges of rape against an instructor at the Delgado Community College (DCC). The instructor (Veller) testified that no one in the educational system had questioned his background. Veller did, in fact, have a variety of prior convictions. Through lengthy court proceedings, DCC was found to have breached its duty by hiring a convicted felon. Furthermore, the court found that Louisiana employers are "vicariously liable only if an employee is 'acting within the ambit of his assigned duties and also in furtherance of his employer's objective.'" (*Id.* at 851.) Because the rape took place during an activity in which the instructor represented DCC, the state was found vicariously liable for Veller's actions. (*Id.* at 852.) (See also *Godar v. Edwards*, 588 N.W.2d 701 [Iowa 1999] and *Brown v. Youth Services International of South Dakota*, 89 F.Supp.2d 1095 [D.S.D. 2000].)

EMS faculty and administrators also must be aware of potential litigation that may result from negligent or inaccurate referrals. The case of *Tarasoff v. Regents of the University of California*, 551 P.2d 334 (1976) established the duty to warn third parties when a dangerous person seeks employment. In *Randi W. v. Muroc Joint Unified School District*, 929 P.2d 582 (Cal. 1997), the courts determined that any person who writes letters of recommendation owes a duty to not misrepresent the person's qualifications or character if such action could result in harm to the prospective employer or third party. Even though these national cases have established standards regarding negligent referrals, EMS educators should determine whether any other laws apply in their own states.

Safe and Drug-Free Schools and Communities Act

The Safe and Drug-Free Schools and Communities Act (SDFSCA) (20 U.S.C. § 7101 *et seq.*) was enacted in 1994. Through this statute, Congress required federally funded K-12 schools to maintain drug education and prevention programs and Drug Abuse Resistance Education (DARE) programs, and to provide education about prejudice and intolerance. Postsecondary schools were mandated "to establish, operate, expand, and improve programs of school drug and violence prevention, education, and rehabilitation referral for students."[22]

Gun-Free Schools Act

The initial Gun-Free Schools Act (GFSA) (18 U.S.C. § 922 q[1][A]) was enacted by Congress in 1990. In 1995, the US Supreme Court determined this law to be unconstitutional. During the time that the GFSA was being Constitutionally challenged, Congress established the Gun-Free Schools Act of 1994. (20 U.S.C. § 3351.) The new law required that each state that was receiving federal funds had to expel students who brought weapons onto school property. Congress determined that any student bringing weapons onto school property would be expelled for no less than 12 actual calendar months. However, Congress also gave power to school superintendents to modify the expulsion and discipline on a case-by-case basis.[23]

A weapon, as defined in 18 U.S.C. § 921, is any type of firearm. The following items fit into this category:

- Any weapon, including a starter gun, that is designed to, or may be modified to, expel a projectile by means of an explosive
- The frame, receiver, muffler, or silencer of any of the above items
- Any destructive, explosive, incendiary, or poison gas bomb, grenade, or rocket having more than 4 ounces of propellant charge, missiles having more than one-quarter ounce of an explosive charge, mines, or similar devices
- Any destructive device that may be used as a propellant or that has explosive action, with a barrel with a bore of more than one-half inch diameter (GFSA, *supra*)

Knives are not specifically identified in GFSA as weapons. However, in accordance with legal standards, laws may be enforced that are more stringent than, but not in contradiction to, a federal statute. Accordingly, state legislators and educators may elect to include knives within their own definitions of weapons.

Jeanne Clery Act

In 1990, the Higher Education Act of 1965 was amended by Congress and renamed the Jeanne Clery Disclosure of Campus Security and Campus Crime Statistics Act (20 U.S.C. § 1092[f]). It is referred to as the Jeanne Clery Act and was named in her memory.

Jeanne Clery was a university freshman in 1986. She was sexually assaulted and murdered in her residence hall. Her murderer was a student whom she did not know. After the investigation, Jeanne's parents learned that 38 undisclosed crimes had occurred on the university's campus during the 3 years before Jeanne's death. Her parents worked diligently to encourage Congress to establish the Campus Security Act, which was later named in their daughter's memory.

All postsecondary institutions receiving federal funds are required to publish an annual report on crime statistics. This must be done annually by October 1. Within this document, 3 years of statistics must be reported. The report must be provided automatically to all current students and employees. Additionally, this information may be provided to prospective students, employees, and the public upon request.

Crime statistics must include data from all campus and local law enforcement agencies, and they must include incidents that occurred on the campus and in public areas surrounding the campus. Crime categories to be reported include the following:

- Aggravated assault
- Arson
- Burglary
- Manslaughter (negligent)
- Murder and nonnegligent manslaughter
- Motor vehicle theft
- Robbery
- Sex offenses (forcible)
- Sex offenses (nonforcible, incest, and statutory rape)
- Other hate crimes involving bodily injury[24]

Occupational Safety and Health Act

The Occupational Safety and Health Act (OSH) was enacted in December of 1970 to "assure safe and healthful working conditions . . ."[25] This Act is overseen by the Occupational Safety and Health Administration (OSHA) and has been amended 10 times since its enactment. In 1992, the penalties for unwillful or repeated violations were increased. The last amendment, which was added in September of 1998, included the US Postal Service as an "employer" subject to this Act.[26] Box 10-2 identifies the basic findings upon which OSH was established.

EMS educators should be familiar with OSHA guidelines as they apply to the educational setting. OSHA "is authorized to investigate—with no advance warning—suspected safety hazards and violations of its regulations for all workplace facilities involved in interstate commerce—which includes practically all colleges and universities."[27] Although OSH is a federal statute, states have been charged to accept responsibility for administration and enforcement of OSHA policies. Not all states have established Occupational and Safety Health Plans. Information about which states have such plans and related Web sites may be found at http://www.osha.gov. EMS educators must be familiar with OSHA requirements within their own states. When no state plan exists, the federal Act provides the level of accountability.

BOX 10-2 Occupational Safety and Health Act of 1970

Congress enacted the Occupational Safety and Health Act upon finding "that personal injuries and illnesses arising out of work situations impose a substantial burden upon, and are a hindrance to, interstate commerce in terms of lost production, wage loss, medical expenses, and disability compensation payments" (PL 91-586). This situation is to be relieved in the following ways:

- Encouraging employers and employees to reduce the number of occupational safety and health hazards at the workplace
- Assuring that employers and employees share in this responsibility
- Creating an Occupational Safety and Health Commission
- Advancing initiatives to provide safe and healthful working conditions
- Providing occupational safety and health research
- Exploring the relationship between diseases and environmental conditions
- Providing medical criteria for safe and healthful working conditions
- Providing training programs
- Establishing occupational health and safety standards
- Enforcing standards
- Encouraging states to assume fullest responsibility for administration and enforcement of OSHA policies
- Creating appropriate reporting procedures
- Encouraging labor and management to jointly reduce employment injuries and disease (*Id.*)

WORKERS' COMPENSATION

To protect employees who are injured on the job, state and federal workers' compensation laws have been established. Formerly known as workmen's compensation, these laws determine who will be eligible for benefits such as medical expenses, wage loss, and family support (in the event the employee is killed on the job.) "Workers' compensation, a type of no-fault insurance, is a mutual arrangement between the employer and the employee in the event of injury or illness related to employment."[28] In such cases, the employer does not admit fault for the injury and the employee agrees to receive benefits without litigation. No federal or state laws provide workers' compensation benefits for persons injured on the job as the result of horseplay, alcohol, or illegal use of drugs.

State Guidelines

Each state is responsible for establishing its own workers' compensation laws. Although they may be similar, state laws do vary. EMS educators should contact their human resources department for information on workers' compensation that is specific to their employment situation. Institutional employees in this department will be familiar with definitions provided in the Federal Employees' Compensation Act (5 U.S.C. §§ 8101-8193) and applicable state and federal laws. Additionally, the US Department of Labor Web site (http://www.dol.gov) provides information on each state's workers' compensation offices.

Coverage

Generally, coverage for workers' compensation benefits is purchased at the state level through insurance policies. Each state determines how employers are required to provide workers' compensation coverage. For example, 47 states do not require small businesses to carry workers' compensation insurance. Texas does not require any private employer to carry workers' compensation insurance.

As with any career and technical education program with laboratory activities, EMS programs have the potential for on-the-job injury. Faculty should be aware of institutional policies and should follow procedures exactly. In many cases, accident or incident reports must be completed within a specified time frame. The injured party may be required to visit a physician who has contracted with the institution or state workers' compensation insurance.

EMS educators also must be familiar with the status of students in their programs in regard to workers' compensation coverage. Some programs may treat students on clinical rotations as they treat employees. Other programs may provide no workers' compensation coverage for students under any circumstances. Regardless of the policy, the EMS faculty member should be knowledgeable and should respond to questions accordingly.

Fraud

Misrepresentation of a work-related injury might result in charges of fraud. Because workers' compensation benefits are determined by physicians' reports, the injured party must provide accurate and detailed information. Previous medical conditions, medications, or any other factors that could relate to the injury must be disclosed at the time of treatment. Most states have laws that require employers, insurance carriers, or members of the public to report suspected cases of workers' compensation fraud. States frequently allow the informer to remain anonymous. Persons fraudulently claiming workers' compensation benefits may be subject to criminal proceedings.

Many workers' compensation cases are related to education. Among the relevant cases are *Board of Education of Alpine School District v. Olsen*, 684 P.2d (Utah 1984) (volunteer injured in woodshop classes denied workers' compensation benefits); *Jefferson County Schools v. Headrick*, 734 P.2d 659 (Colo. App. 1986) (high school shop teacher paid disability benefits for occupational hearing loss); and *Begel v. Wisconsin Labor and Industry Review Commission*, 631 N.W.2d 220 (Wis. App. 2001) (student research assistant who became quadriplegic because of a work-related activity awarded disability benefits).

INSURANCE

Insurance coverage for employees and students generally falls into one of two categories: health or liability. Requirements for employees and students most likely will vary, especially in the area of health insurance.

Employees

Health insurance may be an employee benefit. EMS faculty should speak with appropriate administrative personnel to determine whether this is a covered benefit. Frequently, employees are required to share the cost of insurance with their employers. Benefits will vary based on institutional health insurance policies.

Liability, or malpractice, insurance is generally not a covered employee benefit, so EMS faculty must determine the necessity of carrying such insurance themselves. In some institutions, health educators are required to carry malpractice insurance. As practitioners, EMS personnel may already be familiar with malpractice insurance. The value of carrying malpractice insurance is that it protects the EMS faculty member's certification, registration, or licensure in the event of injury to another party.

Students

Traditionally, students must show proof that they are covered by a personal health insurance policy. If unable to provide such proof, students may be required to purchase health insurance through the educational facility.

Some institutions, clinical affiliations, or certification boards may require that students carry liability insurance in the event that students cause injury to third parties. EMS faculty must comply with institutional expectations in advising students regarding health and liability insurance.

CONFIDENTIALITY

Based on their medical experiences, EMS instructors are already familiar with the rules of patient confidentiality. As educators, the rules of confidentiality extend to the classroom and to student-related activities. The two most important laws regarding confidentiality are the Family Educational Rights and Privacy Act (1974) and the Health Insurance Portability and Accountability Act (1996).

Family Educational Rights and Privacy Act

Originally known as the Buckley Amendment, the Family Educational Rights and Privacy Act (FERPA) (20 U.S.C. § 1232) was passed by Congress in August of 1974. This law, which was enacted in response to concerns that personal information was being maintained and disseminated by the government, pertains to the confidentiality and handling of student records. All educational institutions that receive federal funds are required to comply with FERPA.

Two FERPA presentations were made at the June 2001 meeting of the National Association of College and University Attorneys (NACUA) in San Diego, California. These were *FERPA for All: The Basics Plus* (Footer) and *Recent FERPA Developments (July 2000-June 2001)* (Lynch). Footer and Lynch provided detailed FERPA information and definitions in their presentations. (See, *e.g.*, Hall and Marsh, 2003, and the

NACUA Web site at www.nacua.org.) Information on FERPA is also available on the US Department of Education Web site at http://www.ed.gov/offices/OM/fpco/ferpalist.html.

Guidelines

FERPA guidelines were established to protect students' education records. As cited in the presentation by Hall and Marsh (2003, p 291), student records

- Are to be kept confidential, with access provided to outside third parties only with parental consent (20 U.S.C. § 1232g[b][1], [2]) or adult student consent
- May be accessed on request by the student's parents (for minors) (*id.* at §1232g[a][1][A])
- May be challenged by parents or adult-age students who think that the records are misleading, inaccurate, or a violation of their student privacy rights (*id.* at § 1232g[a][2])

Under federal law, educational institutions must inform students or their parents of FERPA guidelines. Students younger than 18 are considered minors, and their parents or guardians have legal access to their education records. Once students turn 18 or enroll in postsecondary institutions, they are considered to be adults. At this point, parents and guardians have no legal right to access student information.

Education records

Documents maintained at an educational institution that specifically relate to students are considered education records. These records may take the form of written documents, video or audiotapes, films, photographs, or computer files. Lynch and Footer identified five types of documents that are excluded from FERPA regulations. These include the following:

1. Sole possession notes (such as grade books)
2. Medical records of adult students (such as letters from physicians or other recognized professionals)
3. Law enforcement records
4. Student employee records
5. Alumni records[29]

Disclosure

According to FERPA rules, student records may be disclosed in only three ways: (a) directly to the student; (b) to a third party with the student's (or parent's) written permission; and (c) to a third party without written consent. EMS educators must understand the circumstances in which education records have been requested and must be certain to comply with federal regulations (Figure 10-2).[30]

In the adult education setting, faculty members and administrators are frequently contacted by parents who are seeking information regarding the status of their children. This is a difficult situation and must be handled with extreme caution. Education records may be disclosed to parents of minors (younger than age 18). However, educators do not have the legal right to disclose records of adult students (older than 18, or those enrolled in postsecondary education) without written permission of the student. Parents may appear demanding and may state that because they are paying the student's tuition, they are entitled to know how the student is doing academically. Educators must not allow themselves to be caught in this type of a situation. If adult students wish to have parents informed of their progress or be otherwise involved, written permission must be provided.

It is common in the EMS profession for employers to pay for an employee's education. In return, employers expect to remain informed about the student's academic standing. This is a contractual issue between the employer and the employee. It is the student employee's responsibility to provide this release to the educator or institution. The EMS educator must not release information to anyone, including employers, without the student's (or parent's) written permission.

A contract should be established by the employer before the student enrolls in the EMS program. This contract must clearly identify the expectations of both parties and must be signed and dated. For example, the employer might agree to pay for tuition, books, supplies, and all related educational expenses. In return, the student may be expected to provide a record of attendance and/or a transcript at the completion of each grading session. Again, it must be stressed that unless the EMS educator (or institutional representative) has a copy of the signed document provided by the student, no information may be released under FERPA guidelines.

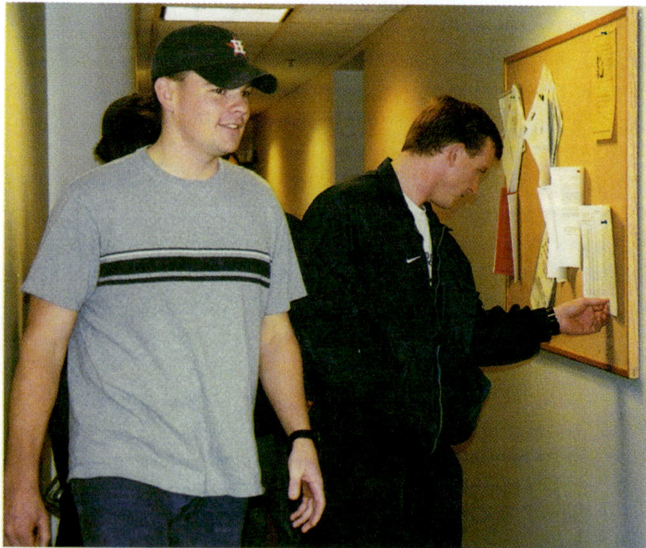

FIGURE 10-2 Educators should obtain student permission before they post grades and must not post them in conjunction with any identifiable student information.

Under the following circumstances, education records may be released without previous written consent:

- Directory information (unless a written request denying the publication of this information is provided by the student or parent)
- Information required by a school official who has a legitimate educational interest. Educators must be careful to demonstrate the legitimate educational interest, or they could be in violation of FERPA
- Information requested from an educational institution into which the student plans to enroll
- Financial aid documentation
- Documents necessary for accrediting bodies. It is best to remove student identification whenever possible
- Information necessary for studies on behalf of the institution regarding financial aid, testing, and other related research. Again, if possible, it is best to remove any personal identification
- Health and safety information necessary to protect other persons in the event of an emergency
- Documents or data required under lawfully issued subpoenas or orders[31]

Legitimate educational interest

As indicated, student records may be obtained by school officials who have legitimate educational interests. Authorized persons may access student records for information pertinent to employment only. Each situation should be handled individually and on a "need-to-know" basis.

Challenges to education records

Under FERPA, parents and adult students have the right to review and challenge education records. Such a request should be made in writing, and institutional representatives must respond within 45 days. Not subject to this review are parents' financial records and confidential letters of recommendation (Footer 2001). (For specific guidelines on challenges to education records, see 20 U.S.C. §§ 1232g[a][1][c]).

Related cases

Several related cases provide direction to educators for dealing with students' education records. FERPA-related cases include the following:

- *Tarka v. Cunningham*, 917 F.2d 890 (5th Cir. 1990) (the courts determined that, under FERPA, students do not have the right to challenge their grades. As long as students' grades in their education records do not misrepresent the educator's intent and are not misleading or inaccurate, the grade stands)
- *Jain v. State*, 617 N.W.2d 293 (Iowa 2000) (university acted appropriately in maintaining the privacy of a student who committed suicide on campus)
- *State Ex Rel. The Miami Student v. Miami University*, 779 Ohio St.3rd 168, 680 N.E.2d 956 (Ohio 1997) (university disciplinary records were not defined as educational records under FERPA)

EMS educators should familiarize themselves with FERPA, so that their actions do not precipitate litigation. Basic knowledge of FERPA is instrumental in preventing legal action.

Health Insurance Portability and Accountability Act

On August 21, 1996, the Health Insurance Portability and Accountability Act (HIPAA) became Public Law No. 104-191. HIPAA was initiated during the Clinton administration and has been considered by some to be an initial attempt to establish a national health insurance policy. HIPAA is of importance to the EMS educator on both a personal and a professional level. As employees, EMS faculty members have the right to expect employers to comply with HIPAA regulations. They also have the responsibility to inform students of HIPAA regulations as part of the EMS curriculum (Figure 10-3).

Purpose of HIPAA

The purpose of HIPAA is to provide specific rules and regulations designed to protect confidential patient information. Standardized data have been developed to enable covered entities to transmit protected health information (PHI), regardless of the process employed (electronic, printed, or verbal). Covered entities include all healthcare providers who deal with patient bills as part of their routine daily activities. This would include hospitals, physicians' offices, pharmacists, and emergency transport agencies, just to list a few.

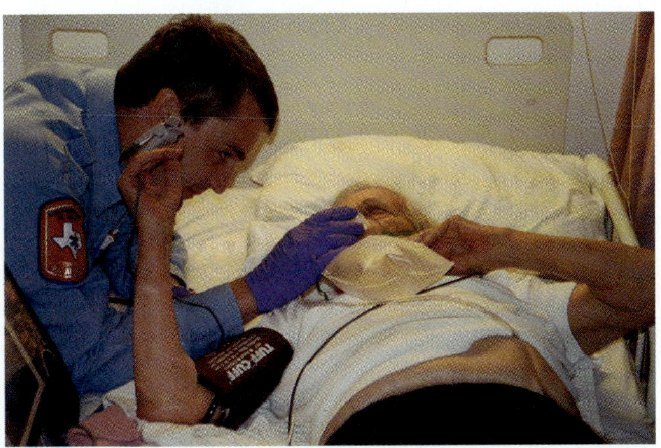

FIGURE 10-3 Students must be very clear about their responsibilities regarding confidentiality of patient information.

All healthcare entities and their employees were required to be HIPAA compliant by April 14, 2003. Covered entities and related personnel may be prosecuted, both civilly and criminally, for HIPAA violations. Penalties for violators may include monetary fines and prison sentences.

Oversight

After Congress enacted HIPAA, the US Department of Health and Human Services (HHS) was charged with refining all regulations. The HHS Office for Civil Rights (OCR) is the regulatory agency responsible for enforcement of HIPAA rules. As the first federal legislation to protect patients' medical privacy, HIPAA established the "norm" to be used throughout the nation. No state may be less restrictive than the national law; however, states may be more restrictive.

Each covered entity must establish written policies and procedures for implementation of HIPAA. Information should "include who will have access to protected health information, how it will be used, [and] when it will or will not be disclosed to others."[32] Whereas all existing personnel were to be HIPAA compliant by April of 2003, new employees must also undergo appropriate education on the rules and regulations. Failure to comply with this requirement may lead to prosecution.

Public trust

In the text *Implementing HIPAA Privacy Regulations in Pharmacy Practice* (Bishop and Winckler, 2002), several incidents in which public trust has been violated by healthcare providers were cited. Among these were identity theft, unsolicited antidepressant medications sent through the mail, and personal health information made public. Healthcare entities and related employees have access to highly personal and private information. "Therefore, patients must be able to trust that the confidentiality of the information will be maintained." (*id.* at p 3.)

Patient rights

Just as with FERPA, persons do have the right to review their personal records. Because of this fact, patients may request access to, and correction of, their PHI. It is best that such requests be made in writing and placed in patients' files. Covered entities have 30 days in which to respond. If they deny the patient's request, an explanation must be included, as well as information on the process for appeal.

Notice of privacy practices

Every covered entity is required to develop a Notice of Privacy Practices. This document must accurately inform patients about how PHI will be used both within and outside the facility. Providers should be cautious to release PHI on a "need-to-know" basis and must diligently strive to protect patients' privacy.

Notice of Privacy Practices information must be publicly posted in a prominent location at each covered entity facility. Likewise, "(p)roviders are required to make a 'good faith effort' to distribute the Notice of Privacy Practices to patients and obtain written acknowledgment of receipt" (Bishop and Winckler, 2002, p 5). According to Winckler (2002), there is a difference between patient notification and patient authorization. HIPAA does not require patient authorization in the reporting of workers' compensation information or in suspected cases of abuse or neglect.

A signed Notice of Privacy Practices must be retained for 6 years from the date signed or from the last date of treatment, whichever is the most recent. It is also wise for the clinician to provide the patient with a copy of the document and to make appropriate references on the original form. Good record keeping is critical for remaining compliant with HIPAA guidelines.

LEGAL RESEARCH

Because this chapter provides limited information on legal issues for the EMS educator, additional research may be of value. When completing legal research, the EMS educator should be cognizant of copyright laws and intellectual property.

Copyright Protection

Copyright protection is afforded to "copyright owners" under Title 17 of the US Code (17 U.S.C. § 101 *et seq.*). Most people think of printed materials when they hear the term "copyright." However, multiple works are protected under copyright laws. See Box 10-3 for works subject to copyright protection.

According to 17 U.S.C., § 302, "copyright protection for works created on or after January 1, 1978 shall endure for the following terms:

- General works (single author): the life of the author plus 70 years after the author's death
- Joint works: the life of the last surviving author plus 70 years after the last surviving author's death
- Anonymous works, pseudonymous works, and works made for hire: for 95 years from the year of the work's first publication, or a term of 120 years from the year of its first creation, whichever expires first"

Fair use

Fair use is a difficult concept to master. No single solution protects both the author of the copyrighted mate-

BOX 10-3 Works Subject to Copyright Protection: 17 U.S.C. § 101, *et seq.*

According to the US Code (17 U.S.C. § 102), works of authorship that are afforded exclusive rights as copyrighted works include the following:

Category	Examples
Literary works	Textbooks, journals, reference materials, research CD-ROMs
Musical works, including accompanying words	Printed music, musical CD-ROMs, videos
Dramatic works, including accompanying music	Plays, dramas, videos, movies, musicals
Pantomimes and choreographic works	Dramatic performances, dances
Pictorial, graphic, and sculptural works	Art, statues, logos, identity marks
Motion pictures and other audiovisual works	Movies (regardless of format)
Sound recordings	Music, radio broadcasts
Architectural works	Buildings, bridges

In no case does copyright protection for an original work of authorship extend to any idea, procedure, process, system, method of operation, concept, principle, or discovery, regardless of the form in which it is described, explained, illustrated, or embodied in such work. (*Id.*)

According to this statutory exception, Einstein would not have been able to copyright his theory of relativity. However, he would have been able to publish an article in which he explained his theory.

From Hall & and Marsh, 2003, p. 442.

rial and the person wishing to copy the document. Copyright owners may sue the person who is violating the law, as well as the institution for which that person works. Penalties for each infringement are extremely harsh. For each separate and willful act of copyright infringement, the court may award up to $150,000 plus attorney's fees, time lost from work, and/or other related expenses.[33]

According to the University of Texas Web site, a person should ask three questions when deciding if permission is necessary for use of copyrighted materials:

1. Is the work protected?
2. If the work is protected, do you wish to exercise one of the owner's exclusive rights?
3. Is your use exempt or excused from liability for infringement? (*Id*) The ability to use copyrighted material is identified in 17 U.S.C. § 107. The four identified factors to consider are provided in Box 10-4.

BOX 10-4 Fair Use Factors: 17 U.S.C. § 107

Fair Use Factor	Generally Accepted
Purpose and character of use	Nonprofit, educational, and/or personal use
Nature of work to be used	Fact-based research and publication
Amount and substantiality of material	Small amounts of copyrighted information
Effect on the potential market	No concrete response as it stands alone. Depends on the use of the previous three factors

With the increased number of distance education programs now available, faculty members and administrators must be cognizant of related copyright issues. It may be tempting to copy sections of text into Web-based courses or for distribution via interactive video. However, educators must be aware that the same potential copyright violations apply to distance education as to the traditional classroom.

TEACHING TIP: When determining whether permission is needed for making copies of copyrighted material, it is best to err on the side of caution.

Digital Millennium Copyright Act

Congress enacted the Digital Millennium Copyright Act (DMCA) (P.L. 105-304) in 1998. "Title II of the DMCA limits the monetary damages available against an on-line service provider (OSP) for copyright infringement by its users under certain circumstances."[34] The University of Texas system document entitled *Complying With the Digital Millennium Copyright Act* is an excellent reference for educators. This may be accessed through the UT System, Office of General Counsel Web site at http://www.utsystem.edu.

Legal Resources

The primary legal resource for any educator should be his or her institution's attorney or risk management office. Those who are working for public or private EMS agencies should have access to their city/county attorney or corporate attorney for private entities. Other legal resources are available in printed and electronic formats. The greatest single access to printed legal resources is found in public law libraries, but not every educator has such a library near where they live or work. Electronic legal research is also valuable. Remembering that educators are not always experts in the field of law, EMS faculty should first and foremost rely upon institutional legal counsel for advice and direction.

Some electronic legal references are available to the general public, and others are restricted to members of the legal profession by subscription only. Several Web sites have been provided in the reference section of this chapter to assist educators in locating legal information.

In this fast-paced era of technology, Web site addresses frequently change. Likewise, court decisions, laws, and other legal information may be established or amended at such a rapid pace that both texts and electronic sites may become quickly outdated. EMS educators should rely on legal counsel for the most current and detailed information.

Understanding Legal Documents

Legal research may appear complicated until the educator becomes familiar with the process and has a basic understanding of legal documents. As with any educational concept, legal research becomes easier to comprehend the more often it is put into practice.

Case citations

Case citations are standardized as to the information they provide. Each citation indicates the name of the case, the location where it is published, the court and jurisdiction where it was decided, and the decision date.

Citation example:

See, *e.g.*, *Cornett v. Miami University*, 728 N.E.2d 471 (Ohio Ct. App. 2000)

- The plaintiff was an individual named Cornett. This person brought suit against the defendant, Miami University. The name of the case is always printed in italics; hence, *Cornett v. Miami University*
- The number 728 indicates the volume of the report in which the case is published. This case was published in the *North Eastern Reporter* (N.E.) Second Series (2d). The second number (471) represents the page of the *North Eastern Reporter* on which the case begins
- This case was decided by the Ohio Court of Appeals in the year 2000

Statutory citations

Statutes are generally cited in a standard format, regardless of the level of enactment (*e.g.*, federal or state). An example of a federal nondiscrimination statute would be

Americans With Disabilities Act (ADA) (42 U.S.C. § 12101 *et seq.*, 1990)

- The name of the law is the Americans With Disabilities Act of 1990
- The number 42 represents the title of the US Code (U.S.C.) in which the statute is recorded. The symbol § identifies the cited section of the Act
- The designation *et seq.* means "and following." Therefore, § 12101 *et seq.* refers to the section of 42 U.S.C. in which the citation begins, then continues

Statutes are originally assigned public law numbers based on the session of Congress in which they were enacted. For example, HIPAA was initially enacted in 1996 as Public Law No. 104-191. The designation P.L. 104-191 indicates that this was the 191st law to be enacted during the 104th Congressional session.

Information on legal documents may prove useful for EMS educators who are pursuing research activities. However, it is rare that faculty members pursue such endeavors on a regular basis. In the event that EMS educators need legal information, their first contacts should be made with appropriate administrators and legal counsel.

SUMMARY

Legal issues affect EMS educators on a daily basis. Educators may not even be consciously aware of the impact that federal or state laws have on their personal and professional lives. Nonetheless, EMS educators need to gain a basic understanding of the legal system and must know how to access appropriate information. Because they are rarely subject matter experts, instructors should not become involved in legal educational matters without the knowledge and support of their administrators and legal counsel.

Statutes, rules, and regulations may be established at the federal, state, or local level. The US Constitution is the "supreme law of the land," and no laws may be in conflict with it. Although federal laws establish a base for national legal standards, state laws may be more restrictive. At no time are state or local laws allowed to be in conflict or of lower expectations than federal laws.

EMS educational standards must be in place and must uphold the integrity of the profession. EMS educators must be familiar with nondiscrimination laws. Students must all be treated the same way from the time of initial recruitment through graduation. All EMS program information must be accurate and reflective of what actually exists. Students have the right to access and challenge their educational records in compliance with FERPA guidelines. Every educational program is required to have formal, published grievance policies in place for faculty and students.

Tort law is especially important to EMS educators. Care must be taken to avoid assault and battery, defamation, misrepresentation, and negligence situations. The best protection against tort liability is to establish strong risk management practices. Some of these practices include waivers (releases), safety instruction, student supervision, and careful clinical site selection. Affiliation agreements must be developed in compliance with legal counsel's direction and should include all necessary components.

Educational programs should be as safe as possible. Federal laws, such as the Safe and Drug-Free Schools and Communities Act (1994), the Gun-Free Schools Act (1994), the Jeanne Clery Disclosure of Campus Security and Campus Crime Statistics Act (1990), and the Occupational Safety and Health Act (1970), provide direction in establishing and maintaining safe educational environments.

EMS educators should become familiar with their own states' and institutions' rules on workers' compensation insurance. Printed information should be available regarding who and what are covered under workers' compensation. False claims of workers' compensation are considered fraud and punishable by law. It is also important for EMS educators to know which health and liability insurance is provided for them, or whether they are expected to provide their own coverage. The same is true with regard to students.

Confidentiality is critical in both the EMS profession and education. The Family Educational Rights and Privacy Act (1974) and the Health Insurance Portability and Accountability Act (1996) clearly define federal guidelines and standards in the areas of educational and health confidentiality.

Copyright issues should always be reviewed with students. EMS educators involved in research must comply with all copyright laws.

Wise EMS educators are familiar with legal issues that affect their programs. Although educators are not expected to be experts, a basic knowledge of legal concepts and an ability to apply them are critical in alleviating potential litigation.

REFERENCES

1. Hall, B and Marsh, R. Legal Issues in Career and Technical Education. Homewood, IL: American Technical Publishers, 2003.
2. Toma, JD, and Palm, RL: *The Academic Administrator and the Law: What Every Dean and Department Chair Needs to Know*. (1999). ASHE-ERIC Higher Education Report Volume 26, No. 5. Washington, DC: The George Washington University, Graduate School of Education and Human Development.
3. Fischer, L, Schimmel, D and Kelly, C: *Teachers and the Law*. ed 5. New York: Addison Wesley, 1999.
4. *Black's Law Dictionary*, 4th Ed. 1972, 1660.
5. Hall and Marsh, 2003, *Legal Issues in Career*, 79.
6. *Black's Law Dictionary*, 7th Ed. 1999.
7. Hall and Marsh, 2003, *Legal Issues in Career*, 73.
8. Hall and Marsh, 2003, *Legal Issues in Career*, 81.
9. Fischer, Schimmel, and Kelly, 1999, *Teachers and the Law*, 80.
10. Hall and Marsh, 2003, *Legal Issues in Career*, 315-316.
11. Hall and Marsh, 2003, *Legal Issues in Career*, 224.
12. National Registry of Emergency Medical Technicians. *About NREMT*. National Registry of Emergency Medical Technicians. http://www.nremt.org/about/nremt_news.asp. 2004.
13. Nordin,V *The Contract to Educate: Toward a More Workable Theory of the Student University Relationship(1981)* Journal of College and University Law, 8(2): 141-81. In Toma, JD and Palm, RL, *The academic administrator and the law: What every dean and department chair needs to know (1999)*. ASHE-ERIC Higher Education Resport Volume 26, No 5. Washington, DC: The George Washington University, Graduate School of Education and Human Development.
14. Toma, JD, and Palm, RL: *The Academic Administrator and the Law: What Every Dean and Department Chair Needs to Know*. (1999). ASHE-ERIC Higher Education Report Volume 26, No. 5. Washington, DC: The George Washington University, Graduate School of Education and Human Development.
15. Davenport, D. (1985). The catalog in the classroom: From Shield to sword? Journal of College and University Law, 12 (2), 201-226.
16. Toma and Palm, 1999, *The Academic Administrator and the Law*, 89.
17. Hall and Marsh, 2003, *Legal Issues in Career*, 405.
18. Hall and Marsh, 2003, *Legal Issues in Career*, 286.
19. Duke University. Center for Academic Integrity Research. 2003. November 20, 2003.
20. Committee on Accreditation of Educational Programs for the Emergency Medical Services Professions. *Standards and Guidelines*, I.D.1.f. http://www.coaemsp.org/standardspolicies.htm (accessed November 21, 2003).
21. Hall and Marsh, 2003, *Legal Issues in Career*, 339.
22. U.S. Congress, *The Safe and Drug-Free Schools and Communities Act of 1994*, (20 U.S.C. § 7101).
23. Fischer, Schimmel, and Kelly, 1999, *Teachers and the Law*.
24. Hall and Marsh, 2003, *Legal Issues in Career*, 289.
25. U.S. Congress, *Occupational Safety and Health Act of 1970*. (OSH, PL 91-596), http://www.osha.gov (accessed November 24, 2003).
26. U.S. Congress, *Occupational Safety and Health Act of 1970*. (OSH, PL 91-596), http://www.osha.gov (accessed November 24, 2003).
27. Toma and Palm, 1999, *The Academic Administrator and the Law*, 115.
28. Hall and Marsh, 2003, *Legal Issues in Career*, 426.
29. Footer, NS. *FERPA for all: The basics plus*, Paper presented at the June 2001 meeting of the National Association of College and University Attorneys, San Diego, CA.
30. Lynch, JR. *Recent FERPA developments (July 2000-June 2001)*, Paper presented at the June 2001 meeting of the National Association of College and University Attorneys, San Diego, CA.
31. U.S. Congress, *Family Educational Rights and Privacy Act of* (20 U.S.C. § 1232).

32. Hall and Marsh, 2003, *Legal Issues in Career*, 293.
33. Winckler, SC (2002, February) HIPAA's privacy regulations: What the pharmacist needs to know. Presentation made at the Idaho State University College of Pharmacy, Pocatello, ID.
34. University of Texas, *Fair Use of Copyrighted Materials*, University of Texas, http://www.utsystem.edu/ogc/intellectualproperty/copypol2.htm, 2004.
35. Hall and Marsh, 2003, *Legal Issues in Career*, 452.

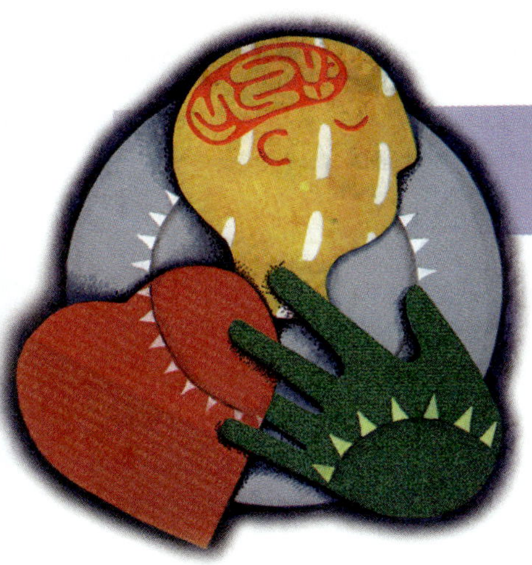

CHAPTER 11

Audiovisual Basics

"Any sufficiently advanced technology is indistinguishable from magic."

—Authur C. Clark

People interact with their environment through the five senses. The more the senses are stimulated, the stronger is the interaction. Likewise, the more senses are stimulated at one time, the more intense is the interaction. Because learning is a process by which a change in behavior is brought about through experience, one could conclude that the more senses are stimulated during the learning experience, the better the educational experience will be. One of the most common means of stimulating the senses while teaching is to use audio and visual aids, more commonly known simply as "AV." The acronym *AV* has come to include almost any tools or techniques used to supplement learning, other than a straight lecture presentation.

This chapter familiarizes the educator with various common AV techniques and equipment. It is not designed to make the educator a technological whiz or graphic designer.

TEACHING TIP: When it comes to using and creating AV equipment and materials, the instructor should know his or her personal limitations. Those who are not computer literate should not plan to use a computer as the main source of AV support. It must be remembered that the primary purpose of a class is to teach the objectives of the lesson, so one must not become distracted by technology or by the creative urge to produce an AV masterpiece.

WHAT IS AUDIOVISUAL?

AV is educational instruction provided by means of supplementary teaching aids, such as recordings, transcripts, tapes, motion pictures, videotapes, radio, television, and computers, to stimulate at least the senses of sight and hearing.[1]

The primary use of AV is to enhance students' understanding of the material by adding authenticity to what the educator is saying, thus stimulating the senses and adding to the educator's credibility.[2] AV also facilitates student learning by adding variety to break up the standard lecture; this helps to capture students' attention.

The most important thing for the educator to remember when planning and using AV is that the material and technology should supplement—not replace—the learning experience. Occasionally, a presentation may be made up extensively of a high-tech AV presentation, which may create the "Wow factor!" However, after the "wow factor" wears off, the basic material presented may also fade. To repeat, AV should merely supplement the basic educational process. An instructor should make sure that his or her use of AV material does not steal the show by evaluating how his or her presentation would be received if he or she could not use the AV portion.

USING AUDIOVISUAL MATERIALS

Here are a few basic guidelines for evaluating, planning, and using AV materials. Generally speaking, AV should summarize information, illustrate, reinforce, and draw attention to the main points. AV should not consist simply of projected copies of the printed text, and it should not be merely read to students. Moreover, transparencies should not be used as handouts.[3]

Regardless of the medium used for AV presentations, use of AV must follow six basic rules:

1. It must meet the criteria of the objective
2. It must provide a positive learning experience
3. It must fit within the allotted time
4. It must be visible to all students

5. It must be cost-effective
6. It must be available

It is important for the educator who is using a complete teaching package (i.e., lesson plans, textbook, AV, handouts, etc.) to review not only the didactic material itself, but also the AV designed for the material. The educator should consider the following when evaluating an educational teaching package, such as those provided by textbook publishers:

- Does the instructor know how to use the AV media provided?
- Is needed AV equipment available at the teaching site?
- Can the instructor present the lesson as planned without using the AV provided or in a different format?
- Will the course sponsor or administrator allow the instructor to change, alter, or customize the AV material? Or, must he or she use the AV material "as is"?
- Can the instructor alter the AV material to suit the needs of his or her students or local requirements?
- Is the AV material of good quality? Does it follow basic AV guidelines? (Commercial preparation does not ensure quality.)
- Is the AV material consistent across lessons and units? This consistency is important if a course is to be taught in modules or by multiple instructors

TEACHING TIP: The instructor must check that AV material is current and consistent with the lesson plan. The two may not be exactly compatible. It is usually cheaper to update lesson plans instead of AV materials. One must be sure to use the appropriate version of AV materials for the lesson plan that is being used. This is especially critical when computer programs are used.

The educator should keep in mind a few basic rules for the use of AV materials and technology:

- Know how to use the technology and the equipment
- Know what to do if a piece of equipment fails during a class; find out where spare parts, such as bulbs, are located and learn how to change them
- Arrive early enough to ensure that AV materials and equipment are in the classroom and ready to go. Don't forget to bring an extension cord and/or power strip just in case
- Find out whether the classroom is arranged for the correct use of the AV technology. Ascertain whether all students will be able to see and hear
- If using a piece of AV equipment later in the class, such as a model or a manikin, cover or hide the equipment so that it is not a distraction for students
- Make sure blackboards or whiteboards are clean and clear of writing from previous lessons
- Have an alternative plan. All technology has the potential to fail, so have a backup plan in the event the material or equipment cannot be used as planned
- Remember: Using AV material takes time. Plan the lesson accordingly, so as not to waste time setting up or operating equipment

CASE IN POINT

This scenario addresses perhaps the most common problem experienced by educators who use AV equipment—the projector bulb burns out! Now what should the instructor do? Regardless of whether he or she is using an LCD projector or a simple overhead projector, the teaching plan has suddenly been altered. The instructor might be lucky enough to have a new bulb available for an overhead, but most likely, he or she won't have a spare, given the cost of such bulbs. So, what can the instructor do to salvage his or her presentation? Here are a few suggestions:

- Cancel the class, but this is rarely a viable option and creates inconvenience for both students and faculty
- Switch to another means of AV presentation. Perhaps 3-mm slides can be substituted for a computer-based presentation
- Convert the media format. If an instructor has time and the right equipment, he or she could print the presentation slides as transparencies. Likewise, if he or she has prepared overheads via presentation software, the instructor could use the file as the basis for a slide show
- Skip the projected slides altogether and have the students refer to handout material. Most likely, the instructor prepared handouts of the slides for students
- Use a chalkboard or whiteboard to present key points, formulas, basic graphics, and so forth. Remember that scores of students were successfully taught this way for years before computers and projectors entered the classroom
- If an instructor was planning to project a video clip or a video, he or she could have the students break into small groups and write a descriptive script of what should be in such a video. This will force them to think of key points and procedures that would have been emphasized in the video
- Teach another lesson that does not require the AV equipment, or change the class to a skills practice and review session

One must remember that technology is the educator's helper—not the educator's replacement! The instructor must be creative and must think simply to find a solution.

TEACHING TIP: If the program does not have its own AV equipment, the instructor should reserve it from the institution well in advance. If AV support is provided from a central AV service, the needed equipment must be reserved in sufficient time to ensure its availability. Also, just because a piece of AV equipment is "always in the classroom or store room" doesn't mean it will automatically be there when needed. This is especially at locations that share resources or for off-site courses. The Saturday that an instructor plans to use an Advanced Life Support manikin may be the same Saturday that an ACLS class is being conducted off-site.

EQUIPMENT

Audio

Audio equipment can include anything from a videocassette recorder (VCR) tape to an audiotape to a compact disk read-only memory (CD-ROM) to a computer to or some type of patient care manikin, and the sounds produced by each. It is important that the volume be loud enough so that everyone can easily hear. If the device cannot produce enough volume, it must be connected to an amplifier and a sound system. Most VCRs, radios, compact disk (CD) players, cassette players, and computers have an "audio output" or headphone jack. A cable is connected from this to the amplifier input so that volume can be boosted and distributed throughout the classroom.

When an instructor uses any form of AV, he or she should consider moving students so they can hear and see properly. If an instructor has an audio device that is not loud enough to be heard throughout the classroom, students should gather around so they can hear. If the class is conducted in a large room such as an auditorium, it may be necessary for the instructor to play the sound multiple times at various locations around the room. A sound recording, such as breath sounds, must be played multiple times to ensure that students not only hear the sound, but understand it. The same applies to video clips.

Microphones

An important first step for the instructor who is planning a presentation is to determine the number and type of microphones needed. Microphones come in a variety of configurations. Those commonly found in the classroom include a wired podium microphone (lectern). This provides clear sound, involves low maintenance, and frees the educator's hands. A wireless hand microphone is sometimes found in areas in which running wires to the podium location would be difficult. This type of microphone allows the educator to move around freely, but it ties up his or her hands. Thus, many educators prefer the wireless lavaliere or lapel microphone. This wireless microphone allows the educator to move within the audience, and to keep his or her hands free to demonstrate skills.

TEACHING TIP: The instructor must be sure to turn off a wireless microphone after the class session. No one wants to broadcast throughout the classroom private conversations or sounds associated with a trip to the restroom.

If more than one audio device is used, an audio mixer must be set up. The mixer allows multiple devices to be connected to a single amplifier and set of speakers, thus causing the sound to be "mixed" to a comfortable level. The AV staff usually sets up the mixer and sound amplifier in a classroom, with the educator merely turning the entire system on or off.

TEACHING TIP: Because of the costs and desirability of microphones and related equipment, most institutions secure these devices in a locked area. The educator should plan to obtain a key or lock combination in advance.

Cassette player

An inexpensive cassette player/recorder can be used in the classroom to play recordings of lung and heart sounds or of dispatch calls from local emergency services to allow students the opportunity to hear items that may otherwise take months to hear in the field.

Audiotapes

Audio recordings can be a valuable tool in the classroom. These tapes are inexpensive and reusable, and can be played back over and over again, enhancing the learning process. A tape can be cued up to ensure that key points are not missed. Students who are audio learners versus visual learners will find tapes a useful way to prepare for exams. For instance, when a student is learning about different heart sounds, what better way than to hear them? Tapes of professional quality are recommended because the volume level on inexpensive brands may not play back well in all tape players. A word of caution with audiotapes: Most attention spans range from 7 to 8 minutes; therefore, this medium should be used in moderation and only when it will be most effective.[4]

Visual Aids

Chalkboard (blackboard)

This less "hi-tech" tool has been a staple since the late 1800s. The chalkboard, or as it is more commonly known, the blackboard, is easily seen and inexpensive, but it is not usually portable. It serves to provide a large writing surface for listing key points, comparing and contrasting information, and highlighting important points.[4] Blackboards are most effective when material is written on the board before students arrive, or for quick drawings or explanations designed to enhance classroom discussion. The material once written can be saved for only short periods and cannot be retrieved once the board has been erased. When using this medium, the instructor is required to turn away from the audience—another downside. Educators may prefer to have the information prewritten on the board, or they may investigate another medium altogether.

Whiteboard (dry-erase board)

The whiteboard is a newer version of the chalkboard, and it has been an integral part of education for years. The whiteboard, as well as the chalkboard, allows the educator to convey spontaneous thoughts, to clarify spelling, and to illustrate ideas.[5] For classroom purposes, whiteboard markers must be erasable.

TEACHING TIP: A presentation board should always be erased entirely. Erasing a small spot in the middle of some old material to write something new does not take the learner into consideration. When finished with a lesson, the instructor should always erase the whiteboard entirely. Leaving marker ink on the board for a long time makes it more difficult to remove later. It's also good form to leave a clean board for the next instructor. Whiteboards should be cleaned regularly with a special cleaner that protects the surface and makes erasure easier.

Electronic whiteboard

This modern version of the whiteboard and blackboard provides a multipage, multiuser drawing application. The user can draw designs or charts on the electronic whiteboard device for display during a presentation. These images can be saved on a computer for future use. Digital images can also be displayed onto the whiteboard.[6]

Flip chart/posterboard

The flip chart is a low-tech, inexpensive, and easily transportable visual aid. Flip charts can be personalized for a particular situation and prepared in advance. They are great for small meetings, allow for spontaneous thoughts, and provide a way to retain information. Flip charts can help facilitate student-educator communication and can reinforce important points. Hanging the pages on the wall allows for quick review of key points. This tool offers a valuable alternative to the chalkboard or dry-erase board.[6]

TEACHING TIP: The instructor must be sure to get approval before taping flip chart pages onto walls or other surfaces. Also, tape that does not damage the finish should be used. IMPORTANT: An instructor should not write on paper that is placed against a wall or other surface. The marker ink may bleed through.

Models and manikins

Not often thought of as AV materials, static displays and interactive devices such as manikins are an important adjunct to EMS education. The instructor who uses models and manikins should follow some simple guidelines:

- A device or adjunct to be used for teaching must be prepared in advance. This ensures that the device is complete and working well and minimizes loss of class time for preparation
- The device must be placed in the classroom in such a way that it is not distracting to the students before they are ready to use it. This is especially relevant for new or complicated devices that students may not have seen before. Students should be concentrating on the lesson—not trying to figure out or study a device they have not seen before. Something as simple as throwing a sheet over a manikin or anatomic model before use is effective
- The instructor must be sure that the model or manikin is correct and is similar to the actual object or patient under discussion. For example, an adult manikin should not be used for demonstration of pediatric interventions
- The model should be large enough that all students can see all parts of its operation
- The model should enhance the educational message—not distract from it
- After the model or manikin has been used, it should be moved aside so it does not become a distraction to students

TEACHING TIP: When a device that has multiple parts or that requires assembly and preparation is part of the procedure to be presented to the class, the use of a checklist will ensure that the device is ready for use in the classroom.

Models may be anatomic in nature (Figure 11-1), such as torso sets, individual organs, and cut-away views, or they may be enlarged versions of devices used in the field, such as syringes or laryngoscopes. Models can also be actual equipment used in demonstrations.

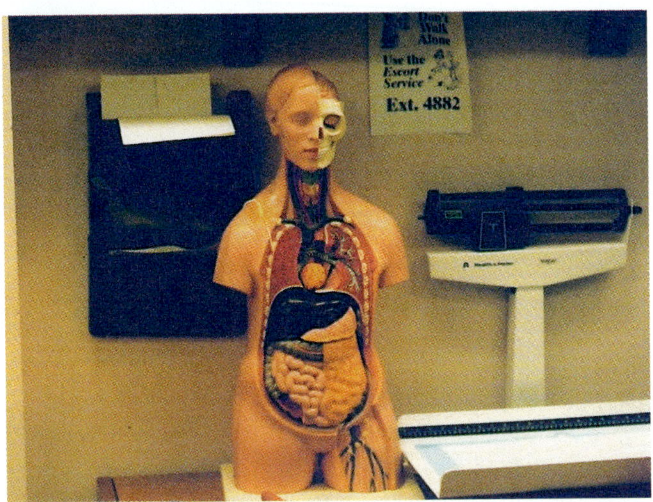

FIGURE 11-1 Models can be a useful instructional adjunct for helping students to see as well as feel.

To be effective, a model should be easy to set up, easy to use, and easy to maintain.

Human manikins, either whole body forms or anatomic sections, are a useful tool in the classroom. Because many EMS skills cannot be demonstrated or practiced on a live "patient," manikins provide a high degree of fidelity to the real thing. They also allow the instructor to alter responses from the manikin in accordance with student interventions.

Many interactive manikins are available on the market. Prices range from $200 for a simple unit to $50,000 or higher for the more complex ones (Box 11-1). The instructor might consider that the simpler the design of a manikin is, the easier it will be to care for and maintain. A manikin should be suited to the skills the student has trained to acquire, and it should be durably constructed (Figure 11-2).

Projectors

Several types of projectors are in use in today's classroom. Each has its own special place and use.

Overhead projectors

The overhead projector is the simplest of AV equipment, and despite its "low-tech" or "no-tech" nature, it is an excellent AV method.[6] The mirrored system projects a transparency of up to a 10-inch by 10-inch size on a flat surface, such as a projection screen or a wall. Despite its simplicity, it is very versatile and portable.[6] Overhead transparencies can be printed in full color, which is useful for projection of anatomic drawings, and they can be printed from most popular computer software on an inkjet or laser printer. They are easy and inexpensive to create, file, and store, and

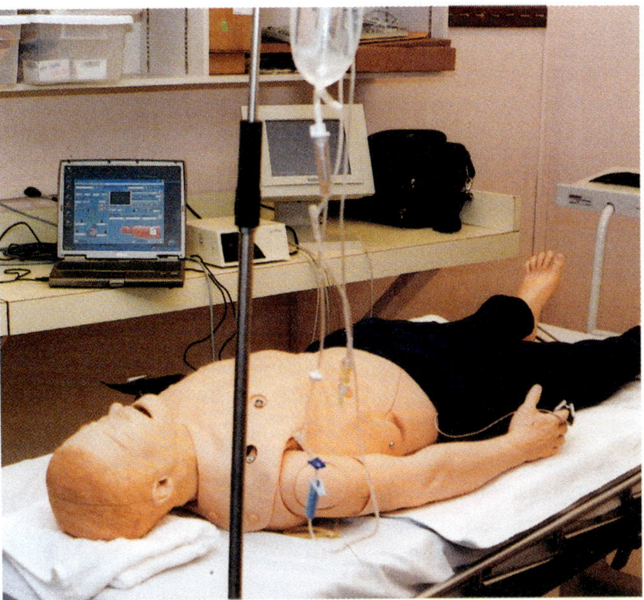

FIGURE 11-2 Simulation manikins can assist students in "putting it all together," or developing critical thinking skills.

they can be edited at a moment's notice, even during class.

The overhead projector allows the educator to face the audience while delivering information in a lit room. It is a good medium for groups of almost any size because it can project a large image that is viewable in normal room light. An overhead provides students with a reliable tool, when it is used appropriately. It also gives the instructor the ability to convey spontaneous thoughts through the use of transparency material and a grease marker or transparency marking pen. An overhead is the ideal AV for displaying a large amount of text, such as a protocol. The instructor can keep the class focused on the content that is being discussed by covering up the portion of the transparency that has not yet been covered.

TEACHING TIP: An instructor can evaluate whether the overhead transparency will be readable in class by placing the transparency between his or her feet and reading it. If he or she cannot read what is written on the transparency, the font is too small.

Overhead media come in inkjet, laser, copier, and write-on formats. One must be sure to select the appropriate type and to print on the correct side. Use of the wrong type media, or printing on the incorrect side, will cause the print to fall off the page if it is bent. One of the major downsides of this medium is the expense of the media and bulbs. Bulbs burn out frequently, requiring that a spare be readily available at all times.

BOX II-1 Simulation: A New Education Tool for EMS

by Kevin L. Parrish, RN, EMT-P

Human simulation training is defined as a team training methodology that utilizes a sensorized mannequin, capable of generating measurable and/or observable clinical parameters, to create realistic clinical scenarios. Simulation training is not new. The airline industry has made use of flight simulators for years. However, medicine lags 20 years behind other industries in the use of simulation as a way to reduce the incidence of error.

Simulators offer a tremendous learning experience. They present the opportunity for students to learn in all three learning domains: visual, auditory, and kinesthetic.

Visually, there's a lot to look at. Human simulators can be equipped with trauma limbs that simulate actual bleeding gunshot or stab wounds. The chest rises and falls in symphony with the breathing pattern selected by the operator. ECG, Pao_2, and capnography readings are displayed on monitors. Realistic airway anatomy offers the opportunity to intubate a "real" patient.

The auditory learner has a lot to listen to. Simulators have the ability to generate audible breath sounds that represent a myriad of functional and dysfunctional lung sounds. Bowel sounds and heart tones are also available. Perhaps the most useful tool is a microphone placed in the simulator's head through which instructors can listen and respond to student's questions and observations, essentially "talking" as the patient. This last feature may influence affective behaviors in student populations.

Lastly, the kinesthetic learner has a lot to feel and do. Features include palpable, anatomically correct pulses, the ability to physically measure blood pressures and compress the chest adds to the realism and practical application of those skills. Psychomotor skills involving defibrillation, starting an IV, intubation, and needle decompression of the chest can be performed. Simulators allow the practice of psychomotor skills that cannot be practiced on student partners or that might otherwise need to be taught and practiced in expensive cadaver labs.

Most significantly, human simulators allow EMS professionals to practice in an environment that presents no risk to actual patients. Here, students can make mistakes that might kill a patient without the requisite risk. Multiple teams and individuals can be trained in the exact same scenario. Also, simulators offer the ultimate in standardized evaluations, presenting each student with exactly the same patient to treat without regard to any personal or professional bias the instructor may, or may be perceived, to have.

Simulators also work in real-world environments. They can be placed in wrecked cars for extrication or at simulated disaster sites. Currently, the military uses patient simulators placed on simulated battlefields. Medics treat these casualties; remove them to field hospitals, and even evacuate them on real troop transports. Entire training planes have been equipped with these simulators to ensure the battle readiness of medical corpsmen.

Yet, in spite of all of these advantages, the use of human simulators and acceptance of simulation training has yet to have widespread application in emergency medical services. Why?

One reason is that human simulators are a new technology. The first simulators appeared on the market in the mid-1980s and were extremely expensive, costing anywhere from $250,000 to $400,000. Large, bulky, and stationary, they were also maintenance intensive, often requiring another full-time person to maintain and run the simulator in addition to the instructor.

Technology has reduced these barriers to entry substantially. Current simulators are available anywhere from $10,000

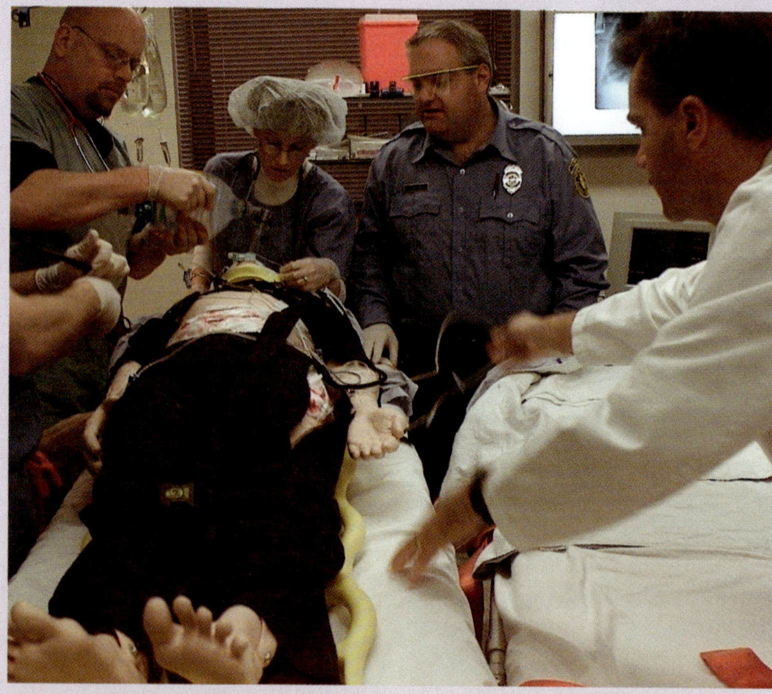

Simulation training allows realistic case scenarios to be presented in the classroom setting without introducing risk for injury or harm during student skills practice. (Courtesy of Laerdal.)

BOX 11-1 Simulation: A New Education Tool for EMS—cont'd

by Kevin L. Parrish, RN, EMT-P

to $75,000. They are smaller, mobile, and have much lower maintenance requirements than in the past (typically, the instructor running the simulator can perform any routine maintenance). Advances in software and hardware allow these newer simulators to run directly from PCs and laptops. Intuitive user interfaces enable instructors to develop customized scenarios and training without programming expense (the interfaces actually perform object-oriented programming while making the process invisible to the instructor-designer).

A remaining issue is the newness of the technology and instructor familiarity with it. Instructors who are new to this educational methodology will require exposure to its philosophy and application. Also, simulation training works best in a team training environment. Since instructors can utilize simulators to create realistic training scenarios to teach good behaviors that reflect the real world, some may feel the need to hone their own skills and knowledge in order to use these simulators effectively.

Then, there are technological fears and phobias. It has taken over 10 years and countless studies to validate the fact that students can indeed learn from computer-based programs. To progress from lecture-based instruction and skill stations on "dumb" mannequins to widespread team training on "smart" simulators will require instructors to embrace technology as never before. Such an embrace may require the development of educational tools like preprogrammed scenarios for use by instructors. Instructors may also require reeducation in terms of how they teach cognitive and psychomotor skills. Certainly, using this technology affords the opportunity to train EMS personnel to work as a team in a realistic setting with a realistic patient without introducing the risk of injury or harm.

Simulation training and the use of a human simulator are new educational tools. These tools present a real opportunity for EMS educators to make a difference in the educational outcomes of their students. More importantly, they may significantly translate educational outcomes into definable clinical practices that reduce the incidence of medical errors in the field. The result may be the increased patient safety that is the goal of all providers.

35-mm slide projectors

The "slide projector" has been a staple of education for years but is now being replaced by the computer projector. Slides are inserted into the carousel-style projector upside down and backward.[4] The slide projector is a line of sight media device (i.e., a clear path from the device to the screen must be ensured). The standard projector works well in a small meeting room with a small group, with the use of a projection screen of 10 feet or less.[6] One limitation of using slides with large groups is that they might require a longer projection distance (up to 90 feet) or a larger screen (12 feet wide or wider). Additionally, compared with newer technology, slides are static in nature and cannot be as easily changed as images from presentation software.

The slide projector can be moved back and forth to increase the size of the image so that all students can view it. If the projector must be moved very far from the podium, one should consider using a wireless remote, use of which allows free movement around the room.

TEACHING TIP: Many publishers offer a 35-mm slide set to accompany their texts. These slides may become rapidly outdated. One solution to this dilemma is to pull outdated slides and replace them with slides that have been prepared with the use of presentation software. Up-to-date slides can be saved and sent to a local photo shop for conversion to 35-mm slides. This allows the educator to continue to use a set of slides for several class terms before they must be replaced.

CASE IN POINT

An instructor is teaching an EMT continuing education class at a local rescue squad. Resources are limited, and he has access only to a commercially prepared 35-mm slide set that was created to match the third edition of the course textbook. He is using the current edition, which is the fifth edition. He knows from using the "old" slides that numerous changes have been made to the information and inconsistencies can be seen between the slides and the current text. What are his options?

- Don't use the slides at all. This will mean that he has to just lecture, or he must prepare his own AV materials
- Prepare his own AV materials. This will be time consuming, and if he doesn't have a computer with presentation software, very difficult
- Edit the slides, and use only those that are still appropriate. Treatments and protocols change, but not so drastically that all of the slides will be useless
- Look for alternative AV materials from such sources as the state EMS office or on the Web at the NAEMSE *Trading Post.* Contact other instructors to see if they have material that can be borrowed or copied. The local public library may be a good source for AV materials. Most libraries participate in interlibrary loan programs, and library staff may be able to locate resources. The same goes for the education office of the local hospital
- He should not, however, use the old slide set "as is." The outdated material will only confuse students, and if he doesn't point it out and discuss it, this will reduce his credibility. He should refrain from making excuses for not having current AV materials

TEACHING TIP: A marking pen should be used for drawing a concentric arc on the tops of the slides in a carousel. In the event a slide, or slides, falls out, it is easy to find where it belongs.

LCD projectors

Both liquid crystal display (LCD) projectors and digital light processing (DLP) are suitable for the classroom. Both project computer presentation software and graphic images through a laptop or desktop computer. The LCD is the more common of the two and the least expensive. It also has the versatility to be placed close to a screen, or as far away as 140 feet. LCD projectors can produce images larger than 40 feet wide. If the audience is made up of more than 100 people, use of an LCD projector should be considered because it has a higher light output.[6]

A disadvantage of the LCD projector is the cost of equipment and maintenance. Although the cost has decreased and the quality of the projected image has increased, some programs may not be able to afford these projectors. Additionally, replacement bulbs can be very expensive, with costs of about $600 for a bulb that lasts approximately 2000 hours (Figure 11-3).

The instructor should consider three main points when shopping for a classroom projector:

A

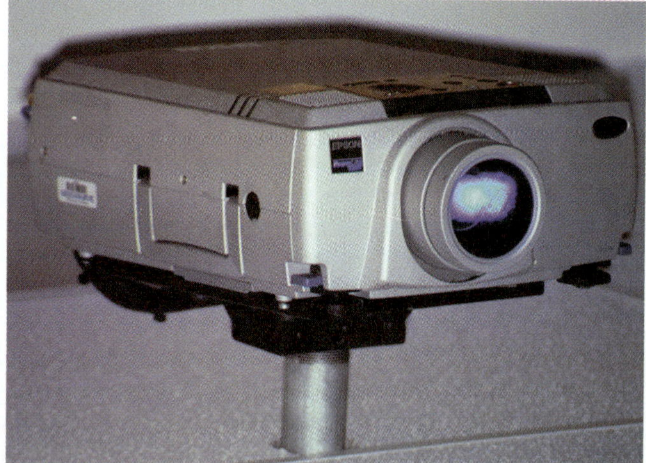

B

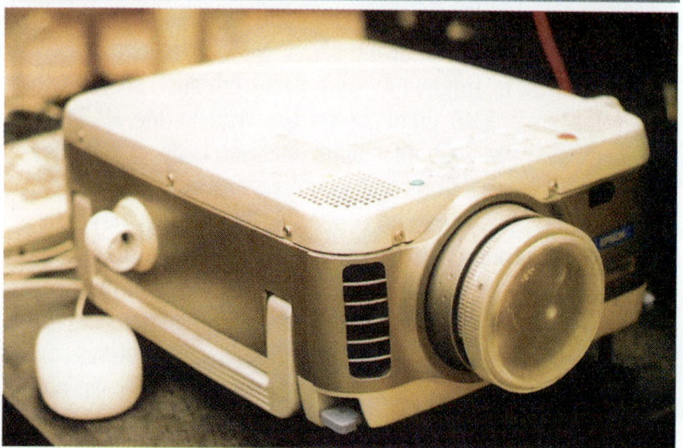

FIGURE 11-3 LCD projectors can be ceiling mounted **(A)** or portable **(B)**.

1. Brightness
2. Resolution (the amount of detail the projector can capture)
3. Features (e.g., ability to project video, remote mouse, speakers)

The minimum brightness for a classroom projector is about 700 ANSI lumens, whereas brightness of 1500 to 2000 lumens is needed for clear projection in a fully lighted apparatus bay. Prices on new equipment range from $1000 to $10,000, depending on size, resolution, and features. Many are available that will fit in a laptop case for transport to off-campus classrooms.

TEACHING TIP: Most modern projectors are compatible with current computer operating systems, including Windows and Macintosh. However, one should always test for compatibility and make sure to have the proper connecting cables. Additionally, computer projectors generate a large amount of heat. Laptop computers must not be placed on top of the projector housing; this might block airflow. The instructor should be sure to follow the manufacturer's recommendation for a cool-down period before turning off the projector.

Projector screens

Choosing the right projector screen for a presentation is as important as choosing the right projector. When deciding which screen to use, one should first determine the size of the room. This will help in deciding appropriate screen size, as will capacity, dimensions, and ceiling height of the room.[6] Once appropriate screen size has been determined, other considerations such as type, format, and material can be addressed. However, a technical discussion of these parameters is beyond the scope of this chapter and is best left to the AV professional.

TEACHING TIP: In determining the screen size to use, one should divide the distance from the screen to the last row of the audience by 8, and use the resulting number as the height of the screen. For example, if the distance between the screen and the last row is 120 feet, 120 divided by 8 equals 15; therefore, the screen should be at least 15 feet high.

Video equipment

Video equipment can be divided into two broad groups: sources and display devices. A piece of equipment that produces a video signal is the source, and the equipment used to view the signal is the display device.[6]

VCR players

The VCR is a true multimedia device, allowing the student to see and hear at the same time information that is in full motion. Videotapes are beneficial to an educator because they are often professionally produced and include examples that cannot be paralleled by still pictures or descriptions.[5] One of the most important factors in the quality of a video recording is the videotape format. Most tapes are Video Home System (VHS) or Super-VHS (S-VHS).

The VHS videotape has replaced the 16-mm film as the standard in almost every classroom. This convenience comes at a price though. Many tapes are expensive, and because the medical field is constantly changing, tapes may be outdated after only one class. Many publishers offer sets of videotapes that cover much of the information in a course. Some videotapes do not follow local protocols, however, and others may have errors in them. It is imperative that the educator review the tape before class and watch the tape with students to point out potential problems. Remember that it's not necessary to show an entire video; select pertinent parts and show only those segments of the tape.

Another matter for consideration when the videotape is used is delivery method. A 25-inch television is the smallest television that should be considered for use in the classroom. Televisions of smaller size would not be seen by students and do not show details clearly enough. An LCD projector can also be used to show videotapes, thus providing a much larger image than is possible on a conventional TV. Newer projectors are cheaper than large-screen televisions, and the size of the image is easily adjustable to the size of the classroom.

DVD players

The Digital Versatile Disk (DVD) is rapidly replacing the videotape, and it is more durable. This disk does not stretch over time, as a tape does. In addition, the picture remains clear even after the disk has been played many times. DVDs can also be played in computers with a DVD drive. Although the DVD medium is currently more expensive than videotape, the price is expected to drop as DVDs become more popular.

A large amount of material can be stored on a DVD; therefore, publishers can provide multiple scenarios and situations for a lesson, as opposed to the typical single example provided with more restrictive formats such as videotape. Some DVDs are now being produced that are capable of being interactive when used in a computer.

Cameras

The most common types of cameras are still (film based), video (camcorder), and digital. A video camera is often used with audiences of more than 1000 to make the educator more visible, because it allows for very detailed images to be seen more clearly on a large screen.[6]

A digital camera does not use film but instead has a sensor that converts light into electrical charges.[7] The resolution of a camera (detail captured) is measured in pixels. The more pixels the camera has, the greater the details that can be captured. Some advantages of a digital camera include that pictures can be viewed immediately on the camera's LCD screen; pictures can be downloaded to a computer for printing, e-mailing, or posting on the Internet; and unwanted pictures can be easily deleted. Furthermore, digital cameras interface easily with printers to produce hard copy images that can be used for review or evaluation.

If the educator will be demonstrating a skill, he or she should consider using a camera that is hooked to a television and can be displayed to the class, or it may be hooked to an LCD projector for a larger image. This is often easier than the "let's gather 'round the table'" approach used in many classrooms. In larger classes, some students will not be able to see the demonstration; in others, students will see it upside-down and backward. The educator does not need to spend hundreds or thousands of dollars for an ELMO camera, which is a digital visual presenter that connects directly to a video or data projector for real-time big screen and monitor viewing of print documents, 3D objects, photos, or slides. It is essentially a digital overhead projector that can be used in the same way as a traditional overhead projector, which is great for a skills demonstration.[8] However, if the educator has a camcorder, he or she can mount it on a tripod, hook the video out to the television or projector, and show the images. If the educator chooses to go the camcorder route, he or she can use it to record student performance in practical settings, then play it back for a classroom critique. When using either the ELMO or a camcorder, the educator can also focus the camera on a book or a sheet of paper and can project it to a television or onto a screen using an LCD projector.

TEACHING TIP: The instructor can ask a student to play the part of a reporter and to capture the images live and up-close with narration.

Computer-Based Equipment

Computer presentations

A newer tool for the educator is the computer. It can provide a powerful and interesting way to present material. Computer presentations are like an adjunct to learning.[4] The most common computer presentation is the slide show, which often replaces overhead transparencies or 35-mm slides.[4] Computer presentations are usually shown on a large computer screen or television, or they may be projected onto a screen.[5]

Presentation software allows the educator to create a presentation with a professional look (Box 11-2). He or she can easily include color and graphics, as well as animation. Modifications or revisions can be made easily. The downside involves the cost of the computer and software and the technical problems that can plague the educator. Although this is a highly recommended format, it is always best to have another medium as a backup. If budget is of the utmost concern, and a projector that displays computer images is unavailable, one should consider printing overhead transparencies from a presentation.

TEACHING TIP: Knowledge and passion for a subject can usually communicate more effectively than a colorful, jazzed-up PowerPoint presentation.

Most publishers offer presentation slides as part of their resource libraries. Slides can be purchased from a textbook vendor or downloaded from a Web site (such as the NAEMSE *Trading Post,* available at http://www.NAEMSE.org), or the educator can make his or her own slides. Each option has its advantages and disadvantages. When slides are purchased from a vendor, they are usually generic and cover the basic points of a lesson. Frequently, material must be added to a lesson so it follows local practice. Because many presentation slides are distributed on CD-ROM, the educator must save the file to the hard drive when making modifications. The advantage to purchasing a full set of slides is that one does not have to start from scratch. If budget and time are both concerns, one should consider downloading a presentation from the Internet. An Internet search on a particular topic usually yields a number of possibilities of free downloads. However, one must be careful to verify the information contained in the slides, and to check that material has not been taken from copyrighted sources without permission.

Educators can also make their own slides and will need a computer and software to produce these. Many slides that are used in the field today can be designed with the use of presentation software (Figure 11-4).

BOX 11-2 PowerPoint Presentation Software Tips

1. Minimize words—use key words only
2. Use no more than six words per line and no more than six lines
3. Font size should be 22 points or larger
4. Use numerals instead of text when possible
5. Abbreviate freely
6. Use simple templates without background clutter
7. Consider using graphs instead of tables
8. Use art only when it helps to say something
9. Never use bad art, even if it's pertinent
10. Use animation only when it helps to make a point; otherwise, it's a distraction
11. Use sound only to support points, not to distract the audience
12. Use high-contrast colors—dark blue or shaded blue backgrounds, with text in yellow or white

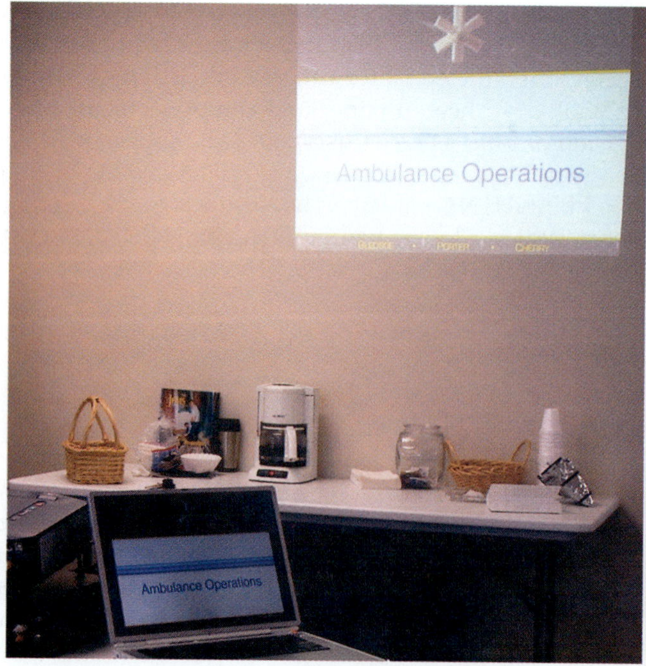

A

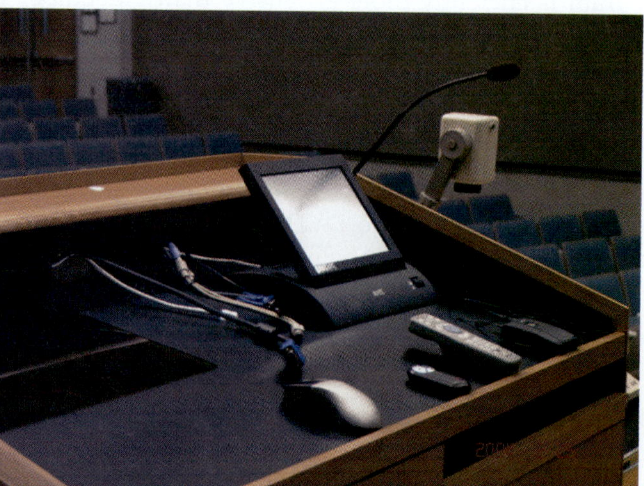
B

FIGURE 11-4 Presentation software can be delivered through a laptop and portable projector **(A)** or through a high-end built-in AV system **(B).**

Presentation programs provide templates that can help the educator to produce visually appealing slides, thus making the task easier for the novice. Medical graphics are also available as packages from vendors or via the Internet. However, the educator is cautioned to understand the legal restrictions involved in downloading and copying graphics and other files that contain copyrighted material.

TEACHING TIP: Although many available programs claim to convert presentations from other formats, some features or formatting may be lost in the conversion process.

Internet

A high-speed connection to the Internet that is available in the classroom provides many opportunities for the educator and for students. The instructor can go to Web sites to show students information firsthand, or he or she can demonstrate the availability of additional information on a topic. Presentations can be used directly, without the need for downloading, especially when graphic- or animation-intensive, large files are used. In addition, sites such as MERGINET.com provide up-to-date information on emerging and important Emergency Medical Services (EMS)-related issues.

In addition to being a resource, the Internet can be used as a tool for course administration. A class Web site can be established that contains course information, as well as the computer presentations used in class. The instructor can post to the Web site additional materials, readings, practice exams, scenarios, and so forth, to assist students in mastering course material.

Multipoint communication (telecommunications)

Three forms of telecommunication have become increasingly popular over recent years: teleconferencing, video conferencing, and Web conferencing. Teleconferencing uses telephones to link persons from around the world. The most common technique is conference calling.[4] Video conferencing uses satellites or cables, along with teleconferencing, which allows for greater interaction between students and instructors. The fastest-growing type of multipoint communication is Web conferencing. This enables two individuals or groups to communicate via the Internet through voice, video, data, or a combination of the three. This technique is not costly, and both students and instructor can participate from the office, home, or classroom.[6]

Accessory Devices

Laser pointer

A common piece of audiovisual accessory equipment is the laser pointer. This relatively inexpensive, small piece of equipment allows the instructor to visually highlight key points during a presentation, without blocking students' view of the material.[6] Some projector remote controls or a remote computer mouse include laser pointers, which allow the educator to handle only one device while teaching. Because the pointer uses a laser beam, the educator should use caution to avoid projecting the beam directly at any person, especially into the eyes. As with any AV device, overuse of the pointer can become more of a distraction than an aid to learning.

TEACHING TIP: If the educator is nervous or doesn't have a steady hand, he or she should use a circular motion when highlighting a word or phrase with the laser pointer. This minimizes the impression of shakiness.

Remote mouse

Radio frequency or infrared remote computer mice are available; these allow the instructor to move beyond the range of a typical hardwired mouse. This option is useful when the instructor wants to move around the classroom, or when the computer must be set up at a remote location.

TEACHING TIP: An instructor who is using a radio frequency remote device must make sure that it doesn't interfere with similar devices that may be in use in adjacent classrooms.

EMERGING TECHNOLOGY

Several new items have entered the AV market. One is the PicShare device, which is a synchronous remote photo-sharing system. PicShare saves the presentation as a series of JPEG files and copies them or saves them to the removable memory in the PicShare device. The device is then connected to a television or projector and the slide show begins, with the use of the remote that is included to control the show. This has eliminated the need for a laptop computer. PicShare retails for less than $50.[9]

The Margi Presenter-to-Go is a device that attaches to a personal digital assistant (PDA) or PocketPC device and connects to a VGA port on an LCD projector. Although slides cannot be created on the Margi device, it does facilitate travel without a laptop.[9]

SUMMARY

The educator's mission is to change students' behavior in a positive way through exposure to meaningful learning experiences. These learning experiences involve stimulation of students' senses to enhance the intake and retention of knowledge, skills, and attitudes needed for mastery of the course objectives.

Audiovisual equipment allows the educator to stimulate more senses in multiple ways to maximize the learning experience. However, the educator must constantly keep in mind that although AV is a useful tool for presenting educational material, it must not overshadow the educational message itself. Proper use of AV requires planning, preparation, and practice on the part of the instructor.

REFERENCES

1. Audiovisual education. Encyclopedia.com [Internet]. Available at: http://www.encyclopedia.com/printable.asp?url=/ssi/a1/audiovis.html
2. The Virtual Presentation Assistant—University of Kansas. Available at: www.ukans.edu/cwis/units/coms2/vpa/vpa7.htm
3. Guidelines for using AV. Available at: www.2myprofessor.com/Common/guidlines_for_using_audiovisual.htm
4. Parvensky CA. *Teaching EMS: An Educator's Guide to Improved EMS Instruction.* St. Louis, Mo: Mosby; 1995:121, 125, 131, 145, 148.
5. AV benefits. Available at: http://www.3.uakron.edu/schlcomm/Turner/avbenfts.htm.
6. Polivka EG, ed. *Professional Meeting Management.* Chicago, Ill: Education Foundation of the Professional Convention Management Association; 2002:199, 226-228, 364.
7. HowStuffWorks: how digital cameras work. Available at: www.howstuffworks.com/digital-camera.htm/printable
8. Presentation available at: http:/www.elmousa.com/presentation/menu/htm
9. Chris Nollette and Mickey Moore, interview.

PART IV

Delivering the Message

One thing is true about the learning process: it is not static. Learning can take on many different shapes, can employ all forms of media, and may involve groups of many sizes and activities of all kinds. One must add to this the fact that Emergency Medical Services (EMS) educators and students must adapt the learning process to some of the most difficult circumstances known to education. The educator must consider the need to coach a single student on assessing pulses with a lab manikin; teach spinal immobilization to a small group in severe heat or in a very cold temperature; explain cardiac physiology through a distance education course; and model compassionate patient care during an actual call for a sick drunk person. In all these situations, EMS educators must tailor their instruction if the best results are to be achieved.

Variety is the spice of life, as the saying goes, and so it is with teaching. The tips and techniques described in these chapters are tools that you will undoubtedly find useful in your practice. This part of the text introduces teaching strategies for individual students, small groups, large groups, distance learning students, and students in field and clinical settings. One must remember that trying a few techniques that are just a bit outside one's comfort zone might just be surprisingly rewarding.

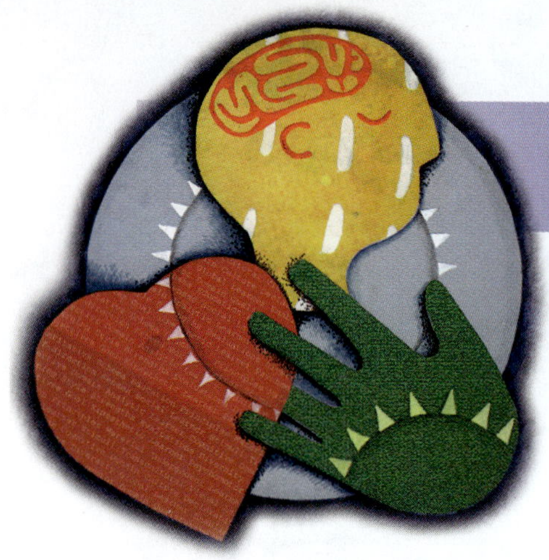

CHAPTER 12

Introduction to Teaching Strategies

"The mediocre teacher tells. The good teacher explains. The superior teacher demonstrates. The great teacher inspires."

—*William Arthur Ward*

TRADITIONAL EDUCATION AND EMERGING TRENDS

Educator-Centered Learning

Traditional education uses as its centerpiece the lecture format, which creates a teacher-centered environment. EMS educators have relied on this presentation style because so much information must be presented in such a short time frame. Although the lecture format itself is not problematic, total reliance on this type of teaching tool can lead to problems because of its teacher-centered approach. Some problems encountered with the educator-centered format include the following:

1. *The lecture and the textbook become the major delivery system of information for students.* Students are expected to listen, read, and be prepared to take and pass tests. Their success is determined by how well they can memorize the information that is presented. This type of instruction places a high value on the cognitive and psychomotor domains with little time placed on the affective domain.
2. *Students are relegated to the role of being submissive while the instructor is all-powerful and all-knowing.* The instructor talks and students listen with only minimal interaction. This learning approach leads to the pouring out of technical information with little understanding of whether students are assimilating the information that is being received. Many instructors feel this is a necessary evil because of the amount of material that must be delivered in such a short time.
3. *Students must be kept in a constant state of fear so they can be controlled.* Instructors do not begin with the idea of trying to create a fearful environment, but a teacher-centered environment by its very nature puts forth this unspoken rule. Should the students become too talkative, it might slow down the quantity of information that the instructor can provide.
4. *The affective component of education is not prized—only the cognitive and psychomotor skills are addressed.* A teacher-centered environment does not provide time for the instructor to facilitate development of the whole person. The focus is on ensuring that students have the information needed to pass their exams.
5. *Students are not allowed to be stakeholders in the direction and scope of their education.* Instructors know best and dictate the pace and focus of students' education. Instructors who subscribe to this philosophy maintain that students who fall behind must not have the aptitude needed to master the information.

The instructor-centered approach as a content delivery method has been the focal point of EMS education because it is the way EMS educators themselves have been taught—instructors teach as they have been taught. Student-teacher interaction may be marked with varying degrees of mistrust, fear, or frustration because this is a somewhat autocratic style. When any type of barrier is raised, learning decreases and both parties do not experience the full benefits of a shared environment. Another teaching approach— one that is effective in EMS and in mainstream education—is a student-centered approach.

Student-Centered Learning

EMS education, similar to mainstream education, involves moving from a traditional, instructor-centered approach to a learner-based approach. In an attempt to meet the varying needs of different learners, instructors are beginning to venture out and explore new ways of teaching and making the classroom as interactive as possible. This change is being driven by an awareness of the need to fully engage students in their learning and to enable them to develop critical thinking and problem-solving skills. In contrast, the traditional curriculum is perceived as reflecting a vast amount of content, which could be construed as a "passing parade of insubstantial content."[1]

A student-centered approach uses innovative teaching strategies that create an active and exciting learning environment. This does not mean that some traditional approaches such as lecture are abandoned; rather, they are only refined for the purpose of creating a more interactive environment in which students can participate in their education. A student-centered approach creates a shared experience wherein the student becomes a shareholder in the educational process. A student-centered approach introduces a sense of community to the learning process. This sense of community creates active learners as opposed to the more passive learners associated with the traditional educator-centered learning process. The following points will assist the instructor in creating an active learning environment:

1. The learning process is fluid and should be engaging for the teacher and for students. The goal is discovery of information and a shared commitment to excellence. Subjects are explored from a variety of sources inside and outside the classroom. Students present materials to the class and have some control as to the pace of instruction and the amount of material that is shared. If students have a problem understanding a module, more time can be committed to ensure mastery of a particular area. This process minimizes the artificial time constraints that are typically imposed on the learning process

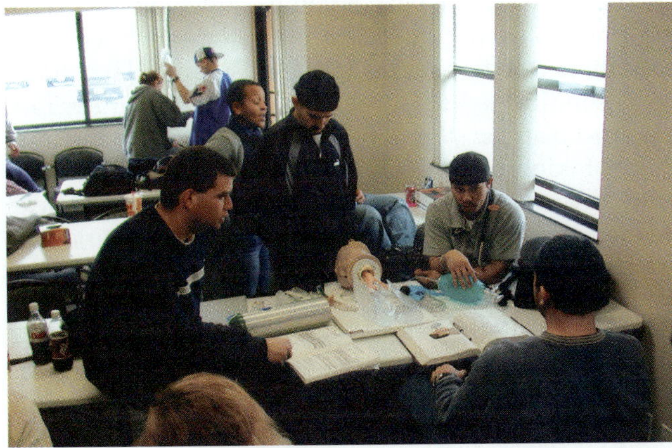

FIGURE 12-1 Learner-centered classes bring a sense of personal responsibility into the classroom.

2. The experiences of students are respected, and the teacher becomes more of a facilitator than the focal point of instruction. Students are viewed as experts who have a wide array of life experiences that they bring to the classroom experience. The students' own experiences are woven into the instruction so that clarity can be achieved from various points of view. Students are encouraged to relate their life experiences to the material that is presented
3. Students are given responsibilities in the classroom, lab, and clinical setting to foster a sense of community, respect, and discipline (Figure 12-1). The profession requires that students be ready to accept leadership responsibilities. The seeds of leadership can be planted in the classroom by assignment of roles that allow students to practice and improve their leadership skills. The classroom experience can be enhanced by appointment of a class representative, a role taker, equipment personnel, note takers, lab assistants, and team leaders on community service projects. Another effective technique is to pair advanced students with instructional staff in the lab to help train and educate students who need more help. This cooperative educational technique is a powerful and productive tool for any EMS institution. Although the intended goal is to build leadership skills, the instructor will also note that many positive and powerful attributes in terms of respect, discipline, and a sense of community are realized. In the final analysis, students become a part of the learning process and are better prepared to enter the profession
4. One of the goals of EMS education is to create lifelong learners and prepare them for a career of self-discovery in a constantly changing and dynamic profession. Students should not view the end of the class as the end of their education. EMS is a critical field in which students must become lifelong learners if they are to be successful. Weekly assignments that require students to read about their profession and present topics of interest to their classmates are crucial in establishing the need for continued education and discovery in a complex and changing profession
5. A concerted effort is made to develop the whole student through equal emphasis placed on values and character as they relate to academic study. Too many instructors believe that the value of an education for students is measured in their success in tackling the cognitive and psychomotor domains. Very little value has been placed on the affective domain, which has the greatest consequence in terms of how a student will perform over the long run. This area is more critical than are all the facts and figures that instructors push students to master. Helping students understand their strengths and limitations in relation to their values and character

can mean more to a student or an employer than has been understood. It is essential that instructors learn and teach to the affective domain to ensure that students can deal with the stress and frustrations that they will face when they hit the streets

CASE IN POINT

Classroom Topic: Shock

Instructor-Centered Method

The instructor tells students to read the shock chapter in the assigned textbook, then provides a lecture to support what is in the textbook. Follow-up consists of a written test on the subject.

Learner-Centered Method

The instructor asks students to take out a blank piece of paper and write down in their own words the definition of *shock*, as they understand it. Once students have had 3 or 4 minutes to formulate a response, they are paired up with another student in the class to compare answers. Each pair must arrive at an entirely new definition based on input from both students. Once each pair of students has developed a revised definition, the instructor requests that each team pair up with another team and repeat the process. The pairing process is repeated until three or four large groups have been formed, each with its own definition arrived at through teamwork and collaboration. At the conclusion of the exercise, each team reads its definition or writes it on the board. The instructor asks the class to compare and contrast the various definitions until final agreement is reached regarding which definition is best.

The Case in Point on shock definition puts students at the center of the learning and places the instructor in the role of facilitating the process. Students remain active throughout the process by formulating responses, arguing their position, practicing compromise, and looking at things critically. This student-centered, active, multidimensional approach is the very "glue" that will help reinforce the subject matter and make it stick.

TECHNIQUES TO ENHANCE STUDENT-CENTERED LEARNING

Several techniques and concepts are common to enhancing student-centered learning, whether this is done in individual student sessions, small groups, or large groups. These include facilitation techniques, group work, questioning techniques, and experiential learning.

Facilitation Techniques

As has been discussed, student-centered instruction places the student at the center of the learning process, and the instructor assumes the role of facilitator. Facilitation is an important teaching strategy, and a better understanding of how it is accomplished is important for the educator.

What is *facilitation?* Creation of a relaxed atmosphere that is more learner-centered constitutes the core of facilitation. In fact, *facilitate* means "to make easier." This strategy allows the educator to create an environment in which student learning is enhanced by interaction. Coaching, mentoring, and providing positive reinforcement represent a variety of techniques that are considered facilitative strategies for learning.

Keys to facilitation

Facilitation has also been called "the *guide on the side.*" Several concepts are important in the process of facilitation, which requires active planning on the part of the instructor. One of the keys is for the instructor to create action in the classroom. This is done, in part, by avoiding lectures when possible and engaging learners in activities, such as writing, role playing, cooperative grouping, and other active learning strategies.

First, the instructor should consider the layout of the classroom (see Chapter 6 for more details). The arrangement of the classroom sends a signal to students about the class session. The use of groups in facilitation may be made most beneficial when the instructor sets up tables and semiprivate work areas so that greater interaction can take place between students and instructors. The goals of this strategy are to take the emphasis off the instructor as the "gatekeeper of information" and to place the burden of interaction with the group. This creates interaction between learners but still allows interaction with the instructor, who will manage the learning activities.

The importance of creating the expectation in learners that they will be participating actively in the learning process cannot be overstated. Students have been conditioned to be tourists in the classroom. They have been conditioned to be passive observers, much like those who are on vacation. Tourists move with the tour guide, taking pictures and having minimal interaction with anyone in the museum, then moving to the next destination. Instructors must work to limit tourists in the classroom by actively seeking student participation in the learning process, which may be foreign to many. Patience, guidance, and positive reinforcement of learners are necessary as they move into this new area. As students succeed, their expectations for learning will change in very positive ways.

Not everyone will agree with or like this new style of learning. Some students will continue to be passive learners despite the instructor's best efforts. The instructor must not be discouraged; it takes effort and persistence to move into the use of facilitation. As the instructor works to include the reluctant learner in the process, eventually the student may choose to willingly participate or may be coerced by fellow classmates to actively participate in the learning process.

Facilitating discussions

Facilitation requires active learner participation; one of the best forms of participatory learning is discussion. This technique is effective for many different types of courses, including recertification or refresher classes in which concepts are reviewed and topics involving opinions are discussed. Facilitation can also be used to motivate a class start-up or a review.

The following tips can be used by the instructor to begin facilitated discussion:

1. *It is essential that all learners be actively engaged in the discussion.* The instructor can accomplish this by having small groups discuss the same idea. This is effective because all students are actively working toward the solution simultaneously. The exception is that some students may become distracted and inattentive, so you must redirect them back to the group for participation
2. *The instructor can keep everyone engaged in the discussion by moving the responses from group to group in an unpredictable pattern.* A prop or some other strategy, such as drawing the name of the group out of a hat, will work just fine
3. *Facilitating takes more time to accomplish than does simply lecturing to the group.* Learners will respond, but one must keep in mind that it is not necessary to comment on each person's contribution; rather, it is more important that students contribute. To check for understanding of the instructor and of the learners, one might paraphrase the responses so that key points can be easily made for the entire group
4. *Everyone likes a compliment, and your students are no different.* The instructor should compliment the student on a good comment and should redirect an inaccurate or incorrect statement for the group, so that students understand what is correct and can avoid becoming confused
5. *A new way can be elaborated or suggested.* Even when learners are correct, the instructor can energize the group by quickening of his or her responses, use of humor, or prodding of students for an answer. The instructor can even disagree, gently, when the learner's response is different from what was sought
6. *Similar to diplomats, educators are often required to mediate differences of opinion in the classroom.* To perform this delicate balancing act, one must try to keep the discussion going without interjecting oneself as the authority—a move that could damage momentum. Students should be encouraged to back up their statements with facts, and everyone must be reminded that differing opinions are important to an active and engaged learning community
7. *Finally, facilitators are essential for pulling diverse ideas together so that everyone is involved in the discussion.* The instructor must close the session by summarizing what occurred in the discussion and by providing follow-up information for additional studying or reading, so that the group knows where they have been and where they are going in the future. These tips may help the instructor who is on a quest to use facilitation successfully in the classroom

Timeline for facilitation

One of the most difficult things for the instructor to accomplish by means of facilitated learning is meeting the timeline for instruction. Despite the many positive aspects of this strategy, one of its biggest downfalls is that it takes a great deal of time to accomplish it in the classroom. Educators can easily meet the objectives of their daily lesson plan by lecturing rather than using facilitated learning. It is important to recall that students retain more information when they practice something repeatedly. Rarely do they argue with the results of their own learning when they discover the answers themselves. If a topic is learned this way, they "own it." The goal of the educator is to assist students in their quest to become critically thinking professionals who think about what they do as they move from lower level to higher level learning. This is impossible to accomplish if learners are not active participants in the learning process.

Classroom control issues

One concern that instructors have about facilitation involves retaining control of the classroom. Certainly, it is easy for the instructor to lose control of the situation in an environment with a high amount of facilitation. Controlling the flow of learning can be difficult for even the most seasoned educator. Use of facilitation in the classroom increases the noise and movement and makes it easier for everyone to become distracted. The instructor must ensure that students stay on task; conversations should be monitored to keep learners focused on the topic.

TEACHING TIP: One way by which the instructor can ensure that students remain focused is to establish times when the group will come together to report back on its findings or progress. With these mini-deadlines in place, students know that they are responsible for giving a progress report and will more readily stay on task. For example, if a set of 10 small cases is provided for students to work through, the instructor should not request completion of all 10 at one sitting. Instead, the class should be divided into groups, with three or four cases assigned to each group. Students work on three cases, then the entire class comes together to discuss those cases. The small groups re-form to work on the next three cases. This keeps the class working together, and if one group is not working as it should, the groups can be reconfigured before they get together again. This can appear to be the instructor's initial strategy so that no student has hurt feelings. This approach also allows the instructor to group students who would not usually work together.

Facilitation is challenging, and with it comes frustration. When students encounter difficulty with an assignment, they may be more willing to give up and quit working than to ask for assistance. The instructor must be careful not to do students' work for them. Rather, the instructor should be ready to offer assistance to help students locate the necessary resources and should keep learners actively involved in the lesson.

TEACHING TIP: One way by which the instructor can maintain learner involvement is to invoke the "3 before me" technique before intervening. This technique requires that when asking for help, learners must inform the instructor of at least three places where they have looked to find the information. They should be directed to the appropriate resources if they have not located enough information on their own. However tempting, it is not in the learners' best interest for the instructor to simply tell them the correct answers, even though this may appear easier. The instructor must stay the course because facilitation is worth the effort.

Job assignments in the class setting

Promoting active participation of class members is another way that educators can increase the success of facilitation in the classroom. One method of increasing participation is to have students assist in some of the day-to-day activities of the course. This may involve something as simple as having them set up the room or bring in equipment. In academic settings, class leaders or a "master at arms" is often appointed to serve a minor disciplinary role or to assist the instructor in maintaining control when breaks begin and end. When not actively involved in a scenario or role-playing exercise, students can act as recorders and note takers. Peer observation allows all learners to gain constructive feedback in a setting that is actively engaged. Stronger students can serve as mentors or coaches when they study in groups or when they assist others in learning and perfecting skills.

Educators may assign roles, such as leader, scribe, and reporter, to various members in the class. Strategies used to assign roles to learners must be creative so they are as fair as possible for students. Techniques include alphabetical order, birth date, hiring date (oldest or youngest), color lottery, random movement (close your eyes and point), random numbers, and a sticker on a name tag or chair. Whichever manner is chosen, duties should be rotated equally among the student body so that favoritism is avoided.

Beyond lecture

Educators must challenge themselves to move beyond strict lecture formats. Doing so builds interest, maximizes understanding and retention, involves participants more actively, and reinforces course content. One might think about an evening newscast that reduces many stories to headlines to gain attention. In effect, the instructor is doing the same thing. The instructor can provide details that will pique the learners' interest by reducing the lecture to major points. A presentation can be altered so that highlights are presented in lecture form to the whole class; then, students can be placed into groups where various instructors can emphasize important areas for which reinforcement is needed. In addition, the instructor can enhance presentations to add more visual appeal, and handouts can be provided that detail pertinent points with a focus on the practical aspects that must be emphasized.

Chapter 16 ("Tools for Large Group Learning") provides more information on enhancing lectures and techniques to make lectures more learner-centered.

Group Work

Individual persons learn best when they learn together. Active learning is most meaningful when it involves group activity. Just as in real life, EMS problems are often solved with a team approach to the situation that is currently being faced.

Because time is precious, classroom groups should be identified in a quick and efficient manner. Some situations dictate that groups should stay the same; others do not. EMS personnel will not always be working with the same partner or crew, and variation among members of groups, as well as among skill levels, can enhance the overall performance of individual members and of the team.

Selection of groups can be difficult; however, it may enable the instructor to creatively assemble the team. Use of randomization techniques such as counting off, drawing numbers, or some other method allows learners to maintain minimal control in the sorting process, although sorting is more random. If the teacher controls selection, it can be done ahead of time based on the instructor's knowledge of the group, keeping in mind student strengths and limitations. Student-controlled selection allows the formation of groups that can be assembled individually or collectively according to the wishes of those in the group. This option offers the instructor less control but may prove to be more effective.

Effective group management

One of the most effective strategies for managing a group of four learners in a team is to add a fifth member. The fifth member is a peer facilitator who is added to guide and mentor the group and to help resolve conflicts. For groups to work effectively, ground rules must be established at the first class meeting. Certain mandates should be assigned by educators, including attending class on time at every session, completing all assignments before class and being prepared to discuss them, notifying other group members in advance if class will be missed, willingly sharing information, respecting the values, views, and ideas of others, and abiding by all other rules as agreed on by the group.

Members of each group must actively rotate roles within the group so that all students can gain experience in all areas of the activity (Figure 12-2). The discussion leader works to keep the group on track and monitors participation of group members. The recorder, or scribe, records assignments, strategies, unresolved issues, and data, and convenes the group outside of class when necessary. The reporter is responsible for reporting the group's findings to the entire class during discussions and writes a final draft of all assignments. The accuracy coach or timekeeper checks for understanding of the group, locates resources, and manages time.

How effective can facilitation be if it is used with inexperienced learners? It can be successful if educators actively plan for its use. Activities must be well defined and must have clearly stated objectives so that learners understand their importance. Time spent in facilitated learning should be short in the beginning of the course, then should build to longer segments as students demonstrate their ability to perform appropriately and stay on task. The class must be brought together for discussion and clarification of issues at frequent intervals throughout the session. In addition, the instructor should plan for individual and group assignments. The opportunity for group members to take the assignment lightly can damage the effectiveness of the strategy. The instructor must remain vigilant for behavior that might diminish the group's strength and undermine it. Peer facilitators can be used to assist both the learners and the instructor in maintaining the integrity of the strategy.

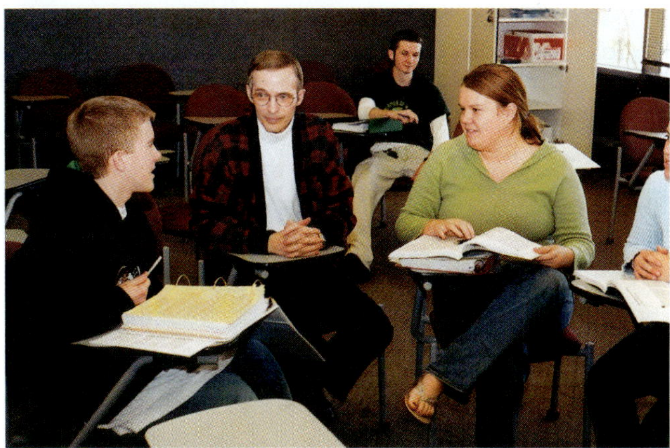

FIGURE 12-2 Creative educators can make learning easier for students by requiring their active participation.

Conflict resolution

Not everyone in a family always gets along with one another, and members of the learning community are no different from a family. In fact, they may actually spend more time with one another than family members do. Tempers often flare when people spend a great deal of time with one another in close proximity. Several levels exist at which the instructor can reduce the likelihood that conflicts will escalate.

1. *The first level focuses on preventing escalation of a conflict.* The instructor should monitor the group for early signs of conflict and should intervene immediately to prevent additional problems. Group evaluations can assist the instructor in monitoring individual student behavior that may need correction, and spontaneous verbal feedback can be helpful in encouraging students to discuss their feelings about all aspects of the class.
2. *The second level of conflict resolution centers on student empowerment.* The instructor must listen to students' concerns and must encourage them to peacefully resolve any conflicts they may be experiencing. Educators can coach students on strategies for possible resolution of conflicts. If a peer leader is involved, this person should not be undermined in front of the other students, or he or she will lose authority among them. The instructor should speak with this leader before confronting students to ensure that they have a game plan in place for resolving the issue.
3. *The third level of conflict requires active resolution of conflicts that may arise.* Ground rules must be established before discussion takes place among those involved in the conflict. Each participant must be allowed to present his or her point while the others actively listen. Students should be asked to define their ideas on an ideal outcome, although no guarantees exist that these will be honored. The

instructor's role is to facilitate the discussion of possible outcomes that will affect those involved in the conflict. If a peer leader participates, the instructor may serve as an observer while the peer leader manages the conflict.

4. *The fourth level requires intervention by the instructor.* Educators must refer to published guidelines for direction, such as those found in course syllabi, student manuals, and other sources. If the infraction is particularly serious, other members of the instructional team may be called upon to assist with handling an issue. Many institutions have staff members who are specifically trained in conflict management who can be used in such situations.

Questioning Techniques

Another way by which the instructor can move toward a more student-centered classroom is through questioning. Questioning is an inquiry that invites a response. Thought-provoking questions used in a lecture can promote active thinking and can stimulate higher level thinking and problem-solving skills. This technique also can increase interaction between the lecturer and the students and may assist with application to the clinical environment.

Socratic method

The Socratic method of questioning is a popular method with instructors. It originally involved instructor questioning during a lecture to check on or test student knowledge to determine whether students had read their assignments or listened to the previous lecture. In this scenario, the instructor selects a student and presents a question that it is hoped the student can answer. If that student cannot accurately answer the question, then another student is selected until one can supply the answer. This method has been criticized because it is embarrassing and favors a small segment of the class (those who can answer the question). Additionally, once a student has been called on, he or she may not listen for a while because it is unlikely that he or she will be called on soon. With variations applied to this technique, questioning can be beneficial for student learning.[2]

Wait time

Wait time is an important concept in questioning techniques. It is important that students be given time to think about questions posed to them and to ponder their response. However, it is not unusual for an instructor to wait only 1 second for students to respond. Waiting for 5 to 10 seconds before calling on a student can increase the number of students who respond and the length of their responses. Before asking a question, the instructor must insist that no one raise his or her hand to answer. This discourages the situation in which the predictable students raise their hands and others immediately quit seeking the answer. By waiting, students are more likely to consider the question. After waiting, the instructor calls on a random student or a volunteer and asks the student to answer. This method allows more students to be involved in the process.[2] The technique is known as "ask, pause, and call (Figure 12-3)."

Other questioning techniques

Another questioning strategy is to use the "wait time" technique, then to ask another student to summarize what the previous student has answered. This technique can promote active listening in that students will listen to each other rather than wait for the instructor to repeat the answer.

Other questioning techniques can be used to engage students. One is the "overhead question," which is given to the whole group without calling on someone in particular. This is also called the "rhetorical question." It may or may not be necessary for this question to be answered out loud at that time. The "relay question" involves calling on different students to add or comment on the previous student's responses until all important information has been obtained. Another technique is the "reverse question," wherein the instructor answers a student's question with another question or asks the class to respond.

Experiential Learning

Another concept that is important to EMS classroom and clinical educators is the use of experiential learning. Carl Rogers was a pioneering psychotherapist who wrote extensively on the concept of experiential learning.[3] He felt so strongly about the role that expe-

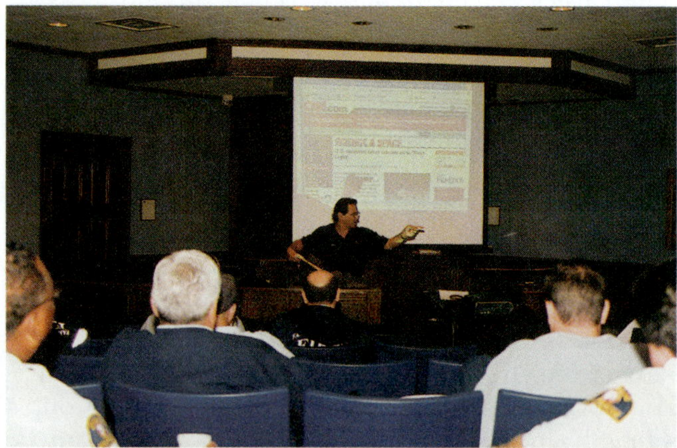

FIGURE 12-3 Effective questioning techniques include the use of thought-provoking questions and of the "ask, pause, and call" technique.

rience plays in how we learn that he distinguished learning into two distinct types: cognitive (which Rogers described as "meaningless") and experiential (which he deemed as "significant"). He wrote that "all human beings have a natural propensity to learn; the role of the teacher is to facilitate such learning." According to Rogers, learning is facilitated when (1) the student participates completely in the learning process and has control over its nature and direction, (2) it is primarily based on direct confrontation with practical, social, personal, or research problems, and (3) self-evaluation is the principal method of assessing progress or success. Rogers also emphasizes the importance of learning to learn and being open to change.

Rogers identified the following five core elements of facilitation that are necessary for successful experiential learning:

1. Setting a positive climate for learning
2. Clarifying the purposes of the learner(s)
3. Organizing and making available learning resources
4. Balancing intellectual and emotional components of learning
5. Sharing feelings and thoughts with learners but not dominating

EMS is the ideal discipline by which the benefits of experiential learning can be maximized because so much of what is done by care providers can be re-created in the classroom through the use of patient care scenarios. In addition, most students will spend valuable time in the clinical and field settings, hoping to apply what they have learned in the classroom. Chapter 18 ("Tools for Field and Clinical Learning") details how instructors can maximize the clinical experience for students. Following are examples of classroom scenarios that can be used to maximize the potential for experiential learning.

For the following examples, an objective has been taken directly from the 1994 US Department of Transportation Emergency Medical Technician-Basic (US DOT EMT-B) National Standard Curriculum; some examples of experiential learning are provided to reinforce the objective.

Example 1: Objective 4-3.46. Explain the rationale for administering nitroglycerin to a patient with chest pain or discomfort

This particular objective comes from the section on cardiovascular emergencies, and it addresses the affective learning domain discussed in Chapter 7.

It is easy enough for the instructor to ask students to read the text, then discuss in class the rationale for administering a particular medication. However, use of this objective to drive a patient scenario can be much more effective.

CASE IN POINT

Live Scenario

Two or three students should be selected to play EMTs; they must step out of the room. Another student should be selected to play the role of the patient; this student should be instructed to present with all the classic signs and symptoms of cardiac chest pain, including a recent history of angina. Additional input should be solicited from the class regarding how this patient should present. The patient is provided with a small bottle of medication labeled as nitroglycerin. Small mints or some similar candy is placed in the bottle to represent the medication. The patient is instructed to "pass out" should the EMTs decide to administer the medication before a baseline blood pressure has been established, or if the EMT fails to determine how many pills the patient has already taken.

The primary objectives of the scenario are (1) to reinforce the need to establish a minimum blood pressure before medication is administered, and (2) to gather an appropriate history before any medication is given. Several secondary objectives will come up during the postscenario critique.

The EMTs should be brought into the room with a simulated dispatch, such as *Rescue 51: respond code 3 to residence for a man with chest pain.* The scenario must be allowed to progress until the instructor believes it has met the stated objective and concludes with a brief critique. Students who are observing are invited to offer their input on how the team did. The instructor's job is to steer the critique along the path toward your intended objective, encouraging students to think critically and experience the learning, rather than just hearing or reading about it.

"The process whereby knowledge is created through the transformation of experience," is how David Kolb, a leading expert in the study of experiential learning, defines learning. "Knowledge results from the combination of grasping and transforming experience."[4] Kolb's theory describes two ways that learners can transform experience into knowledge—reflective observation and active experimentation. Kolb believes that learners transform their previous experience into new knowledge by evaluating and building on this foundation. Many things that are easily done in the EMS classroom can serve as excellent models for these two modes of learning. In the chest pain scenario, students actively engaged in a simulated patient encounter learn through active experimentation. The simulated patient is preprogrammed to provide certain responses to help guide students in performing appropriate steps without providing obvious direction. Observers and participants then benefit from reflective observation by participating in a follow-up critique of how the patient was treated.

Following is another example of experiential learning in which the instructor uses active exploration as a means of reinforcing a particular learning objective.

Example 2: Objective 5-5.15. Describe methods used to assess the pupils

This objective could easily be approached by lecture and is generally covered quite well in the textbook with the use of illustrations. However, allowing students to experience the practice of assessing pupils and having them see and document their findings will help cement the knowledge through experiential learning (Box 12-1).

CASE IN POINT

Experimenting with Pupil Reactions

It is difficult for students to actually see pupil changes in a well-lit room. For this reason, it is best for the instructor to ask students to pair up and take turns assessing pupil response with a penlight or a similar light. First, one student should document pupil size and equality on a fellow student. The lights should be turned out for no less than 2 minutes before students are asked to recheck pupil response with the penlight. Both eyes should be checked several times so the pupils can actually be seen to change in response to light. Students should be asked to record their results for each student in the class, then to compare their results during a debriefing of the activity. Some students should be positioned in a location where side lighting may affect the readings or the ability to assess pupils. Students should be asked to lie on their backs and look up into the overhead classroom lights. When the instructor debriefs this activity, he or she should ask students how the position of the patient in the ambulance and light levels will affect their ability to evaluate pupils.

BOX 12-1 Experiential Tips

Following are just a few examples of experiential techniques that can help reinforce specific learning points:

- Have students feel the pulse of a person with an irregular heart rhythm
- Use a dual-earpiece teaching stethoscope to assist students in understanding what sounds they are listening for when taking a blood pressure
- To reinforce the hands-on aspect of the assessment, have students practice a patient assessment without saying a word or asking any questions. Repeat this assessment in a darkened room

The examples shown in Box 12-1 are just a few of the ways in which an instructor can use an alternative or student-centered method to meet common objectives. Through the process of trial and error, the instructor discovers which methods work best for certain objectives. The challenge for the EMS educator is to identify those objectives with the highest priority and experiment with various methods of delivery. The process of developing a more learner-centered approach to the classroom initially requires more work and adds increased risk to what the instructor does. The rewards for both students and instructor are immeasurable.

MATCHING TEACHING STRATEGIES TO GOALS AND OBJECTIVES

Making the conscious decision to become a more student-centered instructor is quite different from actually making it happen. It may be comforting for the instructor to know that half the battle has already been decided for EMS instructors in that the objectives to which they must teach have been defined by such documents as the US DOT National Standard Curricula, the core content, and the scope of practice for each level of care. The challenge for the instructor is to continue to master current teaching methods while developing new and innovative methods that are best suited for the various objectives.

The task of addressing during class time each and every objective included within the curriculum can be overwhelming. In fact, this is one of the biggest challenges for instructors, given the length of most First Responder, EMT, and Paramedic programs. The Paramedic National Standard Curriculum alone has more than 1800 objectives that must be addressed at some time during the course of the program. Although it is true that many objectives overlap, instructors still must "triage" the objectives and select those most worthy of focus during class time.

Instructors can maximize their valuable time by ensuring that they understand the instructional level required to attain the chosen objectives. Chapter 7 describes Bloom's taxonomy and provides verbs used to describe the behaviors expected at various levels. The important point to remember about this process is that students must progress (and attain mastery) from the lowest levels within a domain to the upper levels. They cannot skip any processes within a level.

The instructor must devise a teaching and evaluation strategy that provides the lower levels of understanding, then allows students to progress toward the upper levels. The old saying, "you must walk before you can run," can be applied here as well. The wisest EMS instructors know that a valuable EMS provider not only understands when to do something, but also knows when *not* to do something. This level of understanding comes only through a thorough immersion into all aspects associated with the particular concepts. Students must understand all appropriate terminology and must be able to see subtle differences between similar terms. Terminology begins in the lowest levels of understanding within each domain. Terminology concepts are then applied as students begin to understand the subtle differences between words and to appreciate their meaning. As students work through problems and scenarios, they use their understanding of the terminology in accurate ways to get their meaning across in words or actions.

For example, many distinct differences can be noted between ventilation and respiration, and students must understand these differences as they evaluate the effectiveness of airway management and adjunct usage. However, many educators may have forgotten the differences, or they may not have learned through their educational process how to make the distinction. Students may experience frustration when they encounter an evaluation process that requires that they discriminate among concepts for which they cannot recall differences. If the instructional process does not focus on students learning the difference between these two concepts but instead focuses on the development of psychomotor skills, students will be unable to effectively problem-solve an airway management issue that differentiates between the two concepts.

SUMMARY

The goals of any teacher are to convey information to students and to make a lasting change in their behavior. To do this, the educator must develop teaching strategies that result in meaningful change. It must be understood that teaching is both an art and a science. Educators must be great performers (the art), but they must also gain expertise in facilitation techniques that involve groups of students, questioning techniques, and experiential learning. The effective educator recognizes the many teaching strategies that are available and chooses which technique will be best for a given situation.

The goal of the following chapters is to introduce both novice and seasoned EMS instructors to a variety of traditional and nontraditional teaching concepts and strategies to ensure a successful and engaging educational experience for both the student and the instructor. Achieving a practical balance between these two approaches is encouraged. It is hoped that the instructor will come away with an understanding of the importance of this balance.

Chapter 13 discusses each domain of learning, along with specific methods for promoting student learning in each domain. Chapter 14 focuses in great detail on specific tools that instructors can use to promote individual and one-on-one learning. Chapter

CASE IN POINT

The medical director, program coordinator, and primary instructor are reviewing the results of a recent module practical examination for an EMT-Intermediate (EMT-I) course. The students had just learned intravenous (IV) and medication administration skills, and this was their first practical examination for the course. The EMT-I course is a new addition to the training program and is under a great deal of scrutiny from the instructional team because team members did not have much time to design or develop the course before it began.

Historically, the program has used outside reviewers for each module practical exam for every course it offers, including First Responder and EMT-Basic (EMT-B). These evaluators are veteran EMS instructors who have not been actively involved in teaching this particular group of students. The program philosophy is that this approach provides an unbiased assessment of student performance that allows students to adjust to the idea of being evaluated by strangers.

Three trends emerged on review of exam results. First, none of the students asked all the pertinent "patient rights" questions, including those that would reveal whether the simulated patient had any allergies. The instructor admitted that she had not focused much attention on this because she assumed that all students carried this knowledge forward from their EMT-B training. The second trend was that many of the students cleansed the site for administration of the IV or injection, then contaminated the site with their gloved finger immediately before performing the skill. This perplexed the instructor, and she stated that she had *never* instructed the students to do it this way. She also stated that they did not perform the skill this way on the day they practiced in class. In reviewing the schedule, students noted that there was never any practice time wherein students performed the skill without direct input from the instructor. The third trend was that none of the students clearly understood the correct order for performing skills when several skills were used in the same scenario. When evaluating class sessions leading up to the exam, the instructional team realized that they had never had a practice session in which students could put several skills together (e.g., starting an IV, drawing blood, and administering IM medication) into a single scenario so that they were forced to think through that process while taking the practical exam. Evaluators reported that many students became frustrated and simply performed the skills in the order listed on the card (which deliberately listed them out of order). The instructional team made several notes on items to review with the entire class. The schedule was reviewed to ensure that more "pulling it all together" practice would be included before the next practical exam was given. The program director made a correction to the schedule for future classes so this would not happen again. The team also agreed to meet on a more regular basis to discuss strategies for teaching the program and agreed to include more hands-on activities for students.

15 discusses methods and tools most appropriate for small groups, including ways to enhance psychomotor abilities and critical thinking skills. Chapter 16 provides insight into instructional methods aimed at large groups, as well as methods used to enhance the lecture approach to instruction. Chapter 17 introduces the many tools and methods used in distance learning. Chapter 18 introduces key strategies for enhancing student field and clinical experiences.

REFERENCES

1. Leeder SR. An Australian approach to medical education: the Newcastle experiment. *Med J Aust.* 1984:158-162.
2. Paulson DR, Faust JL. Techniques of active learning. Active learning for the college classroom. Available at: http://chemistry.calstatela.edu/Chem&BioChem/active/main.htm.
3. Rogers C, Freiberg, HJ. *Freedom to Learn.* Columbus, Ohio: Charles E. Merrill; 1994.
4. Kolb DA. *Experiential Learning: Experience as the Source of Learning and Development.* NJ: Prentice-Hall; 1984.

WORKS CONSULTED

Brereton MF, Leifer L, Greene J, Lewis J, Linde C. An exploration of engineering learning. In: Hight TK, Stauffer LA, eds. *Proceedings of the ASME Design Theory and Methodology Conference, Albuquerque, NM, September 1993.*

Combs AW. Fostering maximum development of the individual. In: Van Til W, Rehage KJ, eds. *Issues in Secondary Education (NSSE Yearbook).* Chicago: National Society for the Study of Education; 1976.

deWinstanley PA, Bjork RA. Successful lecturing: presenting information in ways that engage effective processing. *New Directions for Teaching and Learning.* 2002;89: 19-31.

Galbraith MW. *Adult Learning Methods.* Huntington, NY: Robert E. Krieger Publishing; 1991.

Johnson DW, Johnson RT, Smith KA. Maximizing instruction through cooperative learning. *ASEE Prism.* 1998;7:24-29.

Norman GR, Schmidt HG. The psychological basis of problem-based learning: a review of the evidence. *Acad Med.* 1992;67:557-565.

Nowell L. Rethinking the classroom: a community of inquiry. Presented at: National Council on Creating the Quality School, Norman, Oklahoma. Fort Worth, Tex: Wesleyan University, School of Education; 1996. ERIC Document Reproduction Service No. ED350 273.

Reese AC. (1998). Implications of results from cognitive science research. [online serial]. Available at: http://www.Med-Ed-Online.

Rideout E. (2001). *Transforming Nursing Education Through Problem-Based Learning.* Sudbury, Mass: Jones and Bartlett; 2001.

Springer, Stanne, Donovan. *Review of Educational Research.* 1999.

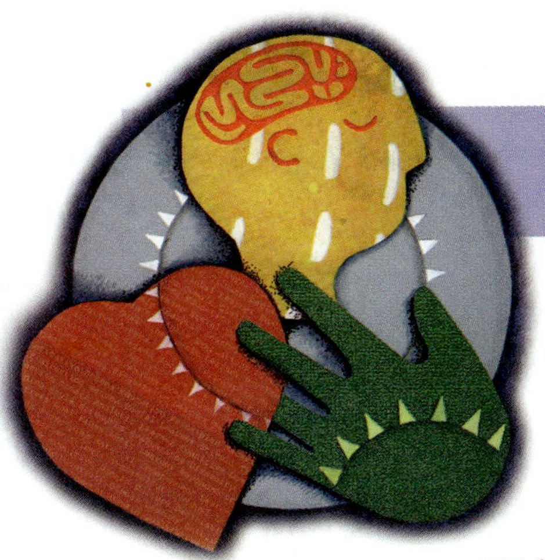

Teaching in All Domains

"Education is not the filling of a pail, but the lighting of a fire."

—*Heraclitus*

Emergency medical services (EMS) education is a complex activity that involves teaching in multiple domains and at multiple levels. It is not enough that EMS educators prepare future EMS responders to be highly skilled technicians who are able to perform flawlessly every basic and advanced skill, nor is it enough that they are able to correctly recite every treatment protocol and every drug dosage and procedure. In addition to these knowledge and psychomotor skills, the EMS provider must be a skilled communicator who is capable of empathy and a deeper appreciation of each patient's social, family, and ethnic background; he or she must also be able to respect and honor patients' diversity. This chapter prepares the EMS educator for the challenge of providing a comprehensive EMS education that will produce competent EMS care providers.

This chapter discusses how to teach critical thinking skills and how to apply them to the knowledge, psychomotor, and affective domains.

TEACHING COGNITIVE AND CRITICAL THINKING SKILLS

Widely regarded as the "father" of modern critical thinking, John Dewey defined critical thinking as, ". . . the active, persistent, and careful consideration of a belief or supposed form of knowledge in light of the grounds which support it and the further conclusions to which it tends." By using the term *active,* Dewey contrasts this method of learning from the more passive method in which the student simply receives information or ideas from someone else. John Dewey believed that the attainment of higher-level thinking skills, sometimes called *critical thinking,* could be nurtured and developed in students. Approaches to teaching that involve critical thinking require the student to think things through, raise additional questions, and explore solutions for themselves. Dewey believed that educators should pay close attention to each student's life experience and should develop curricula that connect with and extend student experiences to real world application. Dewey suggested that school should be less about preparation for life and more about life itself.[1]

It is not enough to simply assume that students will think critically all on their own. Although some do, many must be introduced to this skill in the classroom. By keeping alert to available opportunities, educators can begin to develop more meaningful lessons. In the examples given in this chapter and in the following chapters, the common thread is the element of critical thinking. These examples provide a great foundation for new and experienced educators alike.

Teaching thinking strategies requires a careful and deliberate plan of instruction. Educators must determine which thinking skills students have already mastered and which they have yet to learn. Educators must measure thinking skills on a daily basis and should include thinking skill development exercises and strategies throughout the course. Measuring student achievement is a challenge when the goal is measuring recall of information, but the process becomes even more complex when one adds to it measuring a student's ability to use information to think critically and to problem-solve. This problem is not unique to EMS education. A study on the evaluation of thousands of test items from K-12 education reveals that nearly three quarters of these items tested the recall of information (i.e., a low-level cognitive skill), and very few tested the application of higher-order

BOX 13-1 Keys for Unlocking Higher-Order Thinking Skills

1. Instruction and assessment strategies that promote thinking skills
2. Practice with various methods of thinking that incorporate many strategies
3. Constant and consistent role modeling of the process for students

CASE IN POINT

For example, after a session in which students learned and demonstrated the ability to ventilate a manikin using a pocket mask, the instructor asked these questions:

- How will you know if your breaths are getting into the patient?
- What does it mean if you do not see good chest rise and fall?

Some students immediately shouted the first answer that came to mind without giving it much thought at all. For instance, in response to the first question, one student said, "Because I know I gave a good breath." In response to the second question, a second student said, "The patient has something stuck in his throat." These answers may or may not have been correct; however, other conclusions had to be tested before these responses could be evaluated for correctness. To stimulate higher levels of learning, the instructor began by asking follow-up questions, such as, "How can you be sure that the breath you gave is really adequate for the patient?" and "Is a foreign object the only thing that can obstruct an airway?" By offering additional probing questions, the instructor slowed the class down and encouraged students to process information carefully and thoroughly before responding.

thinking skills.[2] Numerous studies in adult and elementary education have had similar findings.

Three key processes have been identified that enhance an educator's ability to assist students in the development of higher-order thinking skills (Box 13-1). Key Process 1 involves the implementation by the instructor of various instructional and assessment strategies that teach thinking skills to students. To do this, educators must have a fundamental understanding of the thinking process and must possess the appropriate tools and techniques. Key Process 2 requires that students be given ample opportunity to practice these methods. Educators should ensure that they provide opportunities for students to explore various learning styles and preference. In Key Process 3, the educator serves as a role model to be emulated by students.

BOX 13-2 Bloom's Taxonomy: Cognitive Domain

Level 1: Knowledge
Level 2: Comprehension
Level 3: Application
Level 4: Analysis
Level 5: Synthesis

TEACHING TIP: Instructors should provide critical thinking opportunities that appeal to a variety of student learning styles and preferences.

Several valid strategies for grouping and classifying thinking skills have been developed. For example, Costa and associates organized thinking skills into the six R's of thinking: Remembering, Repeating, Reasoning, Reorganizing, Relating, and Reflecting.[3] This model is common to nursing education and is the framework for several of its strategies for the development of critical thinking skills.

Barry Beyer, working with an inventory of operations common to curriculum developers and educators, classified thinking processes into three distinct groups: thinking strategies, critical thinking skills, and micro-thinking skills.[4]

Beyer's thinking strategies include three subcategories: problem solving, decision making, and conceptualizing. Problem solving involves five steps: recognizing a problem, representing the problem, devising/choosing a solution plan, executing the plan, and evaluating the solution. The decision-making process comprises five steps: defining the goal, identifying, analyzing and ranking the alternatives (three steps), judging the highest-ranked alternative, and choosing the best alternative. The process of conceptualizing begins with the identification of examples. The next three steps include identifying, classifying, and categorizing attributes of these examples. Next, examples and nonexamples are identified with the goal of attaining a comprehensive list. Finally, concept attributes and structure are identified.[4]

According to Beyer, the skill of critical thinking consists of ten ordered parts. Steps one and two involve distinguishing between verifiable facts and value claims and sorting relevant from irrelevant information, claims, or reasons. Steps three and four involve determining the factual accuracy of statements and source credibility. Step five requires that ambiguous claims or arguments be identified. Steps six and seven focus on stated assumptions and bias. Steps eight and nine analyze logical fallacies and logical inconsistencies in a line of reasoning. Step ten assesses the strength of an argument or claim.[4]

Techniques for Teaching Critical Thinking Skills: The T.H.I.N.K. Model

A common nursing model classifies critical thinking skills into five modes of thinking: total recall, habits, inquiry, new ideas and creativity, and knowing how you think. It uses the mnemonic T.H.I.N.K. and the processes proceed in the order of the spelling of that word.[5]

Total recall

Total recall is the memorization of facts or remembering where to look for them. As a student practices total recall, it is important to distinguish which information should be recalled instantaneously and which can be looked up.

Using patterns, or *mnemonics,* is helpful in improving recall. An example of recall occurs when a person remembers the following numbers in order: 5553561809. It looks daunting until they are organized like this: (555) 356-1809. Now, it resembles a phone number and is easier to remember. Common EMS mnemonics include PQRST (Provokes or Palliates, Quality, Region and Radiation, Severity, and Time) in obtaining the present and past medical histories in patients with chest pain, and AMPLE (Allergies, Medications, Past Medical History, and Last Meal Eaten) in obtaining a patient's medical history. Another example of recall asks the learner to look at the following list of common words and to try to remember them: apple, car, yellow, pear, bicycle, blue, grapefruit, plane, and green. If the learner sorts the list according to the following patterns, it is easier to recall:

Colors: yellow, blue, green
Fruits: apple, grapefruit, pear
Transportation: car, plane, bicycle

Another method of recall involves the association of facts with an experience. A person may quickly and easily remember a fact because it is associated with a strong emotion or a funny story. For example, will anyone ever forget where they were and what they were doing when they learned that commercial aircraft were being flown into buildings on September 11, 2001? For that matter, has the 9-11 date gained even greater significance since that date? So strong are these emotions that these questions answer themselves.

Habit

Habit, the second process of critical thinking, is any accepted way that works, saves time, or is necessary for the critical thinking process to take place. Habits are thinking approaches that become second nature. Within the psychomotor domain, this level of mastery is called *naturalization.* Driving a car to school illustrates this principle. Have you ever noticed that you arrived at your class without remembering the journey? Habits in the work environment can make performing a job a lot easier, but it is important that a person periodically reevaluate steps taken to ensure that he or she is not taking inappropriate short cuts. For example, students should review whether they always cleanse the top of a medication vial with alcohol before withdrawing any medication from the vial.

Inquiry

Inquiry occurs as the student examines issues in depth and detail and questions what may seem immediately obvious. Although inquiry is often called critical thinking, the nursing model of thinking requires the action of all five modes of the T.H.I.N.K. model for critical thinking to take place. Inquiry is the primary kind of thinking used to reach conclusions, and conclusions are more accurate if inquiry is used.[5]

Inquiry requires the following six steps:

1. Receive information
2. Come to a conclusion, but collect additional information to rule in or out the immediate conclusion
3. Compare the new information with what is already known from past experience
4. Question biases
5. Consider one or more alternative conclusions
6. Validate the original or alternative conclusion

New ideas and creativity

New ideas and creativity is the polar opposite of the habit mode of thinking. Creativity allows the thinker to explore different pathways or alternatives for problem solving. A common phrase attached to this process is "to think outside the box." Creative thinking often leads to many mistakes, which provide additional learning opportunities. Creative thinking allows practitioners of health care to individualize care. When performed at its highest level, the creative thinking process allows for individual choices within the framework of medically acceptable behaviors.

Knowing how you think

Metacognition is the highest of the thinking skills in the T.H.I.N.K. model. "Meta-" means "among" or "in the midst of," and cognition is the process of knowing. A student who attains this level can critically analyze his or her thinking process and make adjustments as needed.

Three major operations occur during the metacognitive process: planning, monitoring, and assessing.[6] Each process has several subprocesses. Planning is considered the most important facet of metacognition. It includes the following parts: stating a goal, selecting operations to perform, sequencing operations, identifying potential obstacles/errors, identifying ways to recover from obstacles/errors, and predicting desired and/or anticipated results.

Monitoring is the second process in metacognition. It includes steps for keeping sequencing in order by keeping the goal in mind, keeping one's place in the sequence, knowing when a subgoal has been achieved, and deciding when to progress to the next operation. Monitoring also involves spotting errors and obstacles and knowing how to recover from errors and obstacles.

The final step is the assessment of goal achievement. It comprises judging accuracy and adequacy of results, appropriateness of procedures, handling of obstacles and errors, and the efficiency of the plan and its execution.[4,6]

BOX 13-3 Distinguishing Between Passive and Active Behaviors

Passive	Active
Quiet classrooms of note takers	Active classrooms of interactive learners
All work done alone	Work done in cooperative small groups
Rare participation in class	Regular participation to some degree
Classroom-guided materials	Creation of new and challenging assignments
Teacher-controlled lesson	Student- and teacher-controlled lessons
All tasks carried by the teacher	Classroom responsibilities shared by students

TEACHING AFFECTIVE SKILLS

Addressing the affective domain begins with the students themselves and the trust that must be placed in them. Creating an affective environment starts by building a student-centered education. This strategy begins with an awareness that students come to us with attitudes, beliefs, emotions, and experiences that are of value to the class.

Educators have long known that the power of emotion can be harnessed to create a powerful learning environment. By tapping into emotion, instructors can build a vibrant classroom that takes students on an exploration of their profession and of themselves. In the end, this active learning atmosphere brings about greater understanding and a more complete student and learning experience. This is why it is critical to begin to change classrooms from passive places of learning to active and engaging ones (Box 13-3).

The affective domain is generally considered to be the most difficult one for EMS educators to address. Many EMS educators believe that the affective domain cannot be adequately reached because of a variety of difficulties centered on beliefs that an instructor cannot change how students think, that it would be too time-consuming to attempt to change student beliefs, that classrooms are too noisy and out of control, that students cannot be trusted, and that information must always be instructor-centered and -controlled. This type of rigid thinking has created too many "student tourists" in the classroom. Student tourists are those who quietly sit in the classroom and try to become invisible. They quietly take notes, ask few questions, and hope that the instructor will not notice them or call on them to participate.

By embracing the affective domain, creating a student-centered environment, and using the technique of facilitation as discussed in Chapter 12, instructors can begin to develop student affective skills in the classroom before students hit the streets. It is simply wrong to assume that the affective domain cannot be effectively taught in the classroom. Educators teach values, whether they realize it or not. Every time an instructor relates a personal experience about how she or he was empathetic to a troubled patient or family member, communicates verbal and nonverbal reactions to student questions or performance, chooses subjects to be tested, and even emphasizes given topics in a lecture or presentation, the instructor is imposing values. The real issue for the instructor, then, is how to cultivate the ethics and values of our profession while setting aside his or her own personal prejudices, beliefs, and emotions. Educators have a much stronger influence on students than they can ever know or appreciate. Students learn from the behaviors that their educators model, including those instructor behaviors that they observe outside the classroom (Figure 13-1).

To appropriately affect a student's progress within the affective domain, an instructor must be consciously aware of the values, judgments, and beliefs that are inherent in the instructor's teaching but that may not be overtly apparent; then, the instructor must monitor changes in students to detect behaviors that indicate that they are adopting desired values and judgments.

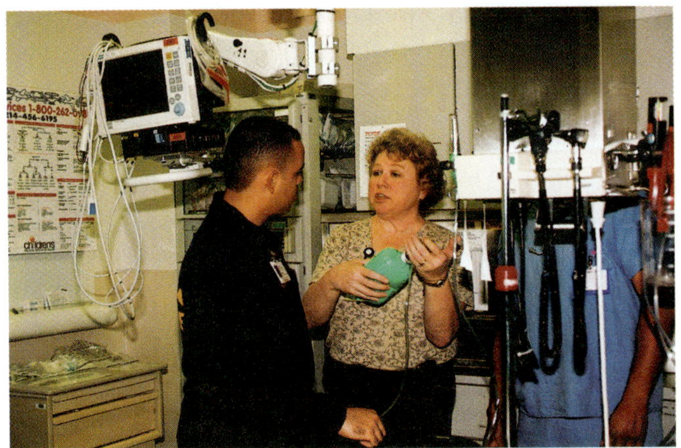

FIGURE 13-1 Educators model values and behaviors by everything they say and do within and outside of the classroom.

BOX 13-4 Bloom's Taxonomy: Affective Domain

Level 1: Receiving
Level 2: Responding
Level 3: Valuing
Level 4: Organizing
Level 5: Characterizing

Levels of the Affective Domain

As has been discussed in Chapter 7, Domains of Learning, Bloom identified five levels in the affective domain (Box 13-4). Each level requires certain steps that normally must be taken before progression can occur through a given level and onto the next. Facilitation is the one overriding technique that can be applied at all levels. In addition to facilitation, other teaching techniques that may help a student achieve a particular level are suggested here. Instructors are encouraged to develop their own techniques as well.

It is possible for a student to skip a level, or insufficiently complete a level, then proceed to the next level. When this happens, problems commonly occur for both the student and the instructor. Behaviors that indicate a problem with level attainment are described to help the instructor identify those students who may need to go back and repeat a level. These are not intended to be all-inclusive, but they are included here to help the instructor recognize problems when they encounter them.

Level I: receiving

Receiving is where the affective domain begins. It requires no more of the student than that he or she be aware of a given piece of information. This is usually cognitive in origin. The student has heard it, seen it, or read it. Receiving is made up of three successive steps. When a student demonstrates any of the actions described by these steps, he or she is operating at the receiving level. These steps include the following:

1. *Awareness*: This step requires only that the student be conscious of the existence of a given piece of information or equipment. For example, the student sees the Hare traction splint in the classroom but does not display any interest in it. Another example might be that the student stays awake during your fracture management lecture. Of course, it may be very difficult to tell if the student was listening or not.
2. *Willingness to receive*: At this step, the student becomes curious enough about the piece of information or object that he or she is willing to devote some, but not all, of his attention to it. For example, the student begins to stop and look at the traction splint before sitting down in the classroom, or the student asks questions during the lecture on fracture management.
3. *Controlled or selected attention*: At this point, the student is so interested in the piece of information or object that it momentarily has top priority, despite the fact that other things are of interest to him at the same time. For example, the student would rather practice with the traction splint than discuss last night's events, or the student is so engrossed in reading his assignment that he doesn't respond to his name when he is called. Exactly why the piece of information or object does or does not have top priority is up for interpretation and may be a function of what goes on in the classroom.

Assumptions of willingness to receive and of selected attention are precarious until the next level, Responding, is demonstrated. The Receiving level, however, forms the basis for all other levels. One must take care not to confuse verbalizations that show understanding of communicated stimuli with responding behaviors. Responding behaviors are demonstrated when "students act out behaviors consistent with . . . a particular value."[7]

Classroom implications

An instructor can promote Receiving by letting students know what is expected of them. This is accomplished first by communicating the course objectives. Many times, it is not enough to just hand out the objectives. The instructor may need to explain what they are and how they can be used to the student's benefit.

Making lectures relevant to the student also enhances the Receiving level. The relevancy of the objectives and of what is being taught may need to be explained. Resources such as equipment, professional magazines and publications, manikins, posters, anatomy charts, and copies of lecture outlines and notes are also invaluable at this level of learning.

Perhaps one of the most important instructor techniques for enhancing the Receiving level can be accomplished by placing the emphasis on course matter where it belongs, and not where the instructor has a personal preference. Students will emulate what the instructor does without realizing that they are doing it, but they will also disregard what they are supposed to be learning if they perceive no clear reason or rationale for what is being taught. Therefore, when emphasis is placed on a subject, it is helpful for the instructor to explain why the emphasis belongs there.

Level II: responding

At this level, the student responds to some degree because of an outside influence. This is the point at which an observable change in behavior can first be seen. Therefore, written objectives now become appropriate. The student has not yet absorbed the value presented but is merely Responding to it. Like Receiving, Responding comprises the following three steps, the sequence of which describes the student's process of value acquisition within this level:

1. *Command response:* This step deals with appropriate responses that the student might not understand or accept the rationale for, and might not perform if certain requirements were not made. For example, the instructor states, "The traction splint must be applied correctly, according to your skills guide, at least once. By the way, you can't leave until you do." The student may call this bribery; the instructor calls this a necessary requirement
2. *Willing response:* This step differs from the first in that the student responds, when asked, without the requirement making it necessary for him to do so. In other words, he will respond, when asked, without bribery. The motive comes from outside the person. Exactly what the motive is isn't known, but what is important is that the desired response was given. For example, the student will apply correctly the traction splint, according to the skills guide, when asked by his instructor. The motive for the action comes from outside the person (i.e., the instructor), and the response is made because the student chooses to accept the instructor's request. Note that the reason behind that acceptance is not known, but what is important is that the action was done
3. *Satisfaction response:* At this step, the voluntary response to apply the traction splint is accompanied by a feeling of satisfaction or some other type of emotional response. For example, you may want to relate this feeling to the one you felt when you satisfactorily mastered the application of the traction splint. It also could be compared with the student who frequently applies the traction splint because he feels a sense of satisfaction when he performs this skill. This step is directly affected by the response of the instructor, and it has a secondary effect on the student's self-esteem. This effect on self-esteem may be positive or negative

This brings up an important point. The emotional element is present at the Responding level in all levels of the affective domain, to different degrees, for the following three reasons: (1) This is the level at which the emotional element most often begins to occur, (2) this is the point where the emotional element becomes part of the motivation (The satisfaction or dissatisfaction gained during the response serves as its own reinforcement. How great a reinforcement it is depends on both internal and external factors), and (3) the emotional element affects the student's overall perception of himself or herself.

Responding (Level II) is directly dependent on successful Receiving (Level I). This means that as Responding is observed, it may be concluded that Level I was attained. The degree to which it was attained may not be readily apparent. The reverse is also true—if Responding is not observed in a particular student, the Receiving level was not acquired or was not completed.

Classroom implications

Because this is the level at which the emotional element most often begins to occur, it has a direct effect on motivation and self-esteem, as has been stated earlier. Techniques directed toward this level include those that enhance motivation and self-esteem. Perhaps none is as important as ensuring a "safe" classroom. A "safe" classroom refers to an emotionally safe environment where a student will not be ridiculed for asking a question, playing with equipment, or failing (Figure 13-2). Being allowed to fail, without recrimination, is one of the most educational experiences a student can have. Although it may be difficult for the instructor to find the positive, giving honest, positive reinforcement encourages progress at this level.

Other techniques for enhancing the Responding level include leaving equipment out and permitting students to experiment freely rather than conducting only formally structured practicums, and passing judgments on how well students are using the equipment. Of course, inappropriate and dangerous uses should be avoided, but the freedom to take equipment apart and put it back together again is invaluable at this level.

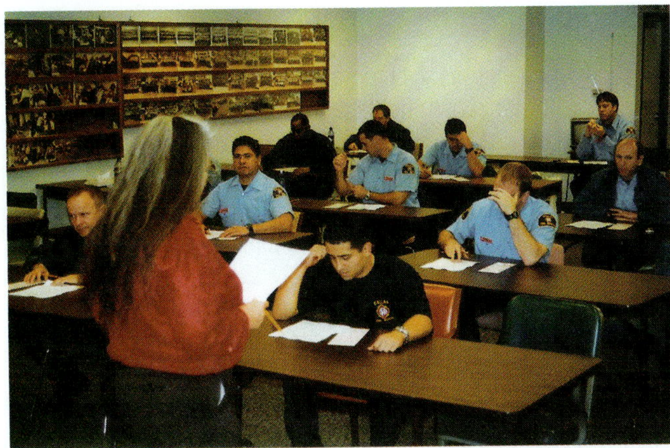

FIGURE 13-2 An emotionally safe classroom where students are freely allowed to ask questions and reveal their failings is conducive to a positive educational experience and promotes the Responding level of the affective domain.

Perhaps no underlying quality of an EMS instructor at this level is greater than respect for students themselves. This attitude of respect will guide and support the instructor's choices and, even when not spoken, will be perceived and communicated by students throughout the entire course.

Level III: valuing

The third level of the affective domain, Valuing, refers to the point at which the student attaches importance and impact to a subject or phenomenon. In this way, a person's values begin to affect their judgment. These values are internalized slowly, a process that occurs through the entire student experience, which includes previous experiences before the class session and interaction with peers, society, and significant others (e.g., instructors, partners, staff of receiving hospitals, and spouses). The following three steps are involved in incorporation of the valuing process:

1. *Acceptance (of a particular value)*: This step is similar to the awareness step of receiving, in that the student has become conscious that a particular action, subject, or phenomenon has worth. The instructor can assess whether this step has been reached by observing a student who makes the same or a similar response concerning the value in question, when confronted with a number of different stimuli
2. *Preference (for a particular value)*: In this step, the student not only has passively accepted the value but chooses to actively pursue it. In other words, when given a choice, the student will choose this value over other values that he or she may hold. The student typically takes every available opportunity to find out more about this value and those things related to it
3. *Commitment (to a value)*: Here, the student is committed to his belief and may be seen trying to persuade or convince others to accept the value. It is at this point that the student has accepted the value without reservation

Simply put, this level is characterized by two things: a choice and, at its best, consistency between choices. At the lowest step in this level, the student is still open to reevaluating his position, so his behavior is still tentative. At the highest step, the student is committed to his value and may be trying to further his knowledge of that value.

As with the previous two levels, this level is dependent on the attainment of Level II—Responding, and Level I—Receiving. The degree of attainment may not be evident until steps (1) and (2) of this level have been explored.

It is important for educators to be aware that both the student and the instructor can get "stuck" at this level.

If an internal valuing process has not developed, students will not progress beyond this level but will appear to do everything that the instructor tells them to do. They will do it the way they are expected to, every time they are observed (i.e., when the instructor is around). What happens when they aren't observed or the instructor isn't there is another thing.

If the student has adopted the values of a significant other, such as a partner or another instructor or mentor, without examining or testing these values for himself or herself, then the values in question tend to be rigid and fixed. This tendency can be observed in the student or in the instructor. In the case of a student, the value may have been developed to gain approval from a rigid instructor, or the student may have lacked the confidence to take a risk. In the case of an instructor, the value may have developed because of lack of field experience or lack of keeping up, or the instructor may have perceived a questioning student as a threat. In either case, values tend to be fixed concepts, rarely examined or tested; as a result, certain values become so rigid that the student or instructor refuses to further his or her knowledge, even when presented with information that is contradictory. Such individuals tend to feel threatened when their value system is questioned. Student comments that suggest that the student or instructor has gotten "stuck" include the following:

"That instructor doesn't know what he's talking about!"

"I've worked in the field for 20 years and I'm not going to change now!"

"It doesn't say that in the book!"

Instructor comments or nonverbal clues include:

"Do it this way because I say to do it this way!"

"Who are you to question me?!"

CASE IN POINT

It was that dreaded time of year when the "last minute crowd" all register for the required refresher courses. The EMS educator always dreaded these refreshers because they are heavily populated with the most experienced and "hardened" EMTs and paramedics, who have waited until the last possible minute to register for their continuing education and refresher courses. To make matters worse, these experienced field providers view instructors as white tower "has been's" who don't do the job any more and don't even remember what it was like being in the field. To cap it all off, the director made improvement of evaluations of the refresher courses one of the EMS educator's performance goals for the year. She was losing sleep over what to do, so she decided to stay up and read the EMS educator's textbook, where she found a few ideas that she thought might help her manage the situation.

As a first step, she set aside 5 days over 2 weeks to get out into the field and ride along with the crews. Second, she decided to show respect for them and their issues. She took the huge step of seeing situations from their perspective. After all, they are doing the job competently on a full-time basis all year, then they have to go into a classroom and practical labs to listen to a rehash of stuff that they believe they already know. Then, they have to pretend to run codes and perform routine skills on plastic manikins. How boring it has to be, she realized. This led her to a breatkthrough concept. She decided to go out on a limb and redesign the presentation format. She kept the same course objectives, the same content, and the same presentation and reference resources, but she changed the way everything would be presented.

On the first day of class, she mingled with the participants over coffee, chatting about the calls that she had been on over the previous 2 weeks. Next, she handed out the course materials and went over the objectives and schedule, but then made an announcement: "I'm not going to do any lecturing for this refresher. Because this is a *refresher* course, you are all very familiar with the content and how to do all the procedures. I'm going to ask you to 'discuss' the topics based on your experiences on calls. The only requirement will be that we all need to discuss every required topic in full. The way we do this will be up to you."

Everyone looked around uncomfortably. Most thought that it was going to be a complete disaster. To everyone's surprise, however, the group became animated, and a lively discussion began. Some participants tried to "hijack" the course and turn it into a social jam session, and others tried to become invisible, but most got on track and drove it in the right direction.

The result was a successful course that covered all course objectives and had a 100% pass rate on the final performance testing. The instructor, of course, was a nervous wreck after it was over, but the excellent course evaluations made it all worthwhile.

In this case, the EMS instructor took some very real risks and allowed herself to be vulnerable. First, she spent very rare and precious time in the field with crews, which helped to dispel the "ivory tower" stigma. Second, she decided that she would respect the responders and trust them. When she communicated this sincerely, they picked up on it and respected her and the process in return. Finally, she gave up the "security blanket" of presenting topics through traditional lectures in favor of letting participants form discussion groups and present their knowledge to each other. She realized that this approach might not work for every group or in every system, but she also suspected that opportunities for nontraditional approaches that incorporated trust and empowerment could probably be found in nearly every course, once she decided to look for them.

For instructors to avoid getting "stuck," they must become secure in themselves. They might, for example, stay active in the field and, if that is not possible, they may talk with those who have done so. Instructors can ask fundamental or complex questions without worrying what others might think. They must be honest about what they do and do not know. They must keep up with changes in subject matter, and they must build their own library and consult it often. The field of medicine changes rapidly, and keeping up with these changes requires that practitioners go to continuing education events and subscribe to professional journals. Keeping an open mind, experimenting with students, and helping students to develop their reasoning skills all work to keep both the instructor and the student "unstuck." By extending one's own personal experiences to students, the EMS educator can ensure that the values she or he holds are continually being reinforced or modified and kept up to date.

Classroom implications

Elizabeth King maintains, "the learning of an attitude occurs when a respected role model makes a verbal communication to the learner regarding desirable choices of action or displays these actions directly."[8] The implications of this are clear. We must think about what we, as EMS educators, say and do at all times. We must display an interest in our students and accept and guide and encourage them while we give them the tools they need to support their own conclusions. If a "safe" classroom environment has been maintained, students will find the freedom to fail, and in that failing, they will explore the values and choices the instructor has given them in the classroom. Students need the chance to analyze and synthesize for themselves, so they can claim values as their own. Students can be helped in this process by an instructor who supplies them with a good background in general knowledge, then forces them to explore new concepts and ideas, to analyze what they are learning, and to synthesize new ideas and concepts on "their own." For example, the EMS educator can ask students, "Why would a patient sweat?" When students arrive at two physiologic reasons—"to cool off or as a sympathetic response"—the instructor can then follow up by asking, "What are the causes of a sympathetic nervous system response that causes sweating?" This leads students to explore the emotional responses (i.e., fear and anxiety), then to relate these responses to the physiologic compensatory mechanisms, all of which are part of the spectrum of shock. Finally, moving up the taxonomy scale to higher orders, the instructor can then ask, "How, at a scene of a motor vehicle crash, when the patient is up, walking around, would you be able to tell if the sweating hands, pale skin, and mild tachycardia are due to an emotional response or due to compensation for organ injury?" This type of progressive, probing questioning leads students to analyze what they already think they know and to synthesize the information they do have to be able to apply it to new and different situations. All of this forms the basis for the next level.

It has been said that good judgment comes from experience, and experience comes from bad judgment. Isn't it best to start the student's experience from bad judgment in the classroom so they can develop good judgment in the field? One way to start this process is to present challenging realistic simulations in the classroom. For simulations to be effective in helping students move through this level, the choices that they will face in the field must be made available in the classroom. Careful planning and coordination are necessary if students are to make the most of this experience.

Students who are "stuck" at this level are often found in continuing education classes. They are the ones who already have a strong value and belief system that they have formed over years of experience and other training. To "get through" to these students and really offer them a worthwhile educational experience, the educator must appreciate their educational experiences from the students' perspective. First, such students not only have ideas and concepts that are already deeply rooted and that work for them, they also frequently are fearful, and fear of failure is the strongest fear for adults. Their fear does not need to be realistic or rational from the perspective of the educator to be very real to the adult student learner. This fear need only involve a perceived threat. The most likely threat is that to the student's esteem and his or her self-perception of competence, as failure is associated with incompetence. Therefore, the ideal strategy for the educator is to calm the fears of these students by removing all threats.

To achieve a change at this level when students are "stuck," the educator can go back to the Receiving level and use techniques that have already been suggested, such as making the information or change relevant by conveying to students why the training is necessary. The educator can then move to Responding by showing examples and asking for student responses to specific situations, then creating activities that require a response. The educator can then move to Valuing, where learners will have a chance to tear the subject matter apart and put it all together again (analysis and synthesis of the value in question). These activities generally are best accomplished through the use of challenging and realistic scenarios.

Sometimes, alleviating the fears of students is not as difficult as the EMS educator might imagine in that instructor reservations about the student's willingness to learn and change to adopt new ideas are frequently tied to the educator's own self-perception of his or her competence. Sometimes, everyone needs to become "unstuck"!

Level IV: organization

During the formation of values and attitudes, students begin to recognize several values that apply to the same situation. Students begin to categorize these by how much worth the new value has in relationship to the other things he values that apply to this situation. By doing this, the student establishes an order of values that he can defend and justify. When this is done, the student is operating at Level IV, Organization. Two steps are required for a student to acquire this level:

1. *Conceptualization (of the value)*: The student identifies the basic concepts of the new value as characteristics that are common to any one value he already holds. He or she then interprets these common characteristics into a subject or "heading" that can easily be recognized for reference purposes. An example is a student who chooses from a group of publications all those with articles that discuss EMS topics
2. *Categorization (of the value)*: At this step, the student organizes his or her own values that have characteristics in common into a relationship or hierarchy based on what has been learned in class, through skill demonstrations, and during personal experiences, as well as through the influence of those the student holds in esteem. This allows the student to defend and justify his or her actions. If Level III has been fully integrated and the instructor has allowed creativity and has supported lectures and demonstrations with adequate and sound medical reasoning, the student will more easily attain this level. The more concretely the student can justify and defend his or her actions, the more confident the student becomes, and the

more secure his or her value system will be. Ideally, this hierarchy of values, or value system, should be harmonious and consistent

To reach this point, the student must have completely integrated Levels I, II, and III into personal thought processes.

Classroom implications

The foundation of this level is set in the quality of supporting information (e.g., anatomy, physiology, pathophysiology, pharmacology) that the student has acquired. The implications for instructors are strong. Instructors must themselves have a good background in basic medical science if they are to help students. The need for the instructor to keep up with information and continue to expand personal horizons cannot be overemphasized. However, it is equally important for instructors to recognize that they cannot know everything. Therefore, making sure that instructors have access to a good library and reliable resources is a must, as is making good use of those resources on a regular basis. Instructors must look up things that they do not know. It is critically important for instructors to remember at all times that they are the students' primary resource, their mentor, and the model that they will be emulating. This is an onerous responsibility for all educators.

Information that instructors provide should allow students to begin to reason out the "why's." Instructors should start the reasoning in the classroom by monitoring and correcting student actions when necessary. For example, the instructor may ask students to compare patient situations, given two patients, both of whom are complaining of abdominal pain; one is a 25-year-old female, and the other is a 65-year-old female. Students can then be asked to discuss the keys of assessment (physical exam and history), explore the differential diagnosis, and compare treatment options. Then, the instructor can make the 65-year-old a patient with diabetes and ask students to explain how this changes their answers and treatment choices.

TEACHING TIP: Exercises that force the student to compare two patients with similar complaints demonstrate to the student how values may apply to similar situations, and how values may differ from one situation to another.

Use of scenarios to force students to examine two values facilitates organization of values according to sound medical reasoning. The reader can consider this example: A patient falls and twists her neck. Upon assessment, she is not breathing adequately. Clearing her airway does not improve her ventilations. The student is faced with immobilizing the patient where she lies, or gently moving her head and neck into alignment. What should the student choose and why? Have students justify their answers. Have discussions involving two value systems, exceptions to the rule, and what takes priority. These all help students to organize their values.

Use of scenarios is especially helpful at this level. Discussions of why certain signs and symptoms appear, what (if appropriate) expected signs/symptoms are NOT apparent and why that may be, and which treatment should be selected and why all go toward helping students justify their actions with the use of sound medical reasoning. "Because it says so in the protocol" is not an acceptable answer from a student at any learning level.

These exercises and others like them prepare students to explain and justify their choices. This type of preparation also helps students become accountable without fear of accountability. How completely students acquire this level varies according to the quality of their background education and their ability to integrate that information into their value organization. If this process is firmly based on sound medical reasoning, students will be able to confidently defend and justify their actions. If this is done in tandem with simulations, students will perform competently in practice.

Level V: characterization

At this level, the value system is so ingrained in students' behavior patterns that it becomes part of their lifestyle, and students' values become integrated into a total philosophy of care. Experience is required to attain this level. Therefore, this level usually is not observed in the classroom unless continuing education is being taught to a group of seasoned providers.

The two steps that constitute this level help describe a person who has attained it:

1. *Consistency*: This means that when the student is confronted with a number of situations that involve a reaction based on the same values, the student's reactions are automatic and consistently predictable. The key here is consistency. When confronted by a situation that demands a choice between values, the student is consistent in his or her choice and is able to consistently defend that choice with sound medical knowledge and judgment based on balancing of values, "book learning," skills, and experience. The instructor is able to predict how the student will act in a given situation
2. *Characterization*: Now, the student is so closely associated with the value in question that people use the name of the value to describe him or her. Here, the student has integrated attitudes, values, and ideas

into a total philosophy. This is most easily seen in the person who carries his or her own pair of gloves in the glove compartment of the car, or a barrier device in the inner pocket of a coat. Typically, this level is associated with a high level of student pride in accomplishments, as well as a high degree of satisfaction in work performed

This level cannot be measured in the classroom. Experience and several months to years are required for this level to fully develop. Experience cements basic values. Progress to this level usually is associated with pride in accomplishments and satisfaction with work.

It is important for the instructor to recognize that students' experiences may greatly contribute to their attaining this level, but only in one area and not in all. For instance, students may attain the level of Characterization with patients with trauma, but they may attain only the first steps of the Valuing level with cardiac patients. This may be so because of the population groups they serve, or it may be a result of where their interest lies. The interest and comfort levels of students dictate choices, such as always caring for patients with trauma while their partner cares for cardiac patients.

Peers, especially partners, receiving hospital staff, administrators, and life events may directly affect attainment of this level. A provider may demonstrate characteristics of this level but then vacillate between levels, depending on what is going on in his or her life. For instance, a provider may be on his way to acquiring Characterization when suddenly faced with the death of a coworker, a divorce, administrative decisions that negatively affect his or her ability to deliver patient care, or a receiving hospital staff whose attitudes are demeaning. If so much stress is introduced that basic value systems are called into question, an individual may revert back to Receiving or Responding. At this point, the important factor to be recognized is that a problem exists and the individual must be referred for more definitive care. Personal stressors may become powerful inhibitors to acquiring or maintaining this level.

Classroom implications

The most important action instructors can take is to model this level. Participating in continuing education as students, belonging to professional organizations, reading professional journals and discussing articles with students, extending their knowledge base to other disciplines, ensuring that classroom topics are relevant and applicable to the field, and being sensitive to what happens to students when they leave the classroom all help to contribute to the acquisition of this level by instructors—not only for themselves, but also for students.

PSYCHOMOTOR SKILLS

Any time that two paramedics from different services meet, two questions will surely be asked in the ensuing conversation. The first is, "How many drugs do you carry?" The second is, "What skills can you perform?" Even though the field of prehospital emergency medicine continues to improve its professional image, it is still tied to a technician-based model of care. Because of this, the learning, mastery, and performance of skills are, and will remain, an important part of the provision of emergency medical services. Therefore, it is imperative that EMS educators be proficient in the teaching and evaluation of skill performance.

Psychomotor skill development is crucial to good patient care. All the effort put forth at the scene of an EMS incident is dependent on the provider's ability to select the right skill, at the right time, and to carry it out in the right manner. In addition, many of the skills routinely performed at an EMS incident are critical to patient survival and leave little or no margin for error. As an example, placement of an endotracheal tube is vital to securing and maintaining an airway. However, this procedure allows no margin for error. The tube must be placed in the trachea, or the patient will suffocate. Thus, teaching paramedics to place endotracheal tubes must be done correctly, efficiently, and in a manner that ensures learner success. This can be accomplished only when the instructor has a solid understanding of psychomotor skill training, mastery, and performance.

Understanding the Psychomotor Domain

The psychomotor domain comprises the skill, action, muscle movement, and manual manipulation related to performing a physical action. Similar to all domains, the physical activities addressed in the psychomotor domain also have affective and cognitive dimensions. A learner who is being taught to start an IV needs not only to learn the physical movements and manipulations needed to insert an IV catheter, he or she must appreciate the discomfort the procedure causes, as well as the why and when associated with the procedure. In addition, the context or environment in which the skill will be performed is important. Many EMS skills and procedures are carried out in a field environment that is very different from that of a hospital or classroom. As one of the basic parts of a behavioral objective, as discussed in Chapter 8, a condition is specified under which the desired behavior is to occur. When psychomotor skills are taught, it is imperative that the instructor stress, and if possible simulate, various conditions in the classroom. It would be unfair for a learner to master a technique while not wearing personal protective equipment (PPE), then suddenly find that he or she is unable to do, or feels awkward doing, the same skill in a field setting wearing PPE. And, as with all learning experiences, modeling plays an important part in the learning experience. It is imperative, therefore, that the instructor and all other instructional personnel carry out skills and procedures in a manner consistent with that expected of the learner.

When teaching psychomotor skills, the instructor must consider learner "prerequisites" needed if the student is to learn the cognitive material. The ability of the learner to actually perform a skill is dependent on a number of parameters. The instructor should consider the following:

- *Physical strength of the learner.* Can the learner, for instance, lift a stretcher containing a 150-pound patient? Can he or she carry equipment and equipment containers up a flight of stairs?
- *Physical endurance.* Can the learner do cardiopulmonary resuscitation (CPR) on a patient in the back of an ambulance during a typical transport to the hospital?
- *Coordination.* Does the learner possess significant coordination, or is he or she "all thumbs"?
- *Sensory acuity.* Can the learner see fine detail? Exhibit sufficient depth perception? Does he or she wear bifocal glasses that make intubation difficult? Can he or she hear well enough to note different heart tones or breath sounds?
- *Composure.* How does the learner perform under stress? Does he or she develop tremors that interfere with delicate procedures? Does the learner become irritated, and thus tend to perform skills too quickly or without proper attention to detail? Conversely, if the skill produces discomfort for the patient, does the student freeze and fail to complete the skill?

The instructor is cautioned that when these parameters are evaluated, measures appropriate to the actual job description of the provider should be followed, as should the requirements of the Americans With Disabilities Act. (For more information on the Americans With Disabilities Act, see Chapter 10, Legal Issues for the Educator.)

Teaching a skill involves more than just correct demonstration of the skill. The instructor must analyze the skill and must recognize that every skill consists of a series of subcomponents. The actual terminology and number of components vary in the literature, but the essential actions include gross muscle movement, fine muscle movement, and spatial awareness. To understand these relationships, one can consider the skill of intramuscular injection. Providers engage in gross muscle movement as they move their arms up and forward toward the injection site. As the needle enters the patient, fine muscle movement adjusts to tactile stimulation to steady the path of the needle and handle gauge resistance. Spatial awareness tells providers where their extremities are in relation to their bodies and the environment. This information allows providers to "aim" the needle and determine when to stop advancement. Because awareness of the environment is so important, sensory acuity and perception also are important aspects of skill mastery. In this example, if the patient had moved, the provider would have to sense this and adjust his or her movement accordingly. Thus, when teaching skills, the instructor must understand not only the steps and sequence involved, but the kinematics of the procedure as well.

Levels of Psychomotor Skill Development

It would be nice if learners could see a skill demonstrated once, then be able to exactly reproduce the skill immediately and permanently. However, this is not the case. Learning a skill and assimilating it into a rote response involves a number of developmental steps. As with the other domains of learning, a taxonomy of psychomotor skill development has been devised. However, unlike with the cognitive domain, for which most educators use Bloom, different taxonomies are reported in the educational literature for psychomotor skill development. For the purposes of this textbook, Bloom's taxonomy of psychomotor skills development shown in Box 13-5 will be used.

Imitation

The most basic psychomotor skill is repeating or modeling a skill that is demonstrated to the learner by an expert. In this "see one, do one" approach, the instructor demonstrates the skill, then asks learners to repeat it. Usually, the instructor talks or guides the learner through the steps of the skill. This method works best for skills that are simple and can be understood easily through observation. For more complex skills, the instructor begins the learning process at the imitation stage by breaking down the complex skill into simpler, more easily learned skills that can be modeled by the beginner. Because learners are receptive to modeling the behavior of the instructor or another expert, it is important that the instructor avoid modeling incorrect behaviors. This can be difficult in

BOX 13-5 Bloom's Taxonomy: Psychomotor Domain

Level 1: Imitation
Level 2: Manipulation
Level 3: Precision
Level 4: Articulation
Level 5: Naturalization

that the instructor has progressed to the naturalization level and may not even be cognizant of how he is performing the skill. The old adage, "Don't do as I do, do as I say" doesn't work for skills training!

Manipulation

The second phase of skill mastery is manipulation. During this stage, learners move away from simple modeling to performing the skill according to guidelines, such as skill sheets. They "manipulate" the various parts of the skill in such a way as to develop their own basis or foundation for doing the skill. Because learners are still exploring the skill, mistakes are common and are to be expected. However, mistakes help learners to better understand the skill through the corrective actions needed. It is important for the instructor to closely monitor learners as they practice skills to ensure that no incorrect actions or "bad habits" are learned as part of the skill. Because each learner is different, some variation in performance may occur, but by and large, the learner must perform the skill as modeled by the instructor. It is also important at this stage for the instructor to explain to learners why a particular action or technique is used. This is especially important if follow-on skills will require this action. For example, proper placement of limb leads in obtaining an electrocardiogram (ECG) may not be critical for a 3-lead ECG, but it becomes more important when a 12-lead ECG is obtained.

This is also the period during which the learner begins independent practice of the skill. It is important that skill sheets or procedures be explained clearly and in sufficient detail. Practice sessions should be observed closely, and any incorrect behaviors should be immediately identified and corrected. Because the learner is discovering the new skill, group practice may provide a supportive environment and can allow learners to explore the new skill together.

Precision

At the precision stage, the learner can perform the basic skill without coaching and with few, if any, mistakes. However, the learner still has not developed the expertise to perform the skill in various contexts. For example, the learner may be able to splint a fractured arm on a simulated patient who is sitting up without angulation. However, any variation of this, such as the patient's lying down, will reduce the learner's precision.

Articulation

This stage blends psychomotor skill development with the cognitive and affective dimensions of a skill or procedure. The learner understands why the skill is done in a particular way and knows when the skill is indicated. The learner can now evaluate the context in which the skill is performed and can adjust his performance to the situation. In the previous example, the learner would now be able to splint an arm, regardless of patient position or other conditions. The learner is now performing the skill without mistakes and without the assistance of props such as skill sheets or instructor prompting. This is the level of psychomotor skill performance that is expected of an entry level provider.

Naturalization

At this stage, the learner can perform the skill flawlessly and without much conscious effort. In a scenario, simulation, or actual patient care situation, the learner will be able to perform the skill while continuing to monitor the context and environment. The learner will be able to multitask effectively (Figure 13-3). The learner has achieved what is known as "muscle memory," that is, the skill has become rote and can be initiated and performed with minimal sensory awareness. A common example of this level of mastery is the provider who is seen performing a manual skill, such as a pulse or neuro-check, while obtaining an oral history from the patient. This level is rarely seen in the classroom learner or entry level provider. It develops later as the provider gains experience on the job.

Teaching Psychomotor Skills

Effective teaching of psychomotor skills involves more than just demonstrating a skill and having learners practice. As with any instructional activity, preparation and teaching technique are important aspects of the overall experience. This is especially true in the psychomotor domain because of the complexity of many EMS skills.

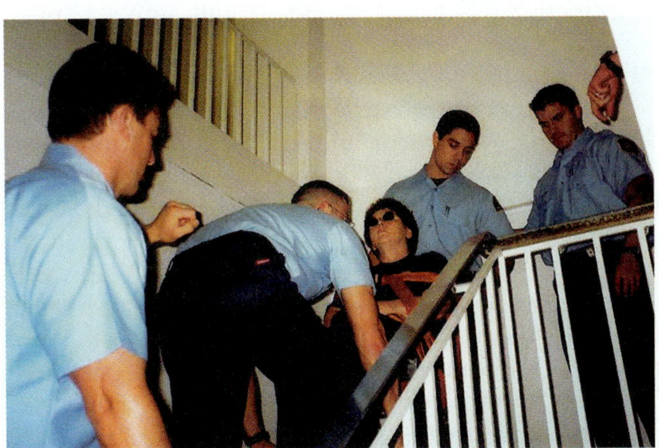

FIGURE 13-3 Naturalization of a psychomotor skill is achieved when the student is able to multitask effectively.

Because EMS skills almost always involve equipment and, to be effectively demonstrated, usually require special teaching aids or manikins, preparation is important. To begin, the instructor must review the lesson goal, objectives, and lesson plan to ensure that he or she is familiar with the lesson. Necessary equipment, supplies, and teaching aids should be identified and secured. The instructor is cautioned not to assume that equipment and materials will be available in the classroom. This is especially true in multiple-use facilities, where different instructors and different classes may meet in the same facility. If the instructor arranges for an in-service unit to provide lesson props, a backup plan should be in place in the event the unit suddenly becomes unavailable. The same applies to lessons planned for outdoors that may be canceled or modified because of weather.

When setting up the classroom or drill ground, the instructor should consider the following:

- *Safety.* The instructor should consider safety, not only in terms of practice by the learners, but as it relates to any inherent danger associated with demonstrating the skill. For example, caution is needed when one is demonstrating auto extrication skills. Vehicles and equipment can shift, or parts may fly off, during certain activities. The instructor should clearly define and mark safe zones
- *Visibility.* For the learner to model and imitate a skill, he or she must be able to see all aspects of the process. Therefore, it is important that the instructor provide visibility. This may involve moving learners or using special, large-scale models or cameras and video projectors
- *Rehearsal.* Regardless of how many times an instructor has performed a skill, or how well he or she can do it, it is always prudent to practice the skill before class. This is especially true when one is using special models or equipment that is different from that routinely used. Nothing kills an instructor's credibility more effectively than an inability to use the equipment that he or she is teaching about. If something is to go wrong, it will surely happen during the class session
- *Classroom preparation.* The instructor should arrange the classroom to ensure visibility and to accommodate the equipment and instructional props. The instructor should check in advance for electrical or oxygen connections, venting, and so forth. Once demonstration equipment has been placed, it should be covered or hidden, if possible. This prevents learners from focusing on the props instead of on the instructor
- *Practice space.* If learners will practice a particular skill, the instructor must ensure that sufficient space is provided, as well as appropriate equipment, at each skill practice area. If learners will rearrange a classroom before they begin practice, the instructor must ensure that this can be done and will not be disruptive to the learning process

WHOLE-PART-WHOLE INSTRUCTION

Various techniques can be used to teach skills. A common approach in medicine is the "see one, do one, teach one" concept. This may work for one-on-one instruction, but for most EMS classes, a method more appropriate for larger groups is needed.

The standard technique used for teaching EMS skills is the whole-part-whole method. To use this technique, the instructor demonstrates the skill three times:

1. *Whole.* The instructor demonstrates the entire skill from beginning to end, while briefly naming each action or step. If possible, the skill should be performed under the conditions specified in the psychomotor behavioral objective
2. *Part.* The instructor demonstrates the skill again, step-by-step, explaining each part in detail. It is important that the instructor select proper size "bites" of the skill. If the information is too specific, the learner can be overloaded with detail. Too broad, and the learner may not be able to make the connection from step to step
3. *Whole.* The instructor demonstrates the entire skill from beginning to end, without interruption, and usually without commentary

This technique provides repeated accurate examples of how the skill is done. If a learner was not completely focused on the skill demonstration the first time, two other opportunities for observation are provided. This approach also provides a rationale for how the skill has been performed. During the "part" presentation, the instructor can integrate affective and cognitive objectives and encourage student interaction and questions. Finally, it has been proved that the technique works well for both analytic and global learners. Analytic learners appreciate the step-by-step instruction, and global learners get the chance to see the skill performed in context.

PROGRESSION THROUGH THE PSYCHOMOTOR DOMAIN LEVELS OF SKILL ACQUISITION

As has been discussed, the learner moves through a progression of increasing proficiency, eventually reaching the mastery level. When teaching psychomotor skills, the instructor must provide an environment that fosters this development.

The instructor should first work with learners to move from novice to expert, that is, being able to perform the skill at the precision level. When moving learners in this direction, the instructor should keep the following in mind:

- Learners should be allowed to progress at their own pace. If learners are moved too quickly, they may not understand what they are doing and will not acquire good thinking skills
- Although the demonstration may provide information on the performance of the entire skill from start to finish, learners should be allowed to learn the individual parts of the skill before pulling it all together and demonstrating the whole skill
- Learners should master individual skills before placing them in the context of a scenario or simulation
- Learners should be allowed ample time to practice a skill before they are tested
- The need for constant direct supervision should diminish as practice time increases and skill level improves

Taking this into consideration, the instructor should plan skill learning to follow a sequence similar to the following:

- The instructor demonstrates the skill to learners
- Learners practice using a skills check sheet
- Learners memorize the steps of the skill until they can verbalize the sequence without error
- Learners perform the skill, stating each step as they perform it
- Learners perform the skill while answering questions about their performance
- Learners perform the skill in the context of a scenario or an actual patient situation (Figure 13-4).

It may be surprising to the reader that one of the most difficult tasks for the instructor is to provide feedback during skill practice. Too often, the instructor tells learners that they are doing something wrong and quickly performs the skill, rather then providing guidance and coaching. When feedback is provided, this must be done in a positive manner—not with a negative tone. However, the instructor should not hesitate to correct incorrect performance. This is especially critical during the early stages of skill development. If incorrect behaviors are not effectively corrected, mastery or muscle memory of the wrong technique will occur, and correcting this later on will be more difficult. The instructor may allow advanced learners to identify and correct their own errors under limited supervision. To reinforce correct behaviors, the instructor should end practice sessions with a demonstration of correct performance.

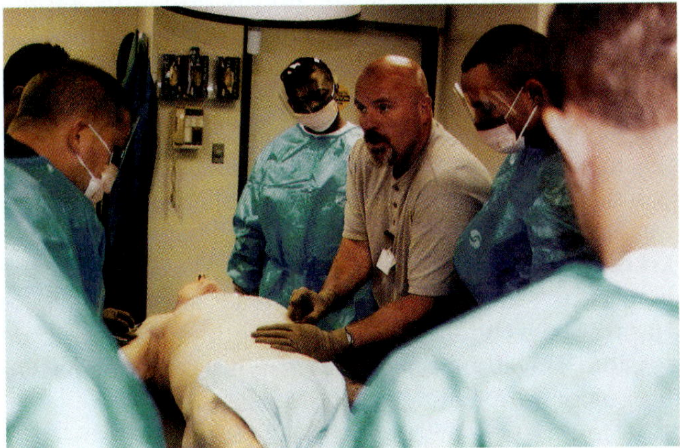

FIGURE 13-4 Learners should move through a progression of increasing proficiency and achieve mastery before using skills on real patients. Shown is a cadaver lab that is used to assist students in achieving mastery.

When the class comprises adult learners, the instructor's role takes on an added dimension. Adult learners exhibit characteristics different from those of younger learners. One such characteristic is the need to look at learning from a variety of angles. Thus, adult learners may spend time trying other approaches and methods of performing skills with the purpose of arriving at a final method. This is not to say that adult learners should be given free rein during skill practice, especially given the precise nature of many EMS skills. However, the instructor should be sensitive to the importance of providing more explanation and guidance to the adult learner than to the younger, less experienced learner. Adult learners also need encouragement and positive feedback to reinforce the correct behavior.

As a learner masters a skill, it is important for the instructor to appreciate the level of mastery required of the learner. Too often, instructors and practical test evaluators expect a learner to perform a skill at a level beyond that attainable by an entry level provider. Some instructors and evaluators expect performance that matches their own level of mastery. This is not only an unrealistic expectation, it is unfair to the learner as well. It is important for instructors and evaluators to accept that many EMS skills may be performed in a number of different but medically acceptable ways. Just because a learner performs a skill in a way that differs from the instructor's performance does not mean that the learner's performance is wrong, unless it is medically incorrect or may harm the patient.

Because most EMS provider certification courses require successful completion of a practical examination, the instructor may insist that learners perform skills one, and only one, way. The intention is to minimize the possibility of confusion for the learner during the stress of a practical evaluation. Although practice is important and is encouraged, the instructor may encourage learners not to practice skills outside the classroom. Again, the instructor is attempting to minimize distracting and incorrect behaviors that the learner may pick up by practicing or learning from others outside the classroom. It is difficult for a novice learner to avoid responding to the seasoned paramedic who says, "Don't do it that way, here is an easier way."

The instructor must determine how best to handle these concerns in each specific teaching situation.

Skill Sheets

When new skills are taught, it is important for the learner to know clearly what is involved in the skill, in terms of both actions and sequence. Although the instructor demonstrates the skill, the use of a skill sheet enhances the learner's comprehension. The skill sheet also serves as a review for skill performance. For visual and concrete learners, it provides the needed framework on which mastery of the skill can be built.

When preparing a skill sheet, it is important for the instructor to clearly list the various steps of the skill at a level consistent with that used in the teaching demonstration. In other words, if six steps are demonstrated in completing a skill, the skill sheet should list six steps. The skill sheet should not be used to break the skill down to a level that is more finite than the one taught, or conversely, to compress actions into fewer steps. It is also important for the instructor to design the skill sheet with emphasis on areas that are critical to proper skill performance and subsequent skill evaluation. If process is important, it should be included. Likewise, if sequence is important, then sequencing should be delineated on the skill sheet, and it should be clearly communicated to the learner that it is important.

Whenever possible, the skill sheet used by the learner should be the same as, or similar to, the one used for evaluation. A common practice is for instructors to provide students with the practical evaluation skill sheets of the National Registry of Emergency Medical Technicians (EMTs) for use during practice. This should not be construed as "teaching to the test" but as a means of (1) ensuring that learners are developing the proper skills and sequence, and (2) reducing evaluation anxiety.

Improving Psychomotor Skill Development During a Skills Session

Skill sessions provide valuable time for the learner to practice and master skills. However, for full support of skill mastery, it is important that the skill session be used to maximum advantage. To accomplish this, the instructor should keep the following in mind:

- Have all necessary equipment set up before the session begins. However, if the setup is complicated or the class is large, the instructor may have the learners retrieve equipment from a storage area and set up the practice stations. In a similar manner, learners can be asked to put away the equipment
- Use realistic and current equipment that is in proper working order. Don't expect learners to master a skill if they don't have the right equipment to use
- Use standardized skill sheets
- Allow ample practice time in class, at breaks, and during other times. However, ensure that all practice sessions are conducted safely and with proper supervision as needed
- Always model correct psychomotor skill behavior
- Keep learners active and involved. This can be difficult, especially as learners become more proficient; they may not wish to engage in repeated practice of a skill
- Insist that learners respect equipment and skills
- Ensure competence in individual skills before using scenarios. Scenarios should be designed to tie together basic skills, once they have been mastered
- Add realism. It is important for the instructor to place skills in the context of on-the-job situations. When using scenarios,
  - Limit the objective of the scenario to three learning points
  - As learners become more sophisticated with the use of critical thinking skills, add dimensions to the scenario
  - Make the scenario realistic, especially in terms of the performance objective and the safety requirements, such as wearing protective equipment
  - Use actual equipment
  - Consider the use of moulage, props, background noises, and so forth

Managing the Skill Session

Skill practice time can be a value commodity for the learner, especially in certification courses like Emergency Medical Technician-Basic (EMT-B). It is imperative that the instructor plan practice time to provide maximum opportunity for the learner to master skills. This is best achieved when some degree of structure is provided during the session. Simply providing a room full of equipment and instructing learners to practice skills will usually result in chaos and little active practice by the learners. This is especially true when skills are being reviewed that the learner believes he or she has mastered. Instructors teaching refresher or renewal courses are often faced with the challenge of motivating learners to perform skills they believe they already know. To ensure maximum use of practice time, the instructor should plan activities to keep the whole class engaged for the entire length of the practice session. This is especially important if only one or two instructors are managing a large class.

A few issues about the use of assistant instructors must be mentioned. Assistants can be a great help to an instructor, and they may provide direct assistance and feedback to learners. However, it is important that the lead instructor and assistant instructors teach the same skill in the same manner. It is also important that assistant instructors do not express their opinions about how the learners are being taught by the lead instructor, and that they do not criticize the quality of learner performance.

Maximizing Skill Session Time

To ensure that practice time is used as efficiently as possible, instructors should plan activities to fill the entire instruction time. Instructors should consider assigning roles to learners during skill practice. In this way, learners will have the chance to practice different skills and rotate through different roles during the skill practice. This approach works well to occupy learners who otherwise would be waiting to practice a skill or to move on to the next skill.

Learners can be assigned to the following roles, depending on the size of the practice group:

- *Evaluator.* Uses a skill sheet or records steps as they are performed. This allows learners to appreciate the challenge of evaluating a skill and reinforces learning through observation of the skill that is being performed
- *Information provider.* Uses a script and provides information as it is requested, for instance, vital signs when they are taken
- *Team leader.* Primary patient care provider and leader of the team performing the skill(s)
- *Partner or assistant.* Assists the team leader and performs care as directed by the team leader. Depending on practice parameters, may be silent or may be able to suggest and interact with the team leader
- *Patient.* Faithfully portrays signs and symptoms according to scenario. May be moulaged for realism. This role also familiarizes the learner with the experiences of the patient and promotes empathy
- *Bystander(s).* Additional practice team members can assume the role of bystanders and can act as distracters or helpers. It is important for the instructor to monitor learners in this role to ensure that they don't get too carried away with their role playing, thereby disrupting the actual practice of the skill in a realistic setting

When designing a practice session, the instructor should distribute a written scenario to practice groups. The scenario should be realistic for the learner's level of expertise and local operational capability. It should also match the performance objective that is being reviewed. Sources of scenarios include actual calls, medical scenario books, EMS textbooks, instructor toolkits, and professional organization Web sites. As always, the instructor should make sure that the scenario stresses safety and appropriate body substance isolation (BSI).

To begin the practice session, the instructor should have the information provider read the dispatch information. Whenever possible, learners should be allowed to complete the scenario without interruption. At this point, the learner should have mastered individual skills, so stopping for correction should not be necessary. Once the scenario has been completed, the group as a whole should evaluate skill performance. This should be a positive learning experience—not a learner bashing. To provide a positive experience, a positive-negative-positive format is used. The evaluation should start off with general statements and positive comments such as, "Good job recognizing the leg injury as a fracture." Instructors should always try to find something positive even if the skill session performance was not up to standard. The instructor should next move to constructive feedback and areas for improvement, citing specific actions or decisions of concern. Comments must be consistent with what learners have been taught, and they must follow the skill sheet. The instructor should end the review with a positive comment such as, "I was especially impressed by how you applied the traction splint, given the location of the fracture."

The various role players should next be called upon to critique the performance. It must be remembered that learners are often their own greatest critics. They should be encouraged to look for the positive aspects of their performance. The patient care provider should comment on what he did correctly, then on what needs improvement. Learners should always be forced to see something positive in what they have done. Otherwise, they may focus on what they perceive as poor performance. The assistants, patient, and bystanders all should take turns providing feedback. Finally, the evaluator should comment on timing, sequencing, prioritization, and skill performance.

Once the scenario has been critiqued, learners should change roles. Sufficient scenarios and time should be provided for all learners to have at least one chance to play each role. This approach keeps all learners active and involved and makes maximum use of the practice time.

SUMMARY

Comprehensive EMS education involves teaching in every domain and at all levels. EMS educators must be conscious of the three domains of learning and must apply appropriate teaching methods for the purpose of developing competent, comprehensive EMS care providers. In addition to giving attention to each domain, the educator must be aware of the multiple levels of learning that students go through in becoming fully competent. Each level requires that the instructor (1) be aware of the signs of progress and

CASE IN POINT

The EMS instructor conducted the cardiac assessment skill session for six EMT-Basic students. He began by asking, "Who wants to be the team leader first?" A lively, bright, and aggressive student jumped up to the head of the manikin and said, "I'll do it." The information provider presented the case of a witnessed arrest on a golf course with bystander CPR and no automatic external defibrillator (AED) when the crew arrives.

"The first thing I'm going to do is BSI and scene safety, and I'll determine whether I need any help. Are there any other patients? Any hazards, like downed electrical lines? He didn't get electrocuted, did he? We have advanced life support (ALS) on the way, right?" He immediately gave out team assignments to check for vital signs, put on the AED, and check the airway and give positive pressure ventilations, if necessary. After a quick airway, breathing, and circulation (ABC) check, the AED indicated a need for shock, and everyone stood "clear" while it delivered a series of three stacked shocks. The AED shock was successful, and the patient had strong and regular carotid pulses at a rate of 90 per minute. The instructor then conducted a brief critique of the session, allowing the evaluator first, then others in the group, to provide input.

Addressing the team leader, he said, "Your initial steps and team management were very well organized and effective. Well done." To the team member who managed the airway, he said, "Your assessment and ventilations were fine, but you didn't use an oropharyngeal airway. I was wondering why not?" After the team member shrugged and looked around for support, the instructor said, "I understand you may have overlooked it, but realize that the oropharyngeal airway is the most neglected adjunct in the basic life support (BLS) tool kit. Everybody should keep it in mind. Can you think of why?" The discussion went on with the instructor providing constructive nonjudgmental feedback in a positive learning environment.

This was a typical cardiovascular skill assessment session in which realistic manikins, an AED, and airway and ventilation devices were provided. The instructor's feedback to participants was nonjudgmental, honest, and helpful. The organized setup combined with a qualified and prepared instructor provided the next best learning environment that we have after actual clinical settings.

(2) know the teaching methods that help move students toward higher levels of learning and critical thinking.

REFERENCES

1. Dewey J. *Experience and Education.* New York, NY: Collier; 1963.
2. Stiggins RJ, Rubel E, Quellmakz E. *Measuring Thinking Skills in the Classroom.* Washington, DC: National Education Association; 1986.
3. Costa AL, Hanson R, Silver HF, Strong RW. Building a repertoire of strategies. In: Costa AL, ed. *Developing Minds: A Resource Book for Teaching Thinking.* Alexandria, Va: Association for Supervision and Curriculum Development; 1985:141-143.
4. Beyer BK. *Practical Strategies for the Teaching of Thinking.* Boston, Mass: Allyn and Bacon; 1987.
5. Rubenfeld MG, Scheffer BK. *Critical Thinking in Nursing: An Interactive Approach.* Philadelphia, Pa: JB Lippencott; 1995.
6. Beyer BK. *Developing a Thinking Skills Program.* Boston, Mass: Allyn and Bacon; 1988.
7. Lorber MA, Pierce WD. *Objectives, Methods, and Evaluation for Secondary Teaching.* 2nd ed. Englewood Cliffs, NJ: Prentice Hall; 1983.
8. King EC. *Affective Education in Nursing: A Guide to Teaching and Assessment.* Rockville, Md: Aspen System; 1984.

ADDITIONAL READING

Krathwohl DA, Massie BB, Bloom BS, et al. *Taxonomy of Educational Objectives Handbook. II: Affective Domain.* New York, NY: David McKay; 1964.

McCombs BL, McNeely S, series eds. *Psychology in the Classroom: A Series on Applied Educational Psychology. Teaching for Thinking.* Hyattsville, Md: American Psychological Association; 1996.

Sternberg RJ. *Beyond IQ: A Triarchic Theory of Human Intelligence.* New York, NY: Cambridge University Press; 1985.

Wlodkowski RJ. *Enhancing Adult Motivation to Learn: A Comprehensive Guide for Teaching All Adults.* 2nd ed. San Francisco, Calif: Jossey-Bass; 1999.

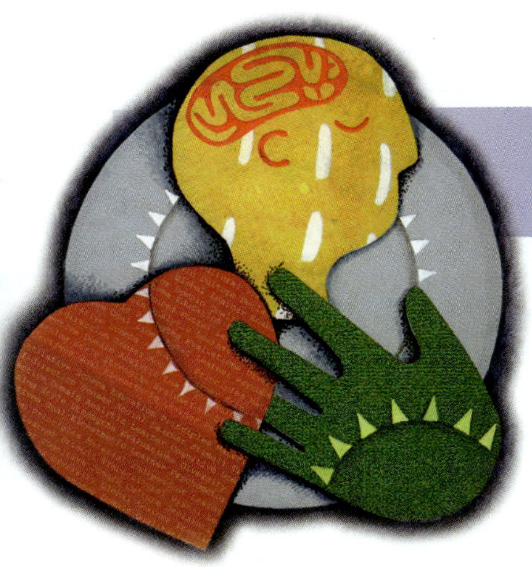

CHAPTER 14

Tools for Individual Learning

"You cannot teach a man anything; you can only help him find it within himself."

—Galileo Galilei

As has been discussed in earlier chapters, adult learners respond best in an environment that offers a variety of learning methods. Adult learners frequently have a motivation for learning that is not present in younger learners. They have consciously made the choice to acquire new knowledge and will often seek out ways on their own to broaden and apply their new-found knowledge. This chapter introduces a variety of methods best suited for individual or self-directed learning.

Individual learning can involve one-on-one learning with an educator or with another student. It can refer to self-directed learning that is indirectly facilitated by an educator, or it may be used in describing an individual who is working on his or her own to further knowledge on a given subject. Additionally, this chapter explores techniques used inside and outside the classroom that encourage self-directed learning.

TEXTBOOKS AS TOOLS

Although the usefulness of textbooks in education is often debated in the literature, a textbook can be an important tool for individual learning if it is used appropriately. Before the educator can begin to maximize the potential of a textbook, however, an understanding of the book and its elements should be reached. Educators should view a textbook as a tool and should study its structure and function, as one would study an anatomy lesson. In keeping with the earlier discussion of a purely lecture instructional format, the textbook should not be used as the sole source of information. Instead, it should provide a foundation of knowledge from which an educator can expand and enhance the student learning experience, and as a tool for answering questions and providing feedback.[1-3]

Know the Textbook

The educator can begin by taking a fresh look at the textbooks that are currently used for the course. He or she can review the table of contents and take note of the order in which the topics are presented. Does this order follow what happens in the classroom, or not? The educator should become familiar with the topics covered within each chapter and should note those topics that might be considered enrichment—that is, material that goes above and beyond the required curriculum. The front matter of most current texts provides a description of "features" or tools included within the book to enhance learning and provide structure to the content. These features are generally highlighted and explained as part of the introduction to students and instructors. Studying each of the features and beginning to plan and strategize how they might be used in the classroom is a good approach. For example, the instructor may want to provide examples and suggestions for students as the class progresses through the book. Box 14-1 outlines some strategies by which learners can benefit most from their textbooks.

Modeling Use of the Textbook

One of the best ways to encourage students to open their textbooks and begin using them is to model the behavior as an educator. Although teaching straight

BOX 14-1 Strategies for Getting the Most From Your Textbook

1. Preview-Connect-Predict

Have students preview content in textbook chapters by working in teams and looking at headings, pedagogical elements, and so forth. While previewing, have students discuss connections to their individual life experiences and knowledge. Finally, have students predict what they will learn in the chapter.

2. Think-Pair-Share

Have students work in teams and take turns sharing knowledge aloud from different passages read silently and individually from the textbook. Imparting or "sharing" knowledge places the student in the role of the educator and demands greater comprehension of the material.

3. Admit-Exit Tickets

Have students enter the classroom with a written-down "fact" that they learned from the assigned reading. This fact "admits them" to the discussion for the day. After the discussion has ended, students can reevaluate what they have learned and list new concepts and thoughts as their "Exit" card. The exit card is their ticket out of the classroom.

Modified from Robb L. Strategies for getting the most from textbooks. *Instructor.* 2003;112.

from the textbook is inappropriate, the instructor can have a positive impact on appropriate student use of the text. How is the textbook that has been assigned to the class used by the instructor in the classroom as he or she teaches? Is the textbook merely used as a means to get students to read outside the classroom? Does the instructor make the class text a living, breathing part of every class session? Or, does he or she refer to it only when providing the next reading assignment? The educator should assign the textbook a role in the overall learning experience, using it as a baseline for knowledge and a reference for questions or clarifications.[3,4]

TEACHING TIP: When students make the inevitable "but that is not in the book" comment, take the opportunity to get students to research the missing or controversial topic, then present to the class the reasons why they think the information in the text is missing or presented in the way that it is. Additionally, textbooks are usually written to a national standard, and information in the text may be incorrect for local protocols. The instructor should use this opportunity to have students research and discuss differences.

Pedagogical Features

Many textbooks have specific elements designed to enhance student learning and retention. Some studies have shown that it is these various elements that are read most frequently by students.[3] Elements such as learning objectives, case scenarios, review questions, and enrichment information all offer opportunities to enhance individual learning. Following are examples of how each learning feature can be used.

Learning objectives

Objectives drive emergency medical services (EMS) educational programs. Whether instructors or students like them or not, they determine what is taught and describe desired outcomes (see Chapter 8). Knowing where they are placed in the textbook, how they integrate with the three learning domains (cognitive, psychomotor, and affective), and what their purpose is will most likely be helpful to many students. The instructor should take the time to explain these resources at the beginning of a program and should describe how all three learning domains will be incorporated into the course.

Students should be encouraged to review the objectives before they read the content. They should refer back to the objectives as they read the text content to ensure that they are identifying the most important information.

CASE IN POINT

This technique can be modeled in class either before or after a lesson is presented. Specific objectives are selected and are reworded as questions. Students are instructed to hold their answers until chosen, then to state the question out loud. Students wait several seconds (20-30) before they select another student, who must give the answer. Students should be encouraged to do the same for themselves as they review the material before an exam. If they cannot confidently answer the objective, they can return to the content to reread the information that was missed the first time around. This may also encourage students to use review of objectives as a reading strategy before they come to class; this promotes individual learning.

In using objectives for individual learning, the instructor should encourage students to review them before taking a cognitive or skills exam. Students should be urged to shape each objective into a question and should confirm that they can confidently answer each of these questions. For objective questions that they cannot answer, students must return to the content of the text or seek answers from other students or the educator.

Case scenarios

Case scenarios are another common element of many textbooks. For example, many texts begin each chapter with a scenario in an effort to put what is about to be read into a meaningful context for the student. The case study also serves as a motivational tool to help the learner identify why the topic is important. Scenarios can be excellent tools for students as they learn to think critically and improve their problem-solving skills. When course material is put into the context of a patient scenario, it frequently becomes more real for the learner and thus more easily understandable.

CASE IN POINT

The instructor is encouraged to begin or end the next lecture using one of these scenarios. If it is presented at the beginning of a lecture, the instructor should read the scenario and ask students to write down a response based on the context of the topic. For example, if it is a scene safety scenario, students should be asked to identify the hazards contained within the scene. Which hazards are the most obvious? Are there potential hazards that currently don't exist at the scene but may appear later? The instructor should allow students just 3 or 4 minutes to jot down some thoughts before asking them to share their comments with the student sitting next to them. Comparing answers is a great way for students to see through someone else's eyes; it opens them up to other possibilities.

In the same manner, the instructor may choose to end a class session by reading or assigning a scenario from the next chapter. Students should be encouraged to think about the scenario and should come to the next class meeting prepared to discuss it.

Review questions

Many textbooks also offer some form of review of the content of each chapter or section. Review questions, for example, are often placed at the end of the chapter in an effort to test or validate that the student has learned or gained some new knowledge from the reading. These questions can become a valuable tool for the student, especially if the educator models their use and incorporates them into classroom discussion.[5]

CASE IN POINT

The instructor can select two or three review questions to either begin or end a lesson to encourage students to discuss or find the answers. This selection of questions from the next class lesson or topic, even though students have not yet read it, may encourage them to complete the assigned reading. If the instructor makes a practice of beginning a lesson with some of these questions, students are more likely to read the questions ahead of time and formulate a response.

Learners can use review questions as a self-evaluation tool to prepare for exams or simply to gauge their understanding and progress as they move through the content.

Enrichment

Enrichment content refers to information presented in a textbook that goes beyond the required curriculum. Enrichment information often presents topics that are closely related to, but not directly contained within, a respective curriculum, and they can be used as a valuable tool for individual learning if this is modeled by the instructor.

Enrichment content can be a great place for a student to begin looking for topics for research papers or extra credit assignments; it can be used to motivate students to think beyond what is "required" of them.

Addition of enrichment information can be detrimental if it is added to an already heavy required learning load. Educators should choose this material carefully so they do not burden students with information of little value, or that will not directly affect how they may care for a patient. For instance, if presented well, the basic pathophysiology of congestive heart failure can help students identify afflicted patients sooner. On the other hand, presenting the details of jellyfish stings to a class of emergency medical technicians (EMTs) in Nebraska may not be the best use of class time.

Textbook Ancillaries

It was not so long ago that textbooks were the one and only tool used to support classroom learning and individual study. Today, the choices of instructional tools are many. Textbook support materials may include items such as workbooks, companion CD-ROMs, companion Web sites, and exam review manuals. All these instructional formats are potentially valuable tools for self-directed learning in initial and refresher training. However, as with textbook use, it is incumbent upon the educator to reinforce the use and importance of these ancillary materials.[6]

Student workbooks

Print workbooks that accompany textbooks typically consist of questions and written exercises that are specific to each chapter. They are ideally suited for individual learning because the workbook material is self-paced, generally follows the format and content flow of the textbook, and promotes active learning through content reinforcement exercises.[6] For example, students can use workbooks for exam preparation, remediation, and reinforcement of concepts (Figure 14-1). Educators can use them for homework assignments and for assessment of student understanding and growth. The disadvantage of the workbook is that it requires an additional cost to the learner, and it can be time-consuming and subjective for educators to grade.[6] At the very least, however, educators should make students aware of such resources and should encourage their use. An example of encouragement may be to offer extra credit for completed workbook assignments, or the instructor can present workbook activities during class time.

Electronic workbooks have also become available. These workbooks are generally available online (not in print format), and they include interactive activities that provide immediate feedback. Again, these are ideally suited for individual learning, and the online feature of immediate feedback can make grading easier for the educator. One study that compared the use of print workbooks and electronic workbooks found that, although learner satisfaction was greater with the electronic product because of ease of use and time savings, no significant difference was noted in posttest performance.[6]

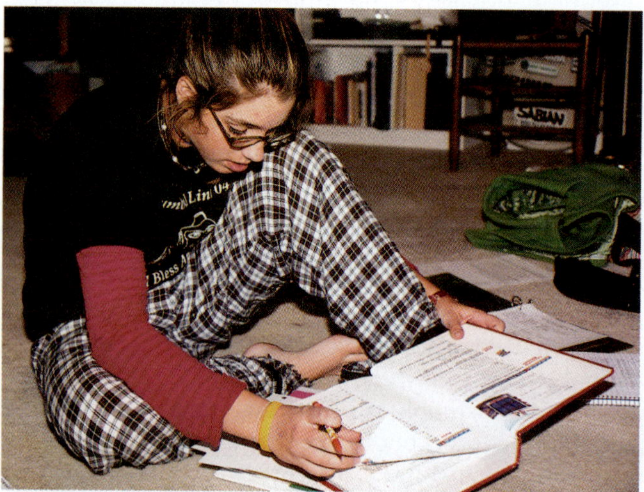

FIGURE 14-1 Workbooks can be a valuable tool for examination preparation and content reinforcement, especially if the content is applied to case scenarios.

Companion CD-ROMs

A companion CD-ROM is defined as a CD-ROM that is packaged with a textbook. Such CD-ROMs use technology to extend the functionality of the textbook by offering such items as review questions, audio glossaries, case studies, and an assortment of games—all designed to encourage independent learning and enhance the content of the textbook. Educators should model the use of these tools in the classroom so that students become aware of their existence and purpose as learning tools.

TEACHING TIP: If technological resources are available in the classroom, once a week or so, the educator can select a feature or topic of the companion CD-ROM to highlight and demonstrate for the whole class. Alternatively, a student can be asked to demonstrate the use of the tool and to begin a discussion on the topic. If resources to demonstrate the companion CD-ROM are not available in the classroom, the educator should make a point of creating an assignment that encourages learners to access the CD-ROM and to use one of the tools.

Not all learners may have convenient access to a computer to use the content on a companion CD-ROM, but with a little brainstorming, some simple solutions can be offered. For example, the CD-ROM activities can be printed out by a fellow student or the instructor and can be provided as a handout. In other cases, learners may have to use a friend's computer or one at the local library or college computer lab. With enough forethought and planning, most barriers to computer access can be overcome in a reasonable manner.

Companion web sites

Many publishers have created online tools that are ideally suited for individual learning and exploration. These tools typically are contained on a Web site that has been developed and is owned by the publisher for a specific book, hence the name "Companion Web site" (Figure 14-2). These sites generally contain information such as learning objectives and various activities that reinforce content from the text. Instructor tools are also available, including instructor manuals, lesson plans, and test banks.

In many instances, companion Web site activities are similar to those found in the electronic workbook, described earlier. They can take the form of simple labeling exercises that are provided along with a variety of quizzes. Additional resources that can

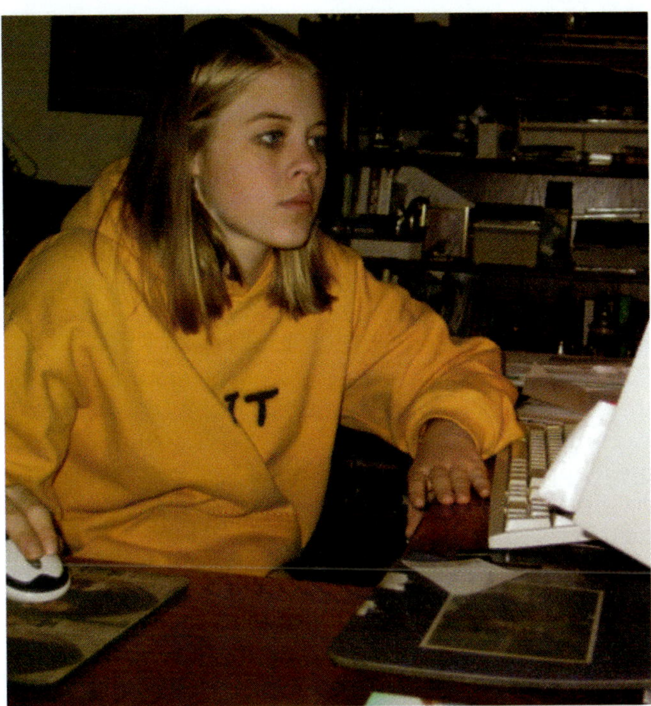

FIGURE 14-2 Studying on a companion Web site may suit the needs of younger students because of the advantages of audio and visual movement.

extend the capability of the book include audio glossaries that allow students to actually listen to a medical term being pronounced, and links to pertinent Web sites that include more information on the specific topic. Most of the tools offered on companion Web sites require very little bandwidth and function well on a dial-up Internet connection. However, as more interactive elements and streaming video become available, bandwidth may become an issue. This can be an important consideration for the educator who assigns some of these more complex activities. More information on companion Web sites and learning management systems can be found in Chapter 17.

INDEPENDENT STUDY

Sometimes the best way to teach is to be seemingly absent from the learning process. In this type of teaching, the educator's role is more that of a facilitator. The educator can assist the learner in setting his or her own educational goals, then can help the learner create a strategy for attaining these goals outside the traditional classroom (Box 14-2). In general, an educator's role in facilitating self-study is to assist the learner in discovering helpful resources and supportive experiences that can serve as source material. Once the learner is in touch with the source material, the educator can assist with identification of key learning elements and can help put the newly acquired knowledge into context.[7] Self-study helps the student to become more independent and to develop skills that will lead to internal motivation to seek out knowledge throughout his or her career.[8,9]

BOX 14-2 Examples of Independent Study Assignments

- Workbooks
- Self-assessment quizzes, puzzles, and games
- Step-by-step tutorials
- Computer-aided instruction
- Library research
- Additional reading
- Guided exercises for reviewing and organizing notes
- Interviewing of and discussion with experts or other individual persons or groups

In a more directed or programmed approach, an educator might construct predetermined goals and clear exercises through which a learner can reach these goals. In the context of EMS education, this type of directed independent study assignment can be a helpful adjunct to learning. It is often a challenge for the instructor to cover all of the curriculum prescribed in EMS courses. Independent study offers options for learning to take place outside a traditional classroom setting.[10]

Adult learners in particular can be well suited to independent learning. Many are mature enough, are internally motivated, and have strong study habits that will allow them to succeed. It should be noted that younger students may misinterpret the customization and flexibility of independent study as an "easy" way to acquire knowledge. Self-directed learning, however, can be difficult. The learner must be self-motivated and, when expert consultation is not immediately available, must have the curiosity and discipline needed to search for a correct answer. Understanding a complex subject without the explanation provided by an instructor in the classroom might be more difficult than some students originally predict.

The proliferation and widespread availability of televisions, videocassette recorders (VCRs), DVD players, computers, and the Internet have given a new look to self-directed learning. It is important to note that although the latest methods for self-study have focused on electronic and audiovisual media, this kind of learning does not have to be driven electronically. Research has proved that reading printed materials, reflecting on the meaning of their content, and writing a summary of what has been learned is an effective educational method.

Note Taking and Reviewing

One way to enhance individual student learning is to encourage note taking during lectures and reading assignments, and while the student is completing other assignments. Taking notes is a cognitive activity that helps students process information and capture key concepts for later review. Students can write or draw notes. Research suggests that the activity of transferring cognitive thought onto paper alone enhances student learning. Future review of these notes and further reading have been shown to further enhance retention.[10-12]

Note taking requires that the learner listen, sort out the more important information, and capture something that will stimulate his or her memory and understanding. This activity alone improves comprehension and retention. The more detailed the notes, and the more often the student reviews these notes, the greater is the likelihood that the student's learning will be enhanced by note taking.

Educators can facilitate and guide effective use of notes by pacing the delivery of lectures and emphasizing key points. They can also prompt students to write down and remember elements that might be critical to an understanding of future concepts or information that will be tested.

Some experts suggest the use of a structured lecture process called the guided lecture procedure (GLP). This allows for a formal 5- to 10-minute pause during which students try to encapsulate what they have just heard, followed by 10- to 15-minute small group discussion during which students can compare notes and discuss lessons learned.[12,13] Chapter 16 discusses guided lecture in greater detail.

A handout with the general outline of the lecture topic or assignment can also encourage note taking and can provide organization and structure to the lesson. When electronic presentation tools (such as PowerPoint) are used, it is possible for the instructor to provide to students a complete lecture summary. It is probably best for the instructor to hand out general outlines and to avoid giving out full slide summaries before the lecture. Studies have shown that review of instructor-provided lecture summaries is effective for short-term recall, but that retention is significantly enhanced when the learner has taken his or her own notes. The combination of taking one's own notes and reviewing these notes between lectures is most effective.[14]

In all cases, educators should encourage active learning techniques to prompt students to review materials. Passive listening is one of the least effective methods of learning.[15]

Independent Assignments

Educators can facilitate independent learning and studying through the use of independent assignments. Box 14-3 lists examples of individual learning strategies. This section highlights the use of flashcards, research, journaling, and portfolios.

Flashcards

The literature on flashcards typically describes their use in teaching children how to read. Although some critics claim that flashcards promote only rote learning and not comprehension, their usefulness has more recently been explored; research shows that flashcards can improve the speed of reading, which then improves comprehension of the subject matter.[16] Accordingly, flashcard use in EMS education may be most appropriate for subject areas that require memorization and learning of another language, such as medical terminology or pharmacology.

The use of electronic media to produce image-enhanced flashcards can also help learners (particularly visual learners) retain information.[17] Commercial products are often available, or the educator or learner can make cards by using blank index cards or programs such as PowerPoint.

BOX 14-3 Individual Learning Strategies

1. A positive attitude should top your list of strategies! Believe you can succeed and you will!
2. Know how you best learn.
3. Plan your study session: plan when to study, plan where to study, do not allow other plans to take your planned study time, take breaks in your study session, and plan how you will use your study session (read the chapter in the text, review notes and handout, work in workbook, answer questions at the end of the chapter, etc.)
4. Plan your reading strategy: skim the chapter to get an overview, read the chapter carefully, read key points out loud, take notes on main ideas, and review chapter and notes.
5. Analyze note taking by listening carefully, organizing notes, reading and thinking about the notes, and writing notes out.
6. Study actively: answer review questions in the book or workbook, use new vocabulary words, use computer-based tutorials or reviews, and form a study group.
7. Use all the resources you can! These include the instructor(s), study partners, study aids, learning lab activities, related articles, and other information.
8. Prepare for tests: use practice tests, stay healthy, keep up with material daily so you don't feel the need to cram, do not take medications that will make you drowsy, and try to get a good night's sleep.

Modified from Patton K *Student Survival Guide for Anatomy & Physiology.* St. Louis, Mo: Mosby; 1999.

TEACHING TIP: Flashcards can easily be incorporated into lectures by the use of features in presentation software such as PowerPoint. A word, phrase, or image can be placed on a single slide, and features such as build and dissolve can be used to place the "answer" on the bottom of the slide or on the next slide.[17]

Research projects

Research is an important component of individual learning, both as a resource for finding information and in the discovery or validation of information. Conducting of research may be required in some educational programs; however, this section focuses on individual research assignments.

Educators should always encourage students to expand their knowledge. One of the best ways for them to do this is through research. With the availability of the Internet and all that it has to offer, students are more eager than ever to do a little "surfing" and expand their knowledge. Research projects can be both fun and informative and should include a variety of formats and styles. In addition to an Internet or library search, research may involve such things as student-led comparisons of products and equipment, or a study of the trend of class blood pressure measurements over the semester to see if readings run higher on testing days. For many students, the difficult part of the research project is not the research itself but the selection of a topic; therefore, it is a good idea for the instructor to provide a list of suggested topics that can be offered to students who wish to complete a research assignment.

Research projects can be given as a mandatory assignment that all students must complete, or they may be used as an optional assignment that offers students the opportunity to earn extra credit. Whichever the case, the instructor must provide clear direction and must outline expectations for the project in as much detail as possible. Details such as the nature and scope of the topic, the length of the final paper, the due date, how much class credit it is worth, and acceptable format for submission should all be spelled out before any research is begun.

TEACHING TIP: Without some guidance and direction from the instructor, students may select topics that are too broad in scope or that do not relate to EMS at all. The instructor should have each student select a topic and submit it for approval before he or she begins the research.

A student may wish to do research on the pay rates of EMTs. If the student's goal is to find a job as an EMT in a local department or agency, it may not benefit the student or the class if he or she begins researching EMT pay scales across the United States. One instructor suggestion might be to focus on EMT jobs within a 100-mile radius of home, thus providing more useful information not only for the student who is conducting the research but for the rest of the class as well.

Another tool that the instructor may use, especially if the research project is optional, is a list of preselected topics that can be assigned as students express an interest in doing a project. Ideas for topics can be gathered from news and magazine articles or from current events. The instructor should keep a running list of ideas that can be used when students come up empty-handed. "Enrichment" topics included in some textbooks may be helpful as well. These topics typically go beyond the curriculum and are of interest to many students.

TEACHING TIP: It is important that instructors spell out what they expect from completed research projects. For instance, stipulating that research projects be typewritten on 8.5 × 11-inch paper, double-spaced in a 12-point font, and that they be 3 to 5 pages long is not unrealistic. Suggesting that students use at least two Internet sources, one journal article, and one personal interview will help even out those who think the Internet is the only place to find information. The more direction the instructor provides, the more successful students will be with their projects.

Journaling

Encouraging learners to write about their experiences during a training program can be enlightening for both the learner and the educator. Journal writing (journaling) is an effective method of allowing learners to reflect on what they have been learning and to put it into words that can be read by or shared with others as appropriate (Figure 14-3). Journaling also provides an opportunity for students to explore feelings about experiences—a task that taps into the affective domain.

Journaling can take many forms, ranging from a formal composition notebook that is submitted for a grade to less formal online discussion boards. Topics can range from a general class experience to specific experiences in clinical and field settings. One example of a journaling assignment is to ask students to track all medications encountered during clinical or field internships. Students must research each medication encountered and must list the most common indications, contraindications, and adverse effects. Another journaling technique is to ask students to document any questions that may arise as they read the text. Students must then seek out the answers to these questions from fellow students. Because the actual task of journaling is conducted throughout an extended class, such as an EMT or Paramedic program, students can use the journal as a reflective tool through which they can observe changes in their knowledge base and can assess how acquired knowledge has affected the way they treat patients. Journals can also serve as a great study tool for major division exams and finals.

As with any appropriate assignment, expectations should be clearly defined at the beginning. What form will the journal take, and what will it contain? Will the instructor accept handwritten journals? Or, must they be typewritten before submission? When will the journal be due, and what point value, if any, has been assigned? These are all questions that must be addressed so that students can begin with a clear understanding. Even with the most explicit of instructions, students may interpret things differently than the instructor intends. For this reason, it may be appropriate for the instructor to inform students that he or she will be sampling their journals on a random basis throughout the program and will offer informal feedback along the way. This helps the instructor in identifying those students who are not doing the assignment at all, or who may be headed in the wrong direction. Anonymous examples of journals from previous classes are also helpful in guiding students to understand what is expected.

Educators can also use journaling as a way to individually explore their own teaching methods and effectiveness.[18]

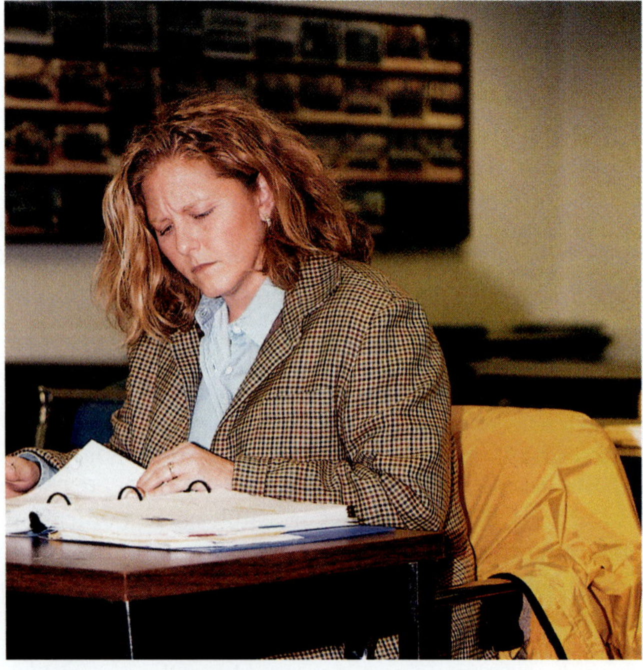

FIGURE 14-3 Journaling allows students the opportunity to reflect on their experiences and explore their feelings.

Portfolios

A portfolio is a collection of student work that demonstrates progress and attainment of educational goals.[7,19,20] Portfolios are not a new idea. The concept is borrowed from the arts, wherein the portfolio is a collection of work used to demonstrate an artist's talent. Portfolios have also been used in other educational settings, including college business programs, high school technical programs, and elementary schools. Portfolios can be used in many ways, depending on their purpose and intended audience:

- *Working portfolios* act as containers through which the student and the instructor interact on progress made through assignments and tasks
- *Showcase portfolios* represent the student's best work
- *Assessment portfolios* document student learning and demonstrate mastery of concepts; they are graded by the instructor

The key characteristic of a successful portfolio is that it is carefully planned and purposeful (Box 14-4).

Topic assignment is an important first step in the creation of a portfolio. The instructor should approve the topic and the forms of expression used. The instructor can provide a list that includes a variety of options, such as oral presentations, debates, original games, visual presentations, flow charts, time lines, demonstrations, role-plays, musical/rhythmic presentations, skits, journals, creative visualizations, poster presentations, and Web pages. This list can guide students as they plan their projects. The instructor should monitor the developmental stages of the project. One method of monitoring student progress is requiring the student to submit intermediary steps for consideration and possible impact on the course grade. For instance, the instructor may require a "check-in" for the following steps: (1) description of title, purpose,

BOX 14-4 Characteristics of a Carefully Planned Portfolio

1. Objectives are determined jointly by the student and the instructor
2. The focus is on student projects and evidence of progress
3. Student strengths are emphasized instead of mistakes
4. Students help decide what will be included
5. Students have access to their portfolios
6. The portfolio should contain a definition of goals, as well as evaluations by the student and instructor

and major points, (2) sources, data, and references, (3) outline, (4) first draft, and (5) final version. Check-ins should be applied to all forms that the student plans to use, whether they involve a written presentation or another style of presentation.

Assembling the portfolio is an active learning and self-reflection process. The student and instructor can select elements that best represent the student's progress. The student then reflects critically on his or her work and the types of elements that will best represent achievements. This activity encourages students to pay closer attention to their own performance and prompts students to work on areas where performance has been weak.[19]

Portfolios can be used to enhance self-reflection and ownership of learning. Assembling the portfolio encourages students to reflect on their own progress and performance as they select the most positive aspects of that performance. Students take responsibility for their accomplishments, and they take on ownership of their learning.

Billings and Halsted[7] warn that this method of instruction may require new ways of thinking on the part of educators. It is important for instructors to teach students how to take advantage of this learning process. Students must see the clear objective and benefit of the portfolio, or it might be viewed as "busy work." Billings and Halsted also suggest specific inclusion criteria for the portfolio so that it doesn't become too bulky. If the portfolio is being used to assess student performance, grading criteria and expectations should also be clearly identified. Students should be required to continually evaluate their own products, and educators should schedule conferences with students during which they can provide feedback and guidance.[12]

For information on evaluation of portfolios, see Chapter 21.

CASE IN POINT

Sample materials to include in a portfolio for an EMS student:

- Summaries of attendance and course completion(s)
- Successfully completed skill station check sheets
- Summaries of clinical hours, locations, contacts, skills, and preceptor evaluations
- Summaries of major exam scores
- Personal mission, oath, or career goals
- Essays, research papers, or review articles

INDEPENDENT LEARNING LABS

Independent learning labs, known as the learning resource center (LRC), provide a variety of learning activities that stimulate students' senses of sight, sound, and touch. Although the LRC originally focused on psychomotor skills, the LRC of today has a wide array of technology and various resources that are made available to students to help them acquire cognitive, affective, and psychomotor skills. Through the LRC, students are encouraged to learn, make decisions, and think critically in a low-stress environment.

Some students do well independently in the LRC. Some institutions have developed various types of modular learning approaches for teaching and evaluating skills. These generally are specific instructional units with pretests, posttests, objectives, structured activities, resources, and evaluation tools. Such learning approaches may be computerized, or they may use multimedia along with models or hands-on materials. One medical school, for example, used problem-based assignments, case studies, and computer-based simulations and exercises to direct individual learning.[21] The LRC approach is self-paced, and assignments can be completed whenever the student is available, as long as the LRC is open. The environment is a nonthreatening one, and the student can linger on a particular topic as long as he or she desires.[7]

TARGETED INTERNSHIPS

A targeted internship experience is a focused area of clinical experience (hospital or field) through which learning is enhanced or remediated. Students who report back on their experiences can enlighten fellow students about a particular specialty area. Such experiences require objectives for the rotation, learning activities, and means of measuring achievement of the objectives. A student who becomes intrigued by behavioral disorders may choose to spend some time in the in-patient psychiatry area to observe how patient behavior changes after an acute episode. A student who is struggling with electrocardiogram (ECG) interpretation may benefit from clinical experience in a cardiac stepdown unit, where he or she can observe many ECGs over time. A student who is interested in rural EMS may be interested in spending focused time with a rural EMS unit.

LEARNING CONTRACTS

Learning contracts serve as a medium through which an adult's experience can be combined with new learn-

BOX 14-5[22] Creating a Learning Contract

1. Diagnose your learning needs
2. Specify your learning objectives
3. Specify learning resources and strategies
4. Specify target dates for completion
5. Specify evidence of completion
6. Specify evidence of accomplishment
7. Specify how the evidence will be validated
8. Review your contract with external sources
9. Carry out the contract
10. Evaluate your learning

ing. Contracts can take a variety of forms (e.g., paper-based, audio, descriptive statements) that can be as individual as the learner. Similar to personal development plans used in the work environment, learning contracts provide a pathway through which learners can personalize their learning and apply it to immediate and future situations and goals.

When a learning contract is arranged, learning objectives are not set by the educator or presented in a textbook; instead, the learning contract provides an avenue by which learners can assess their personal learning needs and set their own goals and objectives. Box 14-5 lists the steps involved in creating a learning contract.

The keys to successful learning contracts include (1) setting measurable, achievable objectives and goals, and (2) changing the contract as time and needs progress and change. Educators can introduce this tool to learners and can help them define their own individual learning goals and framework.

SUMMARY

Students enrolled in EMS programs generally are well motivated and have a sincere interest in what they are learning, especially those who have chosen the path on their own. The instructor must recognize and exploit this motivation for the benefit of the learner. As has been discussed in this chapter, an instructor can use many methods to maximize the benefit of this motivation by providing a wide variety of individual learning opportunities for the student.

The educator should become intimately familiar with the many tools available for individual learning to push students to expand their learning beyond the classroom. In addition, individual learning aids can assist struggling students. Individual learning aids can be tailored to each student's needs. The keys to success for the individual student who uses any of these tools are (1) to establish clearly defined expectations to guide the student through the assignment, (2) to model the use of learning aids in the classroom, and (3) to integrate their use into the curriculum.

Instructors must remember that not all learning occurs within the four walls of the classroom. EMS students often are eager to extend their learning beyond the classroom and to develop critical thinking skills that will remain useful throughout a lifetime.

REFERENCES

1. Lidstone J. Teaching with textbooks in undergraduate geography courses. *Journal of Geography in Higher Education.* 1995;19:335.
2. Robb L. Strategies for getting the most from textbooks. *Instructor.* 2003;112:5.
3. Van Boxtel C, van der Linden J, Kanselaar G. The use of textbooks as a tool during collaborative physics learning. *Journal of Experimental Education.* 2000;69:57.
4. Holmes J. Are textbooks inevitable? *Journal of Geography in Higher Education.* 1995;19:339.
5. Kellum KK, Carr JE, Dozier CL. Response-card instruction and student learning in a college classroom. *Teaching of Psychology.* 2001;28:101-104.
6. Gutierrez C, Wang J. A comparison of an electronic vs print workbook for information literacy instruction. *Journal of Academic Librarianship.* 2001;27:208.
7. Billings DM, Halstead JA. *Teaching in Nursing: a Guide for Faculty.* Philadelphia: WB Saunders; 1998:334.
8. Brookfield S. *Understanding and Facilitating Adult Learning.* San Francisco: Jossey-Bass; 1986:41-75.
9. Yeazel M. Demonstration of the effectiveness and acceptability of self-study module use in residency education. *Medical Teacher.* 2004;26:57-63.
10. Davis BG. *Tools for Teaching.* San Francisco: Jossey-Bass; 2001.
11. Morrison E, McLaughlin C, Rucker L. Medical students' note-taking in a medical biochemistry course: an initial exploration. *Medical Education.* 2002;36:384-386.
12. Toole RJ. An additional step in the guided lecture procedure. *Journal of Adolescent and Adult Literacy.* 2002;44:166-169.
13. Kelly B, Holmes J. The guided lecture procedure. *Journal of Reading.* 1979;22:602-604.
14. Thomas G. (1978). Use of student notes and lecture summaries as study guides for recall. *Journal of Educational Research.* 1978;71:6.
15. Erlendsson J. (n.d.) Learning retention rates. Available at: http://www.hi.is/~joner/eaps/cs_reten.htm. Accessed August 11, 2003.
16. Nicholson T. The flashcard strikes back. *Reading Teacher.* 1998;52:2.
17. Burmark L. Visual presentations that prompt, flash and transform. *Media & Methods.* 2004;40:6.
18. Dicker M. Using action research to navigate an unfamiliar teaching assignment. *Theory into Practice.* 1990;29:203-208.

19. Lyons RE, McIntosh M, Kysilka ML. *Teaching College in the Age of Accountability.* Boston: Allyn & Bacon; 2003:217-220.
20. Orlich DC, Harder RM, Callahan RC, Gison HW. (2001). *Teaching Strategies, a Guide to Better Instruction.* 6th ed. Boston: Houghton Mifflin; 2001:369.
21. Whitaker EM. How we teach physiology. *Medical Teacher.* 1994;16:213.
22. Anonymous. (n.d.) Learning contracts. Available at: http://www.distance.syr.edu/contract.html. Accessed October 25, 2004.

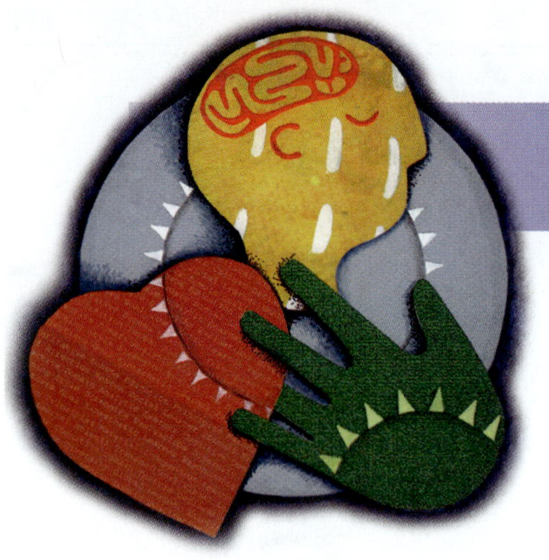

CHAPTER 15

Tools for Small Group Learning

"The dilemma for the humanistic educator was to devise alternative ways of working within an education system characterized by a prescribed curriculum, similar assignments for all students, lecturing as the only mode of instruction, standards by which all students are externally evaluated, and instructor chosen grades as the measure of learning, all of which precluded meaningful learning."

—*Carl Rogers, 1969, Freedom to Learn*

OVERVIEW OF SMALL GROUPS

Small group teaching is well recognized as an important means of facilitating learning. A small group format encourages learners to express their comprehension and compare their ideas with others, thereby improving their understanding of the subject. The basic tenet of small group teaching focuses on teamwork and cooperation; educators and learners work together to solve problems and develop critical and higher-order thinking skills. Educators should facilitate learning within small groups and provide the opportunity for learners to monitor their progress and become more self-directed.[1]

A group can consist of two or more students working together.[2] However, the size of the small group is relative to the educational environment. If an educator is used to teaching groups of 100 to 200 or more learners, then a small group may consist of 40 to 50 students. Alternatively, if a large group consists of 35 to 40, the small group may comprise fewer than 10 learners. For the purposes of this book, a small group is defined as consisting of 4 to 10 learners.

Small group learning has many characteristics that set if apart from other models of teaching and learning in both approach and delivery method. This chapter explores the concepts of facilitation in small groups and provides examples of different strategies that educators can use in teaching small groups.

Advantages of Small Group Learning

Small group learning offers many advantages. It allows learners to bring their own experiences to the learning process and increases active learning. It encourages creativity, stimulates discussion, and has been shown to improve confidence and performance.[3] In addition, small groups encourage and assist students in developing such transferable skills as teamwork, communication, collaboration, and leadership. This is particularly true in the field of health care, where small groups are used outside the classroom in continuing education environments such as journal clubs and case reviews.[4]

Working in small groups allows students to learn from others—from the examples they offer and their insights, opinions, and mistakes. The educator facilitates the learning objective. For example, one learner may learn a task more quickly than the others, then may offer to demonstrate to others how the skill was mastered.

Although some schools of thought claim that small group learning requires more instructor time and preparation, others claim that it actually decreases lecture load and overall workload.[2,3,5]

The primary purpose of teaching and learning in small groups is to develop learners' knowledge, skills, and attitudes so that they can meet desired educational outcomes. This is done in association with the learning outcomes that are described in the curriculum. Because of the intensive nature of the instruction provided with a ratio of one instructor to a small number of students, small groups afford the student the opportunity to learn the finer details of the profession.[6]

Disadvantages of Small Group Learning

Disadvantages of small group learning seem to center on the time it takes to plan appropriate activities and to initiate a "learning change" with learners. Developing a small group learning environment can take time and requires a change from typical educator-centered lectures to learner-centered activities.[3] Learners may resist, and educators may find themselves wanting to give lectures rather than facilitate discussion. Management of group dynamics can become an issue, and workloads within groups may not be equally distributed (see Chapter 12). The small group learning format requires that more time be spent on a lesson, and educators may not be able to cover all subject matter in the curriculum.[5] Some believe that teaching small groups can be very demanding in terms of preparation in that individual student learning styles must be identified, and the instructor must respond to those learning styles by adopting teaching methods that meet individual needs. Facilitation may be complex because of the diverse range of learning styles, as well as variation in abilities and personalities, age differences, and different cultural backgrounds, and because students may be motivated or passive learners.[6]

Most of the cited disadvantages, however, can be overcome with effective planning and time management.[2,5] Box 15-1 lists some techniques for successful small group learning.

BOX 15-1 Creating Successful Small Groups

- Design challenging exercises to be done in a limited time frame
- Ensure that work assignments are clearly defined
- Assess both individual and group work
- Use both peer evaluation and self-assessment
- Monitor and facilitate small group work (remain visible)
- Ensure that the learning environment is suitable to the task

From Cooper et al, 2000; Healey and Matthews, 1996.

Types of Groups

Small groups can be formal or informal. Formal groups typically have a planned purpose, require a formal selection process, and assign roles to each group member (Figure 15-1). A formal small group, for example, may be used for problem-based learning, case discussions, or simulations. Informal groups can work over a much shorter duration without assigned roles (Figure 15-2). For example, breaking up a large class by having learners turn to their neighbors to discuss a concept or problem is one example of an informal small group approach.[5] Having students move between different lab stations to learn isolated skills is another example.

Many educators deliver lectures to larger groups, then subdivide students into smaller tutorial groups to create a manageable environment, particularly when the goal is psychomotor development within practical skills laboratories. These smaller groups often comprise a mix of different types of students (e.g., age, cultural background, personality); the diversity of students adds a dimension of richness to the group.

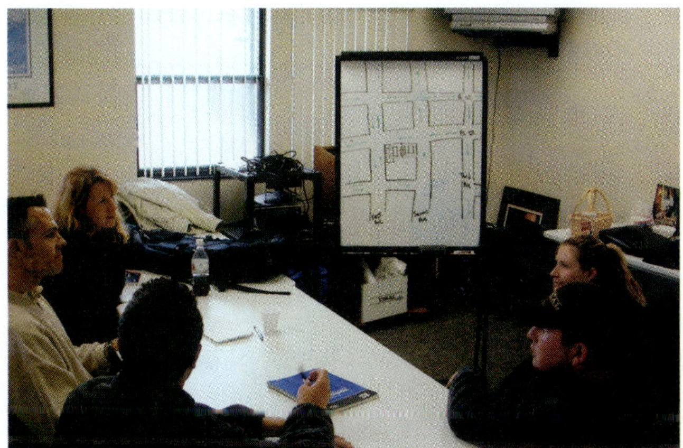

FIGURE 15-1 Small groups can be formal with a planned purpose and roles, as in problem-based learning.

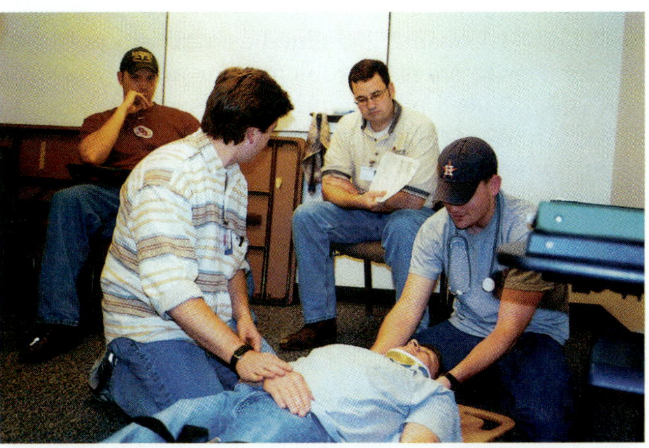

FIGURE 15-2 Groups can be informal, as in a skill practice laboratory. Both formal and informal groups can promote effective learning.

BOX 15-2 Features of Cooperative Learning

- *Intentional group formation*—group members are selected according to predetermined criteria
  For example, a mix of recent high school graduates with older students
- *Continuity of group interaction*—members have regular group meetings to deal with the assignment and, in turn, a social network develops
  For example, the group may elect to meet in the cafeteria, where, over coffee, they can nut out the work
- *Interdependence among group members*—groups work toward a common goal; each member is assigned a specific role associated with the learning process
- *Individual accountability*—students are graded individually to reduce "social loafing"
  Each student makes an independent contribution to the learning; therefore, each assignment is graded on an individual basis
- *Instructor as facilitator*—the instructor circulates among the group to clarify the task and to offer encouragement

From Maughan and Webb, 2001.

CASE IN POINT

The Call Center has received notification of a 28-year-old female patient with severe abdominal pain. The patient is planning to start a family, so she might be pregnant.

To provide appropriate patient care, students must learn about abdominal pain as associated with ectopic pregnancy.

If five students constitute the group, a specific learning task should be allocated to each student, such as:

- Normal anatomy and physiology of the female reproductive system
- Pathophysiology of ectopic pregnancy
- Clinical presentation of ectopic pregnancy
- Clinical problems and complications that may be anticipated
- Patient care required before time of arrival at the hospital

In turn, each student presents his or her findings to the whole group. If additional students are available, then the educator has the option to subdivide tasks (e.g., one student is allocated the anatomy of the reproductive system, and another is asked to find out about the physiology). Alternatively, two students could be allocated to work on a task together.

Cooperative and Collaborative Learning

Cooperative learning and collaborative learning represent two key models of small group teaching and learning. In these types of settings, the educator poses the learning theme, and students work together to find associated details. Cooperative and collaborative learning methods differ from traditional teaching approaches in that students work together instead of competing with each other. Although these two approaches have similarities, they are characterized by significant teaching differences.

Cooperative learning

Cooperative learning is defined as a division of labor undertaken to solve a problem.[7] For any given task, students divide up the work, then come together to present findings. Each student makes an individual contribution. Box 15-2 describes some features of cooperative learning.

Collaborative learning

Collaborative learning, in contrast to cooperative learning, focuses on learners working together and being jointly responsible for successful learning outcomes. It encourages active student participation in the learning process by requiring that individual students do an assigned task and think about the approach they must take. Each student must participate in discussion and justify his or her position. Collaborative learning is one way that students can learn from each other—it is a powerful learning tool in that an element of subliminal peer pressure develops between students when one student is seen to be more knowledgeable than the others. Each member of the group researches a section of the task to find information that assists other members of the group.

CASE IN POINT

The instructor poses the scenario that students are to respond to a caller who states:

"Matthew is wheezing really badly—he's an asthmatic and is having trouble breathing!"

As a group, students research information that explains the following content:

- Anatomy and physiology of the respiratory system
- Causes of asthma—what causes an asthma attack, how asthma develops
- Home management to maintain healthy lifestyle—"reliever and preventer" inhalers
- Pharmacology to relieve the impact of asthma—how these medications work on the body
- EMS medical intervention in asthma crisis/respiratory arrest—oxygenation, intubation, medication, injection
- Hospital treatment of acute asthma

PREPARING FOR SMALL GROUP TEACHING

Within any classroom, the role of the educator is to engage students in learning. Because of the intimacy of small groups, the educator may take on various roles as needed, such as instructional guide, content expert, examiner, facilitator, teacher, learner, advocate, and friend. Each role is determined by the dynamics of the group and the topic that is being presented. On one hand, a firm or semiauthoritative approach may be needed when student requirements for successful completion of the course are outlined; on the other hand, a relaxed, friendly, and casual approach may be used to create a comfortable learning environment when that is the goal.

Planning the Class Session

With any teaching assignment, the instructor must first consider what learners need to achieve so that learning objectives can be identified. Each step of the learning process must include clear tasks so that students can build on existing knowledge and relate new information to previous learning. Each step must be delivered at a level that learners understand, and learners must comprehend relationships at each point.

Chapter 9 provides details on how the instructor should develop lesson plans for a standard class session. Methods of delivering instruction to small groups are consistent with the basic techniques used for a group of any size. The instructional session should begin with an introduction that sets the scene and provides a focus for the learning that is to come. The introduction should include a statement that illustrates the significance of what is to be learned and explains why it is important for students to develop knowledge and skills associated with the learning objectives of the session.

The body of the instruction is set out in logical and sequential manner. The instructor is challenged to design the instruction in such a way that new knowledge is constructed by building on existing knowledge. Various activities that involve students are incorporated into the lesson. Examples of such activities include student identification of cases for discussion, simulations, and role playing.

The conclusion of the lesson brings together its significant features. The conclusion provides an opportunity for the instructor to restate the main components. This statement reminds students of the important things they need to study to consolidate their learning. At the end of the session, it is a good move for the instructor to describe the students' original knowledge base and point out the new knowledge that they have acquired since the lesson began.

Selecting Groups

We learn best when we learn together. Active learning is most meaningful when it involves group activity. To save class time, it is important that group assignments be made ahead of time or quickly if done in class.

TEACHING TIP: If possible, it must be remembered that EMS personnel will not always be working with the same partner or crew all the time. Variation in the memberships of groups, as well as in their skill levels, can enhance the overall performance of individual members and of the team.

The instructor can use several methods to assemble groups. Randomization techniques such as counting off or drawing numbers allow learners to maintain minimal control in the random sorting process. The educator can control the selection before class time based on knowledge of the group and while keeping in mind individual strengths and limitations. Student control of selection allows individual or collective formation of groups based on the wishes of group members. This option offers the instructor less control but may prove to be more effective because learners must actively participate.

COMMON SMALL GROUP STRATEGIES

Various types of small groups can participate in diverse learning activities. Included in this chapter is a discussion of tutorials and seminars, case discussions, role plays, and problem-based learning. Box 15-3 outlines some strategies for small group learning.

Tutorials and Seminars

Lectures presented to large groups of students are usually planned to work hand-in-hand with tutorials

BOX 15-3 Additional Small Group Applications

- Begin class discussion with small groups to motivate learners and set the stage for learning
- Break up a lecture with small groups to deepen and assess understanding
- End class discussion with small groups to summarize the learning tasks of the day
- Use small class format for exam review
- Work in small groups for exam debriefing
- Use small group activities as an adjunct to audiovisual presentations

From Cooper and Robinson, 2000.

and seminars. The lecture provides the formal academic point of view, whereas the purpose of tutorials and seminars is to transfer theory into applications for clinical practice. It is common for tutorials and seminars to be included within the format of the usual class.

The tutorial is achieved primarily through discussion. The educator usually leads the tutorial, and learners are expected to provide input. The tutorial provides a wealth of opportunities through which students can learn. It is in this class that the relevance and meaning of what students are doing become apparent. Effective tutorials require clear guidelines that enable learners to achieve expected learning outcomes, along with expectations that everyone will participate in the learning process and that decisions will be made by group consensus.

In situations in which questions and statements for discussion are drawn from the lecture content, the educator should have an outline prepared in advance. This outline is the road map that guides the learning process. Development of questions for the tutorial requires thorough attention to the preceding lecture content. If another faculty member has delivered the lecture, it is useful for the instructor to liaise with him or her to ensure that the outcome is in accordance with overall curriculum requirements.

TEACHING TIP: The main task that the educator faces is getting the discussion going; this can be a challenge for the new instructor. As with most other teaching methods, getting students involved creates a functional learning environment. One of the most disappointing situations that the instructor can experience is a silent group. If no one offers to start a discussion, then the instructor must take the lead. The instructor should ask students for their opinions and have students share experiences with the group. Students do not always recognize what they do not know. The tutorial provides a means by which students can identify shortcomings, so they can review and work on those areas. For this purpose, the wise instructor pays attention to the tutorial preparation.

Seminars are typically led by students while the instructor facilitates the learning theme. Seminars, like tutorials, are usually associated with a parallel lecture; a seminar provides a forum in which learners can raise learning issues by working through allocated tasks. During seminars, learners and educators discuss a topic that is part of the course content in an environment that does not demand the rigor of academia.

At the commencement of the course, seminar tasks are usually allocated to learners who are required to prepare a theme for discussion. For example, if the focus of the lecture is myocardial infarction, then the seminar could address such topics as physical exercise and nutrition for a healthy heart, or associated physiology of time-related activity of cardiac enzymes after an infarction.

Handouts distributed at seminars and tutorials provide insights into the content discussed. Handouts help the student recall the topic as discussed in class; a reference list of available texts and resources for independent study can be provided as part of the handout. Students are encouraged in this way to read more about the topic than is provided in the handout.

Case Discussion

The relevance of bringing together theory and practice has impact when each learner is asked to describe a particular case that he or she has experienced as part of field internship. The case can be dissected into specific sections for analysis.

A diabetic crisis is used to illustrate how each section can be analyzed. For example:

- *The situation in which the victim was found.* What clues provide information that could assist investigators in determining the cause of the incident?
- *The clinical features of the patient.* What were the clinical features, and how do they relate to the underlying pathophysiology?
- *Associated medical conditions of the patient.* Some medical conditions such as diabetes may be accompanied by retinopathy, an eyesight problem. How and why does this develop?
- *Prehospital care.* What care was provided? Why was this done? What could or should have been included when this care was provided?

Because each learner has a personal interest in the case, the student group and the instructor provide detailed discussion that creates a great learning opportunity. Additionally, case studies can provide a great opportunity for program medical director to become involved in the learning process.

Role Plays

Role playing is a group-oriented process that involves at least two participants in a classroom dramatization. Role plays can involve as many as seven to ten characters but are usually limited in duration and scope. This type of classroom drama can be used to investigate and bring alive almost any topic. The technique is meant to create a situation in which each participant adopts a realistic character, or type of patient, and interacts with others in the role play according to how the character would act in real life.

Adequate preparation and facilitation skills are essential for the successful use of a role play. Box 15-4 lists basic elements for effective role playing. In general, the extent to which the acting performance is realistic determines the degree of learning that will

BOX 15-4 Essential Elements of Role Playing

- *Briefing students.* Explain the subject, goals, and key elements of the situation. If particular physical behaviors are needed, such as facial expressions or body position, the instructor should coach the role players on a realistic way to reenact actual patient presentation
- *Conducting the drama.* Act, or set the stage and environment so others can act
- *Debriefing.* Identify key concepts that have been learned, and facilitate a constructive conversation about the performance of the players

Modified from "Elements of Role Playing" Box, Orlich 2001, p 296.

occur. Instructors should set the stage so that students take the exercise seriously. Giggling, joking, and outbursts of laughter are often related to discomfort on the part of the role players, or students. These outbursts tend to diffuse needed tension and can break the concentration of players, minimizing the importance of the event. It is important for the instructor to remind students that they may face this very situation in an actual patient care environment. Debriefing and discussion are key elements in reinforcing important learning points and integrating the performance into the lesson plan. Acknowledgment of the stress involved in the performance and appropriate use of humor can be encouraged once the goals of the role play have been achieved.

Care should be taken to respectfully diffuse the anxiety of participants so that a safe learning environment is created. Students may try to psychoanalyze the players based on their roles; it is important for everyone to be reminded that these are only dramatizations and improvisations—not necessarily the real feelings or actions of the participants. Inviting guests such as past patients, acting students, local crisis team workers, or graduates to play a role can often lead to a higher level of intensity and learning. Videotaping can enhance this activity, allowing for retrospective group or individual performance review and evaluation.

Role plays differ from scenarios in that very little emergency medical services (EMS) equipment is used. Role plays focus on human interaction, case presentation, symptomatology, interview approaches, de-escalation, and communication skills. Crisis intervention, therapeutic communication, and courtroom testifying skills are particularly well suited to this type of group process.

Some types of role playing include the following:

- *Student-student scripted role play.* A group of two to ten students dramatizes a patient encounter, taking on the roles that would be involved—from patient(s), family members, and bystanders, to first responders and EMS crew members
- *Student-directed improvisational role play.* A group of students creates a situation to which another student (or team of students) must respond. Students prepare the dramatization in advance, researching the signs, symptoms, and possible actions or reactions that might occur during such an event. Students who prepare the role play might anticipate what occurs when a patient is treated inappropriately or is not treated at all
- *Instructor-student role play.* The instructor pretends to be a patient and interacts with two or more students as they try to interview and take care of him or her
- *Guest role play.* A person unknown to the class is invited to dramatize a case. Students are placed in the role of EMS responders who try to take care of the guest

Problem-Based Learning

Problem-based learning (PBL) is an instructional method by which the instructor creates a complex, well-structured problem that a group of students tries to solve. Although the term *problem-based learning* is used loosely as an educational tool for any real life patient problem or situation, the true form of PBL is well defined and structured. The problem presented is realistic and serves as the catalyst for learning. Students first work to uncover the facts and basic science behind the problem. In subsequent steps, students create possible explanations (hypotheses) about the problem and propose ways to solve some of the issues presented.[8,9]

The educator in PBL serves as a coach and helps balance and guide the direction of student inquiry. As a facilitator, the educator sets the tone for a positive and respectful exchange and for critical discussion of ideas. Feedback is essential to this facilitation.[10] The belief behind this method is that by discovering the issues and processes that characterize a problem, students acquire basic knowledge and immediately apply that knowledge to solve the problem.

Research evidence has been steadily mounting to show that PBL improves clinical reasoning skills and helps medical students better organize and apply clinical knowledge. This type of group learning fosters cooperative working and improves assessment skills.[11–14] Some studies have shown that PBL reduces the stress of intense medical education.[11]

PBL is not a new concept in education. Socrates and Plato pushed their students to think and search for answers and debate their hypotheses in an educational environment. In 1968, PBL was more formally established by McMaster University in Ontario, Canada, as a way of helping students apply basic scientific methods to clinical problems.[9]

Advantages of PBL include the development of interpersonal skills, research approaches, communication techniques, prioritization of time and resources, teamwork, and potentially, learner confidence. Additionally, students are motivated by working on a relevant, real life problem, and they are given the opportunity to be self-directed to some extent. Some disadvantages of PBL include the difficulty of stepping back from a traditional information-delivery model, the time and resources needed for setup, and the ongoing need for facilitation.[14] Also, protected time for independent research and study is essential and may not be available because of the requirements of the curriculum.

This type of learning is likely beneficial for EMS students, even though as of this writing, research is lacking in the use of PBL in EMS education.

Parameters for PBL

Although problem-based learning units can be presented in various formats, the following principles remain consistent:

- In a PBL unit, the ill-structured problem is presented first and serves as the organizing center and context for learning
- The problem on which learning centers:
    - Is ill structured
    - Is presented as a "messy" situation
    - Often changes with the addition of new information
    - Is not solved easily or formulaically
    - Does not always have a "right" answer
- In PBL classrooms, students assume the role of problem solver; teachers assume the role of tutor and coach
- In the teaching and learning process, information is shared, but knowledge is a personal construction of the learner. Thinking is fully articulated and is held to strict benchmarks
- Assessment is an authentic companion to the problem and the process
- The PBL unit is not necessarily interdisciplinary in nature but is always integrative

Box 15-5 provides an example of a sample week according to a PBL technique.

Teaching Psychomotor Skills

Teaching psychomotor skills provides an excellent opportunity for the instructor to teach in small groups. Psychomotor skill development is crucial to good patient care. All the effort put forth at the scene of an EMS incident is dependent on the provider's being

CASE IN POINT

Example of a Problem for PBL

Scene

EMS is dispatched on a Saturday evening to an affluent shopping mall for a "girl who is acting strangely and talking out of her head." The dispatcher says that mall security initiated the call, and that the patient is somewhat verbally aggressive. When the crew arrives, they meet a provocatively dressed young woman who is smoking a cigarette and says she is 20 years old and was just pushed by a man she met inside the bar. She says she is "fine" and would be "better if the ? @** police would stay out of her life and leave her alone." Mall security indicates they smell alcohol on the patient's breath. The police officer on the scene states that this could be her cologne, and that she appears to be constantly staring at the floor.

Assessment

The patient admits to occasional drug abuse but says she has not taken anything recently. EMS notes that she has an abrasion on her knee and a medic alert bracelet on her wrist, indicating allergy to haloperidol and benzodiazepines. The police have searched the patient for weapons and have given EMS empty bottles of rifampin, metformin hydrochloride, and valproic acid. The patient is refusing to be treated and states that she is being "set up" for another hospital bill because the "police said the detox unit is full." She just wants to go home. Her blood pressure is 160/90; pulse is 124; respirations are 20 per minute, and SpO_2 is 80% on room air.

In their own defense, the police privately admit that the county detoxification unit is full, but they are willing to arrest her for disorderly conduct if the EMS crew medically clears the patient.

Questions for the First Group Meeting

1. What key elements are included and/or missing in the patient assessment?
2. What physiologic mechanisms might be responsible for the symptoms present?
3. What field impressions should the EMS crew consider?
4. What legal principles are at play? What psychosocial issues are implicated between each of the agencies responding to the call (Mall Security, Police, and EMS)? How would each of those be managed?
5. What is the patient's possible medical history based on the assessment findings?

Complications to Be Discovered After the First Discussion Is Completed

Case Continuation: As the crew questions the patient, she has a tonic seizure (arms only) and then is unresponsive to any stimuli.

- How should EMS manage this patient?
- Should the patient awaken and become violent, what type of physical and alternative restraint systems might be used?

BOX 15-5 Sample Week With Problem-Based Learning Technique

Class Day 1

Morning: Group meeting to (a) review case, (b) review terminology, (c) identify critical data, (d) discuss possible explanations, (e) discuss group action plan, and (f) identify learning issues for group and individual persons.

Afternoon: Lecture or lab to support problem.

Class Day 2

Morning: Independent research to support problem: reading on core issues, writing down individual issues.

Afternoon: Lecture or lab to support problem.

Class Day 3

Clinical experience to support problem.

Class Day 4

Morning: Independent research to support problem.

Afternoon: Lecture or lab to support problem.

Class Day 5

Morning: Group meeting to discuss how new learning applies to the analysis and resolution of the case.

able to select the right skill at the right time, and to carry it out in the right manner. Many of the skills routinely performed at an EMS incident are critical to patient survival and leave little or no margin for error. Details of teaching psychomotor skills can be found in Chapter 13, Teaching in All Domains.

Simulations

Simulation exercises provide an excellent opportunity for students to incorporate cognitive, psychomotor, and affective skills while working in groups (Figure 15-3). The purpose of simulation is to create problem-solving situations that students can expect to deal with during their careers. It is useful to base the problem around student's current learning and clinical experiences to ensure that the scenario is within reach of each student's level of training and degree of expected competence.

Similar to role plays, simulations require a patient actor, a responding crew, bystanders, and a facilitator. They can be used to open a class by stimulating discussion, or to close a class by evaluating student understanding of the covered material. Simulations can be done as remediation during clinical or field rotations when similar cases have been seen. Finally, they can be done during lab time as a "put it all together" activity for students.

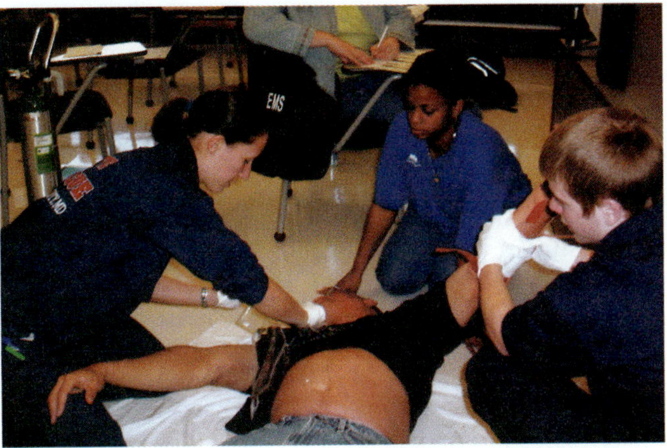

FIGURE 15-3 Simulation exercises are typically popular with students because they give students the chance to practice what they have learned and to self-evaluate.

TEACHING TIP: To make simulations more realistic, move students to a different location such as outdoors, in the hall, or in the bathroom. Use moulage, background noise, and props such as medical supplies, medication vials and bottles, or other products; have students follow a script.

CASE IN POINT

Vehicle extrication is one example of a simulation exercise. Although it might be difficult to acquire or use actual car wrecks, the simulation is effective when a student's or instructor's own vehicle is used. With relevant training equipment, each student takes the role of the victim to be extricated from the vehicle. If different types of vehicles are available, it is beneficial to repeat the exercise in different ones to enhance students' awareness of the problems to be encountered in real life situations.

Different scenarios can be created to dramatize problems of advanced complexity that must be solved—extrication of the patient who has spinal injuries, or a potential leg fracture, or a major hemorrhage and crushed chest. Each scenario will require actions and practices that demonstrate standard competencies of prehospital care.

Simulation exercises offer many benefits. Each scenario can be stopped at any time to draw attention to certain aspects to which the paramedic or EMS personnel must give due attention. Because the demands associated with real life events are not a part of the exercise, each part of the scenario can be discussed at the point of activity, and each can be supportively critiqued at the conclusion.

SUMMARY

For EMS educators, working with small groups is both challenging and rewarding. Not only does the use of small groups help to promote a higher level of thinking and understanding in the classroom, it also fosters "life after class" skills of leadership, teamwork, communication, and accountability. Whether the entire curriculum is designed around small groups, or they are simply used to break up lectures or to teach psychomotor skills, small group instruction can be an extremely effective educational strategy.

REFERENCES

1. Jaques D. Learning in groups. In: *Handbook for Improving Group Learning.* 3rd ed. UK: Kogan Page; 2000.
2. Healey M, Matthews H. Learning in small groups in university geography courses: designing a core module around group projects. *Journal of Geography in Higher Education.* 1996;20:167–181.
3. Sobral DT. Productive small groups in medical studies: training for cooperative learning. *Medical Teacher.* 1998;20:118–121.
4. Jaques D. Teaching small groups. *British Medical Journal.* 2003;326(7387).
5. Cooper JL, Robinson P. Getting started: informal small-group strategies in large classes. *New Directions for Teaching and Learning.* 2000(spring);81.
6. Cooper L, Lawson M, Orrell J. *Raising Issues About Teaching: Views of Academic Staff at Flinders University.* Adelaide: Flinders Press; 1997.
7. Roschelle J, Teasley S. The construction of shared knowledge in collaborative problem solving. In: O'Malley CE, ed. *Computer Supported Collaborative Learning.* Heidelberg: Springer-Verlag; 1995.
8. Center for Problem Based Learning, Illinois Mathematics and Science Academy. Available at: http://www2.imsa.edu/programs/pbl/whatis/whatis/slide12.html. Accessed October 12, 2004.
9. Wang H, Cos A, Thompson P, Shuler C. Problem based learning—PBL quick facts. USC California Science Project Leadership Cohort. Available at: http://www.usc.edu/hsc/dental/ccmb/usc-csp/Quikfacts.htm. Accessed October 12, 2004.
10. Wilkerson. An introduction to problem based learning. Presented at: 2004 National Association of EMS Education Symposium; September 11, 2004; Los Angeles, Calif.
11. Mensink D, Kaufman D, Day V. Stressors in medical school: relation to curriculum format and year of study. *Teaching & Learning in Medicine.* 1998;10;138.
12. Whitfield C, Mauger E, Zwicker J. Differences between students in problem-based and lecture-based curricula measured by clerkship performance ratings at the beginning of the third year. *Teaching & Learning in Medicine.* 2002;14:211.
13. Walters J, Croen L, Weissman Z, Reichgott M. A small group, problem-based learning approach to preparing students to retake step 1 of the United States Medical Licensing Examination. *Teaching & Learning in Medicine.* 1999;11:85.
14. Kilroy D. Problem based learning. *Emergency Medicine Journal.* 2004(July);4:411.

WORKS CONSULTED

Aaron S, Crocket J, Morrish D, Basulado C, Kovithavongs T. Assessment of exam performance after change to problem-based learning: differential effects by question type. *Teaching & Learning in Medicine.* 1998;10:86.

Bertola P, Murphy E. *Tutoring at University: A Beginner's Practical Guide.* Curtin University of Technology: Paradigm Books; 1994.

Billings DM, Halstead JA. *Teaching in Nursing: A Guide for Faculty.* Philadelphia: WB Saunders; 1998:415–416.

Blackman I. *Rasch Scaling—Blood Pressure.* School of Nursing, Flinders University, South Australia.

Cooper JL, MacGregor J, Smith KA, Robinson P. Implementing small-group instruction: insights from successful practitioners. *New Directions for Teaching and Learning.* 2000(spring);81.

Deeny P, Johnson A, Boore J, Leyden C, McCaughan E. Drama as an experiential technique in learning how to cope with dying patients and their families. *Teaching in Higher Education.* 2001;6:99–112.

Maughan C, Webb J. Small group learning and assessment. UKCLE Seminar, "From Little acorns . . ." November 2001. Available at: http://www.ukcle.ac.uk/resources/groupassess.html#top.

Orlich DC, Harder RJ, Callahan RC, Gibson HW. *Teaching Strategies: A Guide to Better Instruction.* Boston, Mass: Houghton Mifflin; 2001:296–297.

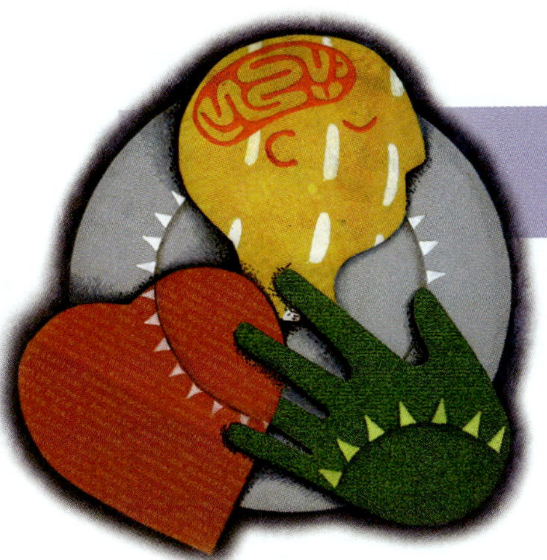

CHAPTER 16

Tools for Large Group Learning

"My play was a complete success. The audience was a failure."

—*Ashleigh Brilliant*

Teaching a large group requires a different approach than is used to teach a small group, but the principles of teaching methods are retained. This chapter offers teaching strategies for instructors to use when they face the challenge of teaching large numbers of students.

What constitutes a "large group" cannot be firmly defined because this is relative to the educational setting and the circumstances of the instructional event. In some situations, a "large group" may constitute 40 or 50 students; in others, more than 100 students may be included. At a regional or national conference, it is not uncommon for a class to be filled with 200 to 400 or more students. Therefore, the concept of "large group" is subject to interpretation. For the purposes of this text, a large group is defined as a greater number than can be easily handled for small group activities (i.e., more than approximately 40 students).

The advantage of teaching a large group is that content can be presented to many individuals at the same time. This saves instructor time, thus reducing costs. One instructor who teaches 45 students is more cost-effective than one who is teaching 15 students over three sessions. On the other hand, teaching a large group requires teacher-centered learning techniques such as lecture, rather than a learner-centered classroom.

Lecturing is the strategy most often used for teaching large groups. Variations of the lecture format and diverse techniques can promote learning and interactivity. Other large group teaching techniques include debate and student presentations. Although a large class can be a challenge for an instructor, effective methods can be identified and applied with careful planning.

LECTURE

Despite the interest of educators in more student-centered techniques, the lecture remains the most widely used teaching method in medical education.[1] Lecture is a teaching session in which the instructor is the principal teacher. Lectures allow the educator to disseminate large amounts of information to learners in a very direct and cost-effective manner. The lecture format has been well described as effective in the literature.[2–4] This method allows the focus to remain on the educator and the educator to be the center of control for the flow of information.

Educators teach as they themselves have always been taught. The model has been the same for as long as anyone can remember. Teaching this way is comfortable for both educator and learner. Lecturing is a traditional strategy to which every student can relate, and it certainly has its place in the educational process.

Advantages and Disadvantages

When used effectively, a lecture can facilitate new learning and clarify complex or confusing concepts that may need special explanation. Lecture can also be used to organize thinking, promote problem solving, and challenge attitudes.[5,6] It may be used as a change of pace from other teaching strategies, or for delivery of material that is not otherwise available to students.[4] The lecture can also stimulate student thought and questions that can then be used with smaller group teaching strategies.[7]

Cooper and colleagues[8] note the consensus among university faculty members that transmission of knowledge through lecture is an important educational strategy, and that there is an interdependent relationship between lectures and other modes of teaching. Most instructors would agree that lectures are significantly more valuable when complemented by tutorials and student-to-student interaction (Figure 16-1).

Many have questioned the role of the lecture in teaching. Some educators believe that lecturing is a poor method for developing thinking skills or attitudes because students are passive, unengaged learners.[4] Certainly, decreased student involvement is a disadvantage. Lecture alone without the use of visual aids favors auditory learners and may easily result in the lost attention of visual and kinesthetic learners.

Clearly, the lecture method entails both advantages and disadvantages. However, thorough preparation and knowledge of methods of enhancing the lecture can make it an effective learning experience.

Basics of Lecture Preparation

Once the learning objectives of the lecture have been identified, preparation is focused on developing the lesson plan to ensure that the lecture content meets those objectives. Previously used lectures should be updated periodically to reflect current protocols and procedures. Educators can take the following steps to enhance lecture preparation:

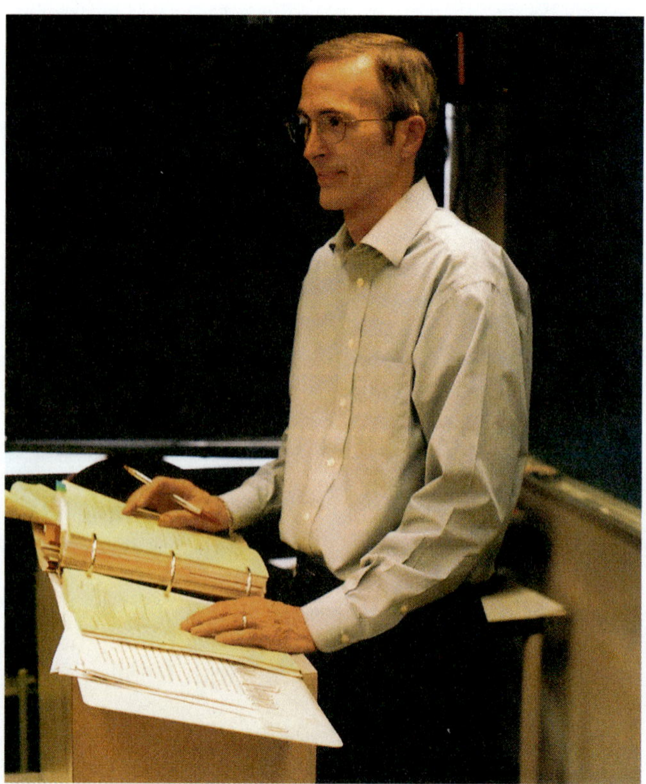

FIGURE 16-1 Techniques can be used to enhance the lecture format and contribute to student learning.

- Conduct research to find the most recent information, statistical data, and clinical practices that relate to the lecture content or objectives
- Identify the most important points that students must understand and retain. Key points are intended to encourage higher levels of thinking
- Distinguish between knowledge and concepts that are essential and those that are not part of the core message. The aim is to focus on the most important aspects of the topic, rather than to synthesize a large amount of material. If the topic is not part of the core learning objective, it can be included in the supplementary readings or identified to the students as "nice to know"
- Create lecture notes and/or an outline in an effective format so as to keep on track and deliver the content in a sequential and logical manner
- Be prepared with more material than needed so as to maintain a degree of security; however, it is important not to *over*prepare. The goal of the lecture is to teach students relevant information—not to prove how much the instructor knows
- On the day of the lecture, educators should prepare for their best personal presentation and should prepare the environment itself

Instructors must assess their own personal attributes to evaluate how they project themselves as teacher, role model, and professional. Due attention to dress and grooming allows the instructor to present himself or herself to the audience as a professional and reflects a professional approach to his or her work. Stage fright is frequently related to insecurities about physical appearance. Modest, conservative clothing is always appropriate. For men, not wearing a tie when the men in the group will likely be wearing them can convey disrespect. Looking one's best helps one to be confident and comfortable in front of the class. Comfortable clothes and shoes are helpful. Hair should be styled in such a manner that it does not create distractions (such as flicking long hair out of one's face). Being clean and tidy works every time. Reciting positive affirmation statements to himself or herself can boost the instructor's self-confidence.

Some lecture classrooms have fixed seating; others are furnished with stackable chairs. If chairs require setup, the instructor should position them in an arrangement that offers the greatest possible degree of interaction. A warm day with no air movement throughout the lecture room will likely cause students to lose concentration. The heating and cooling controls should be checked and windows adjusted to promote airflow and comfort. Ensuring the physical comfort of students significantly aids their attention span.

Instructors should arrive early to set up equipment that will be used. Many institutions do not have technical personnel to attend to this requirement, so it becomes the instructor's responsibility. At the podium, materials should be organized so that the lesson plan and any other needed materials are readily accessible.

Parts of a Lecture

After research and identification of key points to be delivered during the lecture, the instructor develops the three parts of the lecture: introduction, body, and conclusion. These parts are common to any instructional activity. Although most lecturers begin with the development of the body of the lecture, this discussion proceeds in presentation order and begins with the introduction.

Introduction

The purpose of the lecture introduction is to capture students' interest and attention. The lecture should be started with a thought-stimulating statement, an analogy, a thought-provoking challenge, or a question that arouses curiosity. This approach grabs students' attention and focuses their mind on the topic of the lecture. Some examples are as follows:

- "After cardiac arrest, very few patients walk out of the hospital neurologically intact . . ."
- "Patients who require long-term or ongoing institutional care are often the result of a life-saving efforts by paramedics . . ."

The introduction should establish the intention and relevance of the topic and should identify how this piece of information fits into the "big picture," such as, "Strokes are a leading cause of death in America. Disability from strokes alone costs society millions of dollars. Early recognition and management of the patient with stroke can significantly decrease the devastating disability that results from strokes."

Another effective introduction is a case study, that is, information from a real emergency medical services (EMS) call. Some lecturers choose to use a portion of the case study as an introduction, then to complete the case study, perhaps with the patient outcome and diagnosis included, as the conclusion.

The introduction can provide the ground rules for the lecture. Students should be told whether it is appropriate to ask questions during the lecture, or if they should wait for a question-and-answer session at the end. Also, students should be told whether comments are allowed during the class session. The lecturer can identify an approximate time until the next break, which should occur approximately 45 to 50 minutes after the lecture begins.

TEACHING TIP: Students should be given index cards so they can write down questions that they may have during the lecture. These are handed in at the end of the session, and the instructor can discern themes or areas that need reinforcement or clarification. This allows a student to ask questions without having to interrupt, speak up in class, or fear being accused by fellow students of asking "dumb questions."

Some presenters find it helpful to write out the complete introduction so that in the first few minutes of public speaking, they can rely on that as a crutch if necessary. This reassurance can assist the instructor in overcoming initial nervousness.

The introduction should not include an apology for the lack of time or the amount of information to be covered. These statements indicate poor teacher preparation.

Body

The body of the lecture must present key points to be discussed in achieving the learning objectives. Although the instructor has some freedom to select an approach for delivery of information, the lecture must follow a logical order and must be well organized. One example is as follows:

- Describe the cause of the medical condition; discuss incidence of the condition
- Explain relevant medical terminology that is used
- Identify the major clinical features of the illness
- Discuss the pathophysiology
- Explain the prehospital care that should be provided, and relate this to the pathophysiology
- Provide an overview of in-hospital care
- Offer strategies related to health and safety issues (e.g., reducing risk of personal injury or contamination)

Although it may be necessary for the instructor to provide more detailed information during the lecture, it is important that the main principles and ideas are not lost. At regular intervals during the lecture, it is useful for the instructor to summarize the main points. Students do not retain every detail that is presented; therefore, repetition brings focus to the message and reminds students of what they have learned.

TEACHING TIP: The lecturer should provide commercials! Today's generation has grown up with television, with material routinely presented in a half-hour- or hour-long format interrupted by commercials every 15 minutes. So lecture material should be presented in segments, then a "commercial" should be added, such as a summary or illustrative point. This allows students to process information in chunks, and it gives students who are taking notes the chance to get caught up.

Conclusion

The lecture requires some form of closure. This can be achieved in various ways, such as the following:

- Summarize the main points of the lecture by providing a new example that illustrates the main points of the material. This new example provides students with an opportunity to confirm their learning
- Make a statement that identifies what the instructor expects the students to gain from the lecture
- Ask a student to provide a summary of the main points
- Relate the lecture to previous and future learning
- Direct students' attention to additional learning resources related to the lecture
- Hand out 3 × 5 cards on which each student can summarize key points before returning them to the instructor. Through this technique, the instructor receives important feedback on his or her effectiveness and identifies concerns that can be clarified in the next lecture
- Conclude the lecture by asking for questions and answering them

When a student asks a question, it may be important for the lecturer to repeat the question so all students can hear it. After the question-and-answer session has concluded, a second powerful closure to the lecture can be used.

Another closing technique is to complete a case study that was begun as the lecture introduction. The actual patient diagnosis and outcome can serve as the ending of the lecture. Some teachers end the lecture with something memorable such as a motivational story or a challenge. The ending can strongly influence what information students take home.

Techniques for Enhancing Lectures

Because the lecture format has some disadvantages, instructors must develop methods by which to enhance the lecture to promote the acquisition of knowledge. Various techniques can be used, and instructors can explore which of these works best for their style and that of their students.

Humor

Humor can be an effective teaching tool when used correctly. The purpose of integrating humor into a lecture is not to have the lecturer receive high evaluations or to entertain the class. Laughter can be a valuable learning tool that reinforces the learning experience. It helps the lecturer connect with students and arouses interest. Laughter can help people relax and gain or keep attention. Humor can make information more memorable and can highlight an issue. Visual humor can facilitate learning and combat short attention spans. Students can look up at the picture or cartoon or prop and refocus on the lecture. The humor used should always be relevant to the topic under discussion.

Instructors must be careful about how they use humor in the classroom because it may be perceived in a very personal way. Attempts to emulate people from television or others who have a great sense of humor may not translate readily to an instructor's style. As a result, attempts at using humor may not be effective. Caution is encouraged when one uses humor in the classroom because one person's humor may be another person's insult. Instructors should be safe if they use gentle and quirky humor in the classroom setting.

CASE IN POINT

One method of using humor in a lecture is to make a point, illustrate the point with a short humorous illustration, then remake the point. An example is as follows:

> Clear communication with the patient and with his or her family is essential. It's like the EMT who responded to the scene of a shooting. Wanting to be able to quickly assess the injury, the EMT asked the patient where he was shot. The patient responded "over on Hatcher Street!"
>
> Clear communication is an essential component of patient assessment.

Storytelling

Relevant stories can enhance lectures. Stories can effectively illustrate and elaborate points. "War stories," or personal stories of a real EMS call, can assist students in applying information to patient situations. Stories based on actual cases provide an element of realism that reinforces the notion that students will one day encounter the difficulties associated with similar patients with similar problems. Storytelling can be a powerful and effective teaching tool because it can be used (1) to analyze and problem-solve certain elements of the patient care that was provided and (2) to stimulate critical thinking about patient care decisions made in the field. Inconsequential details should be eliminated so the story is not too long and student interest is maintained. Stories should be spaced throughout the presentation to provide a change of pace and to reemphasize the message. Storytelling should not allow students to digress into nonpurposeful discussion.

Case studies

A case study is an analysis of a real life patient situation as a way of illustrating information. Case studies help students learn to apply information to patient care situations. Cases used in lecture should be well designed and should illustrate the important points of the class. Such cases, especially when used with interactive methods, can stimulate critical thinking and problem solving.

Handouts

Handouts can be an important learning aid. Handouts provide a summary of the key points of the lecture and supporting instruction, but they do so without exhaustive explanation. Handouts provide to students the opportunity to reflect on the lecture topic and to expand their understanding. A handout allows many students to reflect on what the presenter is saying instead of worrying about taking notes. Careful listening allows students to think about the applications and implications of the lecture. In addition, the learner can review and reflect on the class at a later time to better integrate learning.

Although speakers typically say 120 to 180 words a minute, most audiences think at a rate that is 10 times faster. A handout can keep the learner focused on the spoken material rather than allowing time for the mind to wander. Handouts can also provide more in-depth information that is not included in the lecture, along with references through which students can enrich their learning.[9]

In general, handouts should be provided to learners at the beginning of the lecture, so they can follow the sequence of the lecture. Although lecturers may state, "don't worry about taking notes—it's all in the handout," conscientious students may find themselves worried that it is not all there and may wish to write down information "just in case." If the handout is not an exact version of the presentation, then the lecturer is more likely to keep student attention. However, in this case, the handout should be given out at the end of the lecture.[9]

Instructors should encourage students to study the lecture material beyond the content provided in the handout because handouts usually are abbreviated to focus the theme of the required learning. Students will find handouts helpful if they include a list of reference materials for further reading.

In addition to outlining or listing key points, handouts may include a glossary with definitions of unfamiliar terms; a list of steps such as a skill task analysis sheet, diagrams, or flow charts; and a reference list.[9]

Audiovisual aids, props, and models

Audiovisual (AV) aids are instructional media such as recordings, projected visuals, audiotapes, video-related technologies, radio, television, and computers that are intended to stimulate the senses of sight and hearing. Props and models are additional visuals that can be used during a lecture. These tools are used primarily to accompany a class presentation, particularly a lecture, for the purpose of enhancing learning.

AV aids offer many benefits, especially when a combination of more than one medium (multimedia) is used. Multimedia presentations can be applied to a variety of learning styles and may facilitate learning. Use of multimedia can reduce the costs of teaching and learning and may improve learning effectiveness. This is accomplished through increased learner motivation, improved retention of learned material, and enhanced interactivity.[10] The instructor should ensure that all students can hear and see the AV aids, model, or prop. A document camera may be helpful in facilitating this. For more complete information on the use of audiovisual materials, see Chapter 11, Audiovisual Basics.

Guided discussion and questioning techniques

Teacher-led discussions help students develop strong thinking skills and gain a sound understanding of the course material. In a large group, it is not always possible for the instructor to use a teaching tool that encourages students to discuss a particular learning point among themselves. However, teacher-led guided discussion allows students the opportunity to have their learning challenged. Guided discussion is designed to give students the chance to develop critical thinking and to increase student's comprehension by exploring an area of learning that is currently unfamiliar to them. The instructor poses a question to the whole class, and learners offer responses or additional questions to broaden the scope of the discussion (Figure 16-2).

Although questioning techniques can be used in a large group just as in any group, these techniques must be more carefully controlled in a large group setting. Discussions initiated within large groups can yield great results that assist students in learning; however, for a new instructor with limited experience in managing very large groups, this can readily turn to chaos. In some cases, two or three students may wish to dominate the discussion and argue their perspective as the model to be followed; they may even become argumentative. Members may not listen to each other, and each faction can become deferential toward the instructor. Discussion may tend to focus on one section of the group, and the rest may stop joining in. Additionally, when a student who is called on speaks, other

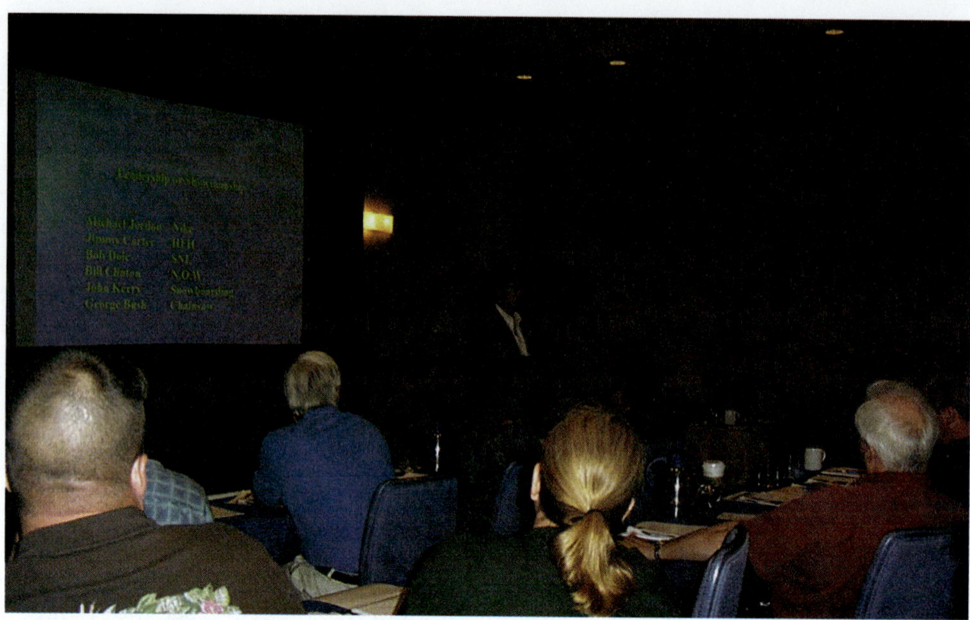

FIGURE 16-2 Effective questioning techniques can be used in a large group. However, the instructor must be prepared to manage the discussion.

students may begin talking among themselves, which can be very disruptive in a large classroom. Students should be instructed to remain silent until they are called on. Large group discussion must be undertaken with careful planning and caution.[7]

During a large group discussion, it is important for the instructor to make sure that the acoustics are adequate or that students use a microphone, because otherwise, only those in the immediate vicinity of the responding student may be able to hear. Presenters should come to the podium and use the microphone to present their findings. Additional information on questioning techniques can be found in Chapter 12, Introduction to Teaching Strategies.

Activities

Lecture content can be reinforced by an activity that is used to review material. By putting forth an application problem, the lecturer challenges students to find solutions to problems in ways that they must do so in the field—by actively participating with others in the group. Under the instructor's direction, learners may conduct a review or even play games that have been structured to allow students to apply the knowledge they have gained in ways that they may never have imagined. Movement from passive to active learning is what makes facilitation such an exceptional educational strategy.

Many instructors would be aghast at the idea of having large groups of students participate in activities during the lecture. Students in this situation become noisy, and the instructor must worry about whether students are actually undertaking the task at hand or are using the time for social chatter. Instructors may be concerned that time will be wasted if students are permitted to become involved in an activity. Despite these concerns, some simple activities have been designed that can readily be worked into a lecture.

CASE IN POINT

Sample student activities that can be used in a lecture format include the following:

- At a key point in the lecture, the presenter can summarize learning by posing some multiple-choice questions. Students must hold up a card with A, B, C, or D on it,[11] or four different-colored papers can be used to represent choices A through D. Obviously, the instructor must prepare the cards or paper before class time
- A multiple-choice question can be presented on the screen so that all students can see and read it. The presenter can invite students to identify the correct answer, then can call for volunteers to justify why the other options are incorrect

Work sessions and guided lecture

Another way that the instructor can modify the lecture format is by pausing every 12 to 18 minutes for a short 2- to 3-minute student "work session." This session assists students in clarifying and assimilating material just presented. Activities may be varied and can include the following:

- Students or student groups of two or three write down everything they can recall from the material just presented with special attention to the main points
- Students working with a partner or two write down everything they can recall from the class, then reconstruct and discuss the lecture (students may not take notes during the lecture).
- Students or student groups develop test questions and answers from the previously presented content.

During the work session, the instructor should be available to clarify any issue that may arise. These short "work sessions" can be followed by a brief student discussion and clarification of material as a large group.[12]

Interactive lectures

Available technology now assists instructors in changing a passive lecture to one that is interactive. Public area display systems (PADSs) are remote control units from which the audience is able to interact with lecture content through a computerized visual display. The instructor poses a question that has several potential answers, and from the remote monitor control unit provided for each participant, one response is selected. Data can then be manipulated to provide immediate feedback that reveals participants' responses. An example of this type of technology is television game programs in which the opinion of the audience is sought.

Considerable content within EMS education programs can be enhanced through a "talk-show host" approach. The instructor poses a general question or statement, and student group members offer responses that describe how they would deal with the scenario. This approach works especially well in sociologic situations for which no answers are absolutely right or wrong.

The new instructor may feel anxious about using this method for the entire lecture period; however, it is advantageous to schedule a 5-minute section that incorporates this method into the lecture. This allows the instructor to develop experience in this teaching approach. Box 16-1 offers several tips for effective public speaking techniques that instructors can incorporate into lecture sessions.

BOX 16-1 Essentials of Public Speaking

- **Preparation.** When instructors know that they and their materials are well prepared, their self-confidence is boosted; this can help reduce the amount of anxiety that new lecturers experience. Although practice delivery of the lecture in private surroundings is encouraged, actual delivery on the day provides vital experiences for the new lecturer
- **Voice modulation.** Lecturing requires the use of one's voice; lecturing to a large group requires additional attention to the speaking voice. Instructors who have not used a microphone before should practice using one. A natural speaking voice should be adopted, and enunciation should be clear. The pace and pitch of voice should be varied; this increases students' attention to the topic and reduces the likelihood that students may lose concentration through a hypnotic monotone. Timely pauses should be included to give students time to write notes
- **Enthusiasm and personalization.** Instructors should keep in mind that they have already put a lot of work into developing the lecture. Conveying enthusiasm for the material through use of colorful language and dramatic adjectives enhances the core concept of the material. First- and second-person pronouns (I, we, you) should be used because these personalize the instruction and lend status to and emphasize the importance of the topic
- **Eye contact.** Eye contact is key to effective communication and is an important aspect of lecturing and teaching. Even with a large group, students should sense that the teacher is looking directly at them at some time during the lecture. With fewer students, it is a worthy goal to look at each student during the course of the lecture. The speaker's eyes should be alert and should convey emotion, enthusiasm, and passion for the topic. As the speaker looks at students and into their eyes, he or she should observe clues from students' body language. Boredom, sleepiness, confusion, and frantic note taking can all speak to the teacher who listens. Alterations can then be made in the style or pace of the lecture, or a break in, or addition of, an activity may be needed
- **Gestures and body language.** Effective lecturers use gestures and body language to help convey their message. Nonverbal clues can speak much louder than spoken words can, so it is important that they match. A lecturer who says he is excited about the ability of EMS providers to positively affect the outcomes of patients with the use of new equipment is difficult to believe if his body language does not say the same thing. The key to using gestures is to use those that come naturally. Natural gestures come more easily when the lecturer is relaxed, comfortable with the topic, and prepared for the class. As the lecturer becomes more at ease with speaking, it also becomes more natural to move from behind the podium and change places in front of the class. Some lecturers change positions when they change subjects or emphasize points

Guest Lecturers

Many instructional organizations invite people who are knowledgeable about a particular topic to deliver a lecture. An invited guest lecturer must realize that preparation is crucial to the success of the lecture. Preparation is vital in ensuring that content stimulates student learning. The following focal points require significant attention to ensure that delivery meets the expectations of both the institution and the students:

- *Find out how the lecture topic fits with the course curriculum.* It is important for the guest lecturer to find out as much about the context of the lecture as possible, and to identify where it fits into the overall course program. The guest lecturer should meet with the course coordinator to clarify how the lecture should reflect course learning objectives. Topic learning outcomes should guide the guest lecturer in that these are the working documents that describe the topic content. The lecture is expected to address each outcome
- *Find out a little about the students.* Knowing about the age range of students, as well as their educational levels and cultural backgrounds will assist the lecturer in preparation and will allow the guest lecturer to use relevant examples
- *Find out what knowledge the students have about the topic.* The course coordinator and teaching colleagues will be able to provide insight so that the appropriate pitch of lecture delivery can be achieved
- *Find out how students will be assessed.* Knowledge of how students are to be assessed should affect lecture preparation. In contrast to assessment conducted through a major essay paper, assessment performed through multiple-choice questions or short-answer information recall questions requires helpful study resources and handouts that specifically address examinable material; these should be made available to students at the time of the lecture
- *Find out the scheduled duration of the lecture.* Although many institutions allocate lecture periods of a "50-minute hour," lecture length should be confirmed in advance with the course coordinator or program director

At least a week before the lecture delivery date, the guest lecturer should check out the venue. He or she must learn how to get there and must become familiar with the location of egress and exit doors and the room's physical layout. Information should be obtained about technical equipment provided within the lecture theater, and each piece that will be used should be tested to ensure that it is in working order. The lecturer must determine which equipment must be ordered from another location.

Instructors and guest lecturers should make sure they know how to confidently use the technical apparatus needed for their presentation. Practicing each function of the equipment before commencement of the class builds confidence, so instructors know that when the time comes for delivery of the lecture, the equipment can be used with no hitches. If microphones are available, the lecturer should test his or her voice against volume control, pitch, and clarity. The best advice: Be prepared in case the technology fails!

DEBATES

In the course of their work, paramedics encounter a variety of situations that differ from their own personal standards, beliefs, and social values. Another teaching strategy for large group settings is debate, or structured controversy. A debate is a structured contest of reason and logical arguments aimed at identifying truth. The session is bound by predetermined rules and can be used any time that the topic is open to opposing points of view. Debates are best used for higher-level cognitive thinking concepts. As a teaching strategy, the debate can foster critical thinking skills and reveal complexities of healthcare issues. Often, in many of the sociologic situations that confront EMS providers, no definite right or wrong decision-making actions can be identified, as each case requires individual attention. Numerous factors may have an impact in compounding patient care decisions. Therefore, classroom debate on those issues encourages students to critically think about the consequences of their actions when they deal with patients in real life situations. Debate can facilitate understanding of the points of view of others and can promote development of communication skills. The basic structure and format of a debate should be introduced far enough in advance that students can adequately prepare. Structure and techniques should not be the focus of the session, as relevant material may be lost in the process.[7]

The primary disadvantages of the debate approach are student anxiety and the need for adequate preparation time. Some students become anxious because of the public speaking skills required and the confrontational nature of debate. Some students do well with this strategy. Debate generally requires that students engage in research.[7] Participants require clear guidelines about the topic that they are to debate, and these guidelines must reflect the learning objectives of the course. It is useful for students to meet with the instructor before the time of the event so that each team can incorporate key learning themes into the debate.

Debating teams require information to be used in developing and printing handouts for the student group, as well as other resource material that can be used within the debate presentation; they also do well when they use available AV technology to enhance their presentations.

Typically, a debate involves five to seven students: two to three to present the "pro" side, two to three to present the "con" side, and one who acts as a moderator. Students must have knowledge of both sides of the issue if they are to argue intelligently. Generally, each side presents opening comments for a specified time, then each side presents its viewpoint, followed by a rebuttal from the other side. The debate ends with a summary from each side. Time limits are clearly defined, are equal for each side, and are strictly enforced by the moderator. At the conclusion of the debate, the class can vote for the best presented argument.

STUDENT PRESENTATIONS

Collectively, students are incredibly creative. They usually enjoy the challenge of demonstrating their ingenuity. Student presentations offer an effective teaching method. In turn, and at allocated times, each student is required to present information to the group on a predetermined topic. This approach has advantages and disadvantages. The strength of this approach lies in the empowerment that it gives each student to research and learn about the theme to be presented. The weakness is that many students are distracted by concern for their own presentation and do not concentrate on material presented by other students. New instructors may need to liaise with the program director to determine the logistics involved with having a large number of students make individual presentations in a timely and effective manner.

CASE IN POINT

At some time before the event, a group of four or five students can be asked to collaborate in developing a short presentation that demonstrates a concept that complements the lecture topic. Three examples are shown here:

1. Discuss methods to effectively communicate with hearing impaired patients
2. Discuss a chronic neurologic disease such as multiple sclerosis, and explain its prehospital care implications
3. Illustrate polarization and repolarization of the cardiac conduction system

Although each of these presentations need take only a few minutes, it is wise for the instructor to allow more time for the audience to reflect on the learning point and to regain composure before the instructor proceeds with the lesson.

SUMMARY

Teaching to large groups is an effective method of instruction when attention is given to the finer points of development, delivery, and management of the event. Mastery of the skill of lecturing takes considerable time and effort; with collegiate assistance, encouragement, and practice, the task becomes easier.

Effective teaching to large groups requires the attention of the instructor in learning how the lecture fits with the overall course curriculum. Armed with this knowledge, the instructor takes the next step: identifying the process for planning and preparing the lecture. The method by which the lecture is delivered and the resource accessories used are integral for the success of instruction.

When instructors are assigned to teach a large group, they should accept the task with enthusiasm because it provides an additional dimension of learning experience relevant to professional self-development, as well as an opportunity to impart knowledge to students.

REFERENCES

1. Nasmith L, Steinert Y. Evaluation of a workshop to promote interactive lecturing. *Teaching and Learning in Medicine.* 2001;13:43–48.
2. Cox K, Ewan C, ed. *The Medical Teacher.* 2nd ed. Edinburgh: Churchill Livingstone; 1988.
3. Laidlow JM, Hesketh EA. Developing the teaching instinct. *Medical Teacher.* 1995;24:364–367.
4. Newble D, Cannon R. *A Handbook for Teachers in Universities and Colleges.* 3rd ed. London: Kogan Page; 1995:378.
5. Gage N, Berliner D, eds. *Educational Psychology.* 5th ed. New York: Houghton Mifflin; 1991.
6. Saroyan A, Snell L. Variations in lecturing styles. *Higher Education.* 1997;33:85–110.
7. Rowles CJ, Brigham C. Strategies to promote critical thinking and active learning. In Billings DM, Halstead JA, eds. *'Teaching in nursing: a guide for faculty.* Philadelphia, WB Saunders, 1998.
8. Cooper L, Lawson M, Orrell J. *Raising issues about teaching: views of academic staff at Flinders University.* Adelaide, Australia: Flinders Press, 1997.
9. Pike RW. *High-impact presentations.* West Des Moines, IA: American Media, 1995.
10. Zwirn EE. Media, multimedia, and computer-mediated learning. In Billings DM, Halstead JA, eds, *Teaching in nursing: a guide for faculty.* Philadelphia: WB Saunders, 1998.
11. McKeachie WJ, Pintrich PR, Lin Y, Smith DAF, Sharma RA. From teaching and learning in the college classroom: a review of the literature. In: Feldman KA, Paulsen MB, eds. *Teaching and Learning in the College Classroom.* Needham, Mass: Ginn Press; 1994:75–114.
12. Seeler DC, Turnwald GH, Bull KS. (1994). From teaching to learning. Part III: Lectures and approaches to active learning. *Journal of Veterinary Medical Education.* 1994;21.

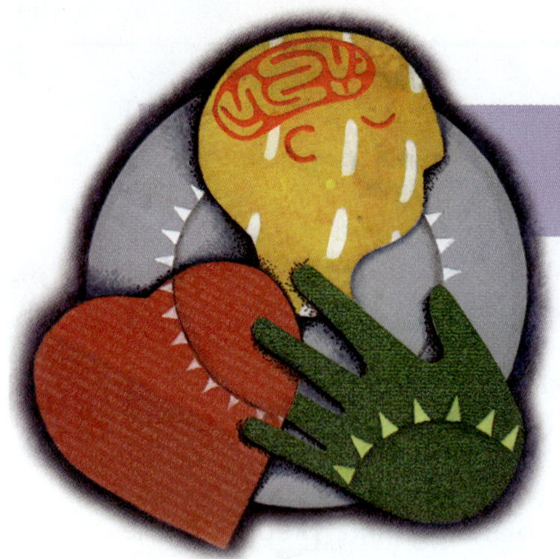

CHAPTER 17

Tools for Distance Learning

"Tell me and I will forget,
Show me and I might remember,
Involve me and I will understand."

—*Chinese Proverb*

Internet-based distributed learning is rapidly expanding across the health professions as an accepted and valuable educational delivery system. By removing the constraints associated with time and distance, the technology provides opportunities for emergency medical services (EMS) providers to build on their education.

Distance education is not a new concept. It offers access to students who otherwise might not enroll into educational programs. For people who have lived and worked in rural or remote locations, distance education via print materials delivered by the postal service has been the mainstay of available education in past decades. Times have now changed! The information and technology revolution has broken barriers and removed obstacles that previously restricted those who wanted to further their education with formal course work. Geographic distances, scheduling conflicts, shift-work rosters, work schedules, and family commitments are no longer a hindrance to those who wish to pursue their education.

Technology has mobilized the way humans communicate and has revolutionized the way they work and learn. With personal computers (PCs) in more than 50% of US homes, the PC has become accessible, commonplace, and readily available to a receptive domestic market.[1] Technological advancements, along with rapid expansion of the Internet, have brought about a proliferation of opportunities for learning at a distance.

This chapter offers insight into the realm of distance education; it describes different model combinations and provides tools to help instructors focus on teaching and learning within the classroom that has no walls.

DISTANCE EDUCATION IN PERSPECTIVE

Distance education (DE) is a system of education whereby students and teachers are separated by time and distance, so students are not necessarily in the actual classroom at a scheduled time. DE has several name tags which aim to capture the "classroom without walls" philosophy: "distance learning," "distributed learning," "open university," "open and distance learning," "e-Learning," "correspondence school," "flexible delivery," "external study," and "virtual education" are some. Although many of the names are interchangeable, a significant difference must be noted here: *distance education* is the term we use when we talk about the *process* of delivering education, and *distance learning* is the desired *outcome* of that education process.

As a delivery system, DE has been around since the beginning of written language! In the late 1800s, the University of Chicago in the United States offered education via postal service; in Australia, the School of the Air was established in 1944 in an effort to reach children and families in the Outback via two-way pedal radio link; and in 1969, the Open University of the UK began offering programs that used print and multimedia resources. Technology has played a significant role in the development of each of these programs.

Today, courses can be developed with the assistance of a wide range of technologies, often in combination, brought together to meet the requirements of the subject. Web-based applications, interactive CD-ROMs, audiotapes, videotapes, videoconferencing, teleconferencing, and computer conferencing all provide excellent means of bringing life to learning. Lectures may incorporate auditory descriptions, color, and animation to deploy a rich learning environment either on their own or in combination with print-based courses. The technology is available for instructors and students to take advantage of fantastic communication tools—both synchronous (at a scheduled time) and asynchronous (nonscheduled time). Although students who are enrolled in a course may be geographically scattered across the suburbs, the state, or the nation, or throughout the world, communication technology enables distance learners to meet with the instructor and discuss educational concepts through the computer (Figure 17-1).

Advances in telecommunications-based technology have leveraged DE programs to use methods that only a decade ago were thought to be futuristic. Satellite, microwave, and fiberoptic communications coupled with video- and audioconferencing and computer conference tools are part and parcel of the technology interface. The online distance learning market is growing annually by 30%, with more and more students choosing to enroll and study online.[2]

The Internet has become the most common method of information delivery, and across the globe, educational institutions are offering a wide range of programs with most courses coming from the disciplines of education, business, and humanities—which include the health sciences.[3] Within the healthcare spectrum, online programs for allied health sciences, paramedical science, nursing, health education, and health management are common. Web sites that offer or describe such programs include the following:

- Medscape at http://www.medscape.com
- Nursing Continuing Education Directory at http://www.nurseceu.com
- CMEWeb at http://www.cmeweb.com

Many other sites can be found through online searches and in journal, newspaper, and magazine advertisements.

Online teaching and learning have demonstrated proven performance with student achievement in the university sector.[4] A multitude of studies have been conducted over the past decade to find out about the effectiveness of online learning as compared with traditional face-to-face student classroom learning. These studies have also measured student perceptions and satisfaction with level of knowledge and with various delivery modes. Sufficient documentation has shown that no differences in exam scores have been seen between distance learners and students who have pursued their learning in the traditional classroom. In fact, emerging research indicates that the grades of distance learners are 5% higher than those of students who undertake face-to-face classroom learning.[5-7] These findings are supported by scientific studies.[8]

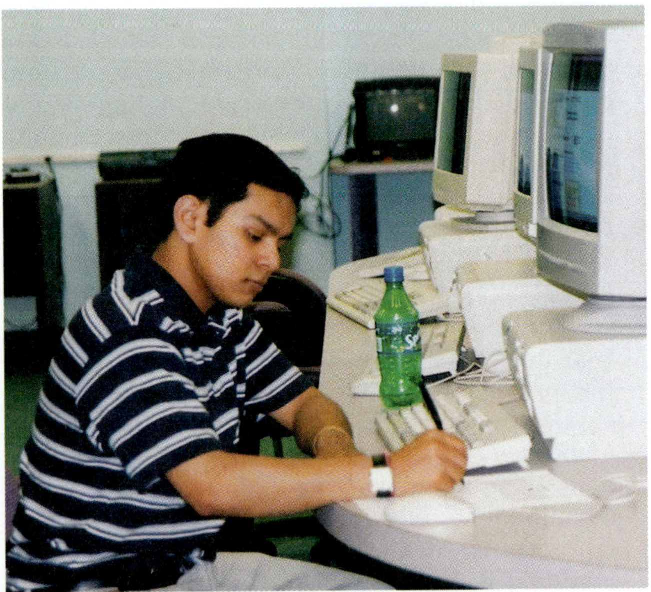

FIGURE 17-1 Geographic barriers to education are eliminated by Internet program delivery.

LEARNING AT A DISTANCE

As has been discussed in Chapter 4, Learning Styles, it is well known that learning is highly individualized, and that people learn in a multitude of different ways. It is also well known that instructors must employ various teaching methods and techniques to ensure that students understand what they are learning. Similarly, online teaching and learning have specific features that differ from teaching and learning in the traditional classroom and that require due attention.

Online Learning: Student-Centered Learning

The traditional classroom tends be teacher centered; that is, the teacher controls what is to be learned, when it is to be learned, and how it is to be learned. One of the significant differences between learning in the traditional classroom and online learning is the change of focus between learner and instructor—online learning is student centered. The student becomes the controller of his or her own learning. Within DE, some general basic themes underpin all student-centered learning.

The role of the instructor changes

The instructor becomes a guide or facilitator; the instructor guides students through their studies. The focus is on the student's development, interests, and needs.

Students take responsibility for their own learning

Students must be self-regulated to meet the demands of learning in isolation, if they are to adhere to task time lines. Although many distance learners are very good independent students, others need a tremendous amount of encouragement to get their work completed on time.

Learning is enhanced through discussion

Although the customary lecture has disappeared in DE, many opportunities are available for talking, sharing, and collaborating with other students.

The instructor manages student learning

The learning process is a shared process; the instructor and the students within the group share information and findings. Learning is ongoing, and students take an active part in the process.

Students construct knowledge through critical thinking and problem solving

This encourages independence and cooperation and promotes understanding and thinking for oneself.

Teaching and assessment are entwined together

In the classroom setting, teaching is often focused on preparing students for the final test. Online teaching focuses on the learning process.

Collaborative Learning

Learning online promotes, and is ideal for, collaborative learning—that is, an instructional method in which two or three students work together toward a common goal. Although this method is a common practice in the face-to-face classroom with small groups who work together, the virtual classroom uses e-mail, discussion boards, and chat rooms to foster collaborative learning online. Students can become responsible for each other's learning, and they may nurture mutual success. The collaborative approach to learning is a stimulus for the active exchange of ideas, which, in turn, promotes critical thinking.

Asynchronous and Synchronous Learning

Any student enrolled in a Web-based course will find that most time spent on course work is done asynchronously, that is, independently, and without assistance or direct instruction from the teacher. The Web site or lecture materials provide a study guide and comprehensive instructional steps that outline the requirements for course completion.

Technology is now available to provide synchronous teaching and learning; with this approach, students are in different locations, yet may meet at a prescheduled time to participate in a videoconference, or they may log onto a Web site for real time discussion with the instructor. Synchronous learning can be achieved through computer conferencing, during which students and instructor are stationed at their computers. With headsets and microphones, they are able to talk to one another, share documents, and use the whiteboard function to brainstorm ideas or to draw up a model. More commonly, message boards and chat rooms are used for synchronous discussion. Internet-based DL through the computer is causing a reduced need for other modes of conferencing technology, such as telephone conferencing and videoconferencing.

CHARACTERISTICS OF THE DISTANCE LEARNER

Although it is not possible to regard distance learners as a group with same likenesses, many students share demographic and situational similarities from which a profile of the learner can be typified. Their characteristics are varied; however, their commonalties include the following:

- *Age*—As cited by Thompson, Holmberg reports that the DE learner is usually older than the typical undergraduate student.[9] The 25- to 35-year-old age group tends to dominate, and the 35- to 40-year-old age group is a close contender
- *Sex*—More female than male students are enrolled in external programs; 60% to 70% are women[9]
- *Geographical distance*—As cited by Thompson, Gibson and Graff report that most distance learners reside between 100 and 200 miles (150–350 km) from campus.[9] However, because of the proliferation of online education programs, students who commute a round trip of less than 30 minutes are enrolling into online courses as a preferred alternative[3,9-11]
- *Life roles*—As cited by Thompson, Fjortoft reports that more than three quarters of students who were undertaking a DE postbaccalaureate program worked more than 40 hours per week, and most were married.[9] Other studies by Eastmond claim that up to 90% of students who undertake external studies are employed on a full-time basis[9]
- *Motivation and autonomy*—O'Shaughnessy states that intrinsic motivation and desire for career advancement are significant characteristics of distance learners.[12] Most DE students are self-regulatory, that is, they set aside regular time for study, establish schedules to meet their learning tasks, and don't need regular reminders to get their work

completed by the due date. They are autonomous learners

Therefore, it can be anticipated that the distance learner will most likely have an existing vocation and may be looking to expand vocational interests or gain qualifications that will facilitate movement into a different career path.

DISTANCE EDUCATION WITHIN EMS

In terms of distance, time, and work schedules, the cost of training EMS personnel is high. The use of distance learning coupled with provision for psychomotor skill practice and clinical experience can be effective and minimize educational costs. EMS training staff make it possible for personnel to attend classroom lectures, so that all operational requirements of an ambulance or fire department service are met.

CASE IN POINT

Shepherd Community and Technical College in Martinsburg, West Virginia, is conducting a basic paramedic training program for students who live and work 2 hours away at Keyser. Two-way audio and video are used for didactic instruction; this is supplemented by Saturday Skills classes for psychomotor skill development.

Paramedic education by distance is well established in Australia, as is evidenced by the following:

- Victoria University, Victoria, offers EMS conversion courses that are totally Web based. Students who have an in-service qualification are able to upgrade to an academic baccalaureate degree, then continue on to a master's or doctoral qualification through the use of Web-based technology[13]
- Charles Sturt University, New South Wales, offers distance education for baccalaureate conversion courses. These programs combine print and Web-based content with a residential school setting for development of psychomotor clinical skills[14]
- Flinders University, South Australia, offers several topics within the ambulance baccalaureate course in online or print format.[15] Additionally, several topics within the master's course are available online

Distance education is a viable option for the volunteer sectors. When one considers volunteer training, ongoing training, repeat lectures, and turnover of volunteers, DE provides a valuable alternative, especially for those who reside in rural areas. The training of volunteers often requires that both instructor and students travel. This may incur added costs for both the instructor and the students that can be saved by distance education. However, courses that are offered totally online may not meet the psychomotor needs of students; therefore, provisions within the course structure should incorporate "day-long" skill workshops.

STRUCTURING DISTANCE EDUCATION FOR EMS

The structure of DE courses within EMS requires unique conceptualization. Technology can be incorporated in many ways into models for EMS DE programs. Although the choices are numerous, it is very clear that Internet-based instruction has become the leading DE delivery mechanism. Many factors must be identified and figured out before a course can be set up. A very important early step is to gather together a group of interested and experienced people to explore suitable possibilities for a particular educational organization.

Determining Course Topics for Distance Delivery

DE can be structured to meet the learning needs of EMS agencies. Many components of Basic Life Support (BLS) and Advanced Life Support (ALS) courses can be readily conveyed through distance modules. For example, topics that relate to the prehospital environment, EMS systems, and the sciences of anatomy and physiology, as well as instruction on significant illnesses such as croup, asthma, or pneumonia, lend themselves well to online delivery.

Continuing education courses can be adapted readily to delivery by distance. The student has already developed fundamental skills within the paramedic practice. Additional distance education expands existing knowledge, reviews past learning, and introduces new practices.

Deciding the Structure of the Course

Deciding how the course is to be structured can be challenging. Different topics must be treated differently. The requirements of the curriculum will influence the course design. For example, it might be decided that students will learn the theoretical information online, then gather together for practical skill workshops to develop competence in psychomotor skill performance. Bringing students together for in-class work acknowledges the importance of the social nature of learning.

Decisions must be made about the use of synchronous and nonsynchronous communications. Will the course be primarily nonsynchronous, with some scheduled synchronous computer meetings? Table 17-1 presents some ideas about how different combinations can be used creatively to optimize student learning.

Mode of Delivery

The choice of delivery mechanisms relies heavily on available resources, administrative support, comfort

TABLE 17-1 Models Combining Different Forms of Technology[15]

	Primary Distribution Mode	Supporting Modes
Model #1	Online audiovisual lectures, discussion board	Classroom workshop for hands-on practical skills.
Model #2	Online text	Audiovisual lectures though CD-ROM, e-mail, telephone conference
Model #3	Print based	Online activities, discussion board, videotaped lectures
Model #4	CD-ROM	Online discussion board, videoconferencing, classroom workshop
Model #5	Print-based, interactive CD-ROM	Telephone conferences, e-mail

level with the technology, and level of available technical support. Each of these considerations is important, no matter what mechanisms are involved. Although Internet-based distribution is new and exciting, like other forms of educational delivery, it can be done well or poorly. A quality Internet-based program requires that many significant aspects are considered, including the following:

- Are technologists available to set up and maintain the technological aspects of the program?
- Do instructors have appropriate instructional expertise?
- Is enough administrative support available for the ongoing needs of the course?

When the Internet is the chosen mode of delivery, a number of technical and administrative decisions must be made. Some questions that arise include these:

- Will the course be located in the public domain?
- Will the course be housed within a learning management system (LMS)?
- If so, which LMS should be used?

Therefore, it is vital for instructors and administrators to get advice from experienced professionals on these important decisions.

TECHNOLOGY FOR SETTING UP AN ONLINE COURSE

According to the literature, online courses outweigh other delivery methods as the preferred method of pursuing distance education.

Learning Management Systems

Learning management systems (LMSs) facilitate the creation of online course work in a World Wide Web–based educational environment. An LMS is a software program that can be used to create entire online courses, or to provide interactive tools that supplement existing courses. Numerous LMSs are on the market. Organizations are encouraged to find one that best suits their needs. A quality LMS performs three functions:

- *Course structure*—Instructors are able to create course material by uploading lectures, activities, links, and tests onto the Web site
- *Course tools*—These are used to assist the student in participating in the course. Examples of course tools include a message board, a chat room, document sharing, a calendar, password changes, and exams
- *Course management system*—Administrative features needed for password authentication, automated grading and test results, student tracking, and generating of statistical data related to the course

For best results with an LMS, the instructor should use a Pentium-class computer with the latest Netscape or Internet Explorer browser version. The browser must be set to enable Java Script, and a high-speed Internet connection is highly desirable. Additionally, QuickTime, Adobe Acrobat Reader, and Real Player software programs may be required.

Course Communication Tools

Course communication tools are essential with any Web-based Internet delivery program. Many students say that these tools provide a sense of "belonging" to the class group and reduce the feeling of isolation. The LMS will have tools built into the software.

Types of tools include the following:

- *E-mail*—Electronic mail is a commonly used tool within the home; e-mail capabilities can link students to Web sites, and documents can be attached. E-mail is useful for asynchronous communications, such as for sending information to a group of recipients, and for sending and receiving course assignments
- *Message board*—Allows asynchronous communication between instructor and student, and between students. The communication is posted to a specific forum where each of the students enrolled in the course is able to read the communication. This tool is useful for sharing ideas and thoughts about a discussion topic
- *Chat room*—Allows instructor and student to communicate in text form in real time. Users must be online at the same time when they communicate (synchronous). This tool is great for immediate interaction and feedback

INSTRUCTIONAL DESIGN

Instructional design, the most important part of DE, progresses much in the way that buildings are constructed. An instructional course must be designed in a very specific manner, so that each task is clearly identified with the curriculum and the exact roles and functions of participants are delineated. Schiffman's model (Figure 17-2) provides a clear pathway that identifies each significant design step that must be addressed at preproduction meetings.[16]

Conceptual Map for Instruction

Instructional design incorporates the need to draw up a conceptual map of the course instruction. The conceptual map should include a series of annotations and links that provide an overview of how the instruction will be constructed and presented. The conceptual map helps developers to think through each element and make decisions about how the content will be presented online. Learning outcomes taken from the syllabus guide the development of the conceptual map, and each of the learning outcomes must be addressed by the instruction. Developers determine the mechanism by which learning outcomes are to be distributed. Figure 17-3 provides an example of the conceptual structure of a pediatric course. It expands to detail the pediatric emergencies section. The conceptual map is influenced by the type of media selected for delivery of the instructional material and by the resources available to produce the material.

Methods for Assessing Learning Online

Learning is assessed according to the processes of the educational institution, and content is determined by the curriculum. LMSs have a range of in-built tests and quizzes that can be used for formative and summative exams. Assignments are usually contained within a secured site. Some examples of test types include multiple-choice, ordering, true/false, and short answer questions. When cleverly constructed, each of these types of testing methods is capable of testing knowledge and comprehension of course work.

Many instructors raise concerns about supervision and exam conduct when the student is required to take the exam from a remote location. Institutions must develop policies to state how this can best be done. Several mechanisms can be put into place to ensure that the right student is taking the right test.

- *Exam pass codes*—An LMS can provide specific exam pass codes that authenticate that the right person is taking the exam
- *Timed exams*—The exam is scheduled to occur within a specified 24- or 48-hour period. The time is determined at the commencement of the course, so that students are able to schedule the event. Additionally, timed exams are usually of a duration that doesn't permit the student to look up texts or references
- *Proctored exams*—The student is required to take the exam at a predetermined location such as the local library. Instructions are provided, and arrangements are made with an overseer before the day of the event. Photo identification may be required
- *Range of assessment formats*—Course work assessments can be divided into several sections, each of which accounts for a percentage of the overall grade. Online tests, essays, collaborative work, projects, and online discussions can be incorporated into the student's overall assessment

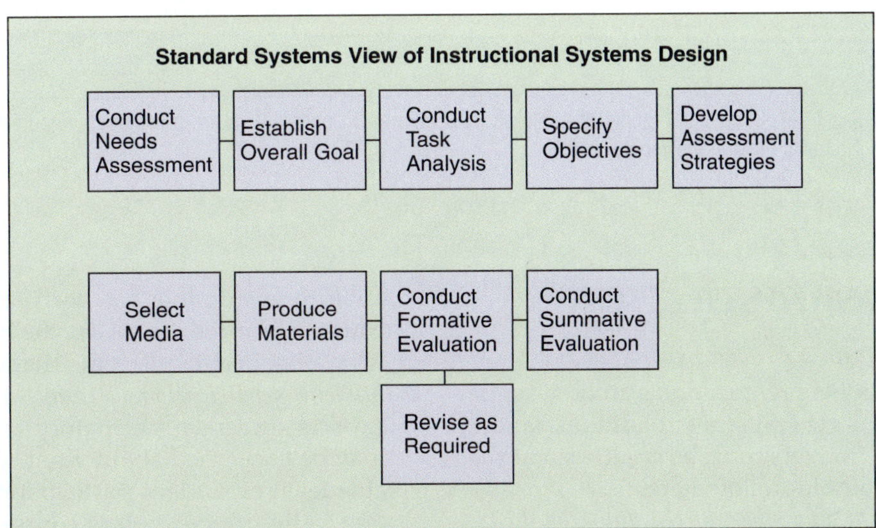

FIGURE 17-2 Schiffman's model of instructional design. (From Schiffman SS. Instructional systems design: five views of the field. In: Angin GJ, ed. *Instructional Technology: Past, Present and Future.* 2nd ed. Englewood: Libraries Unlimited Inc; 1995.)

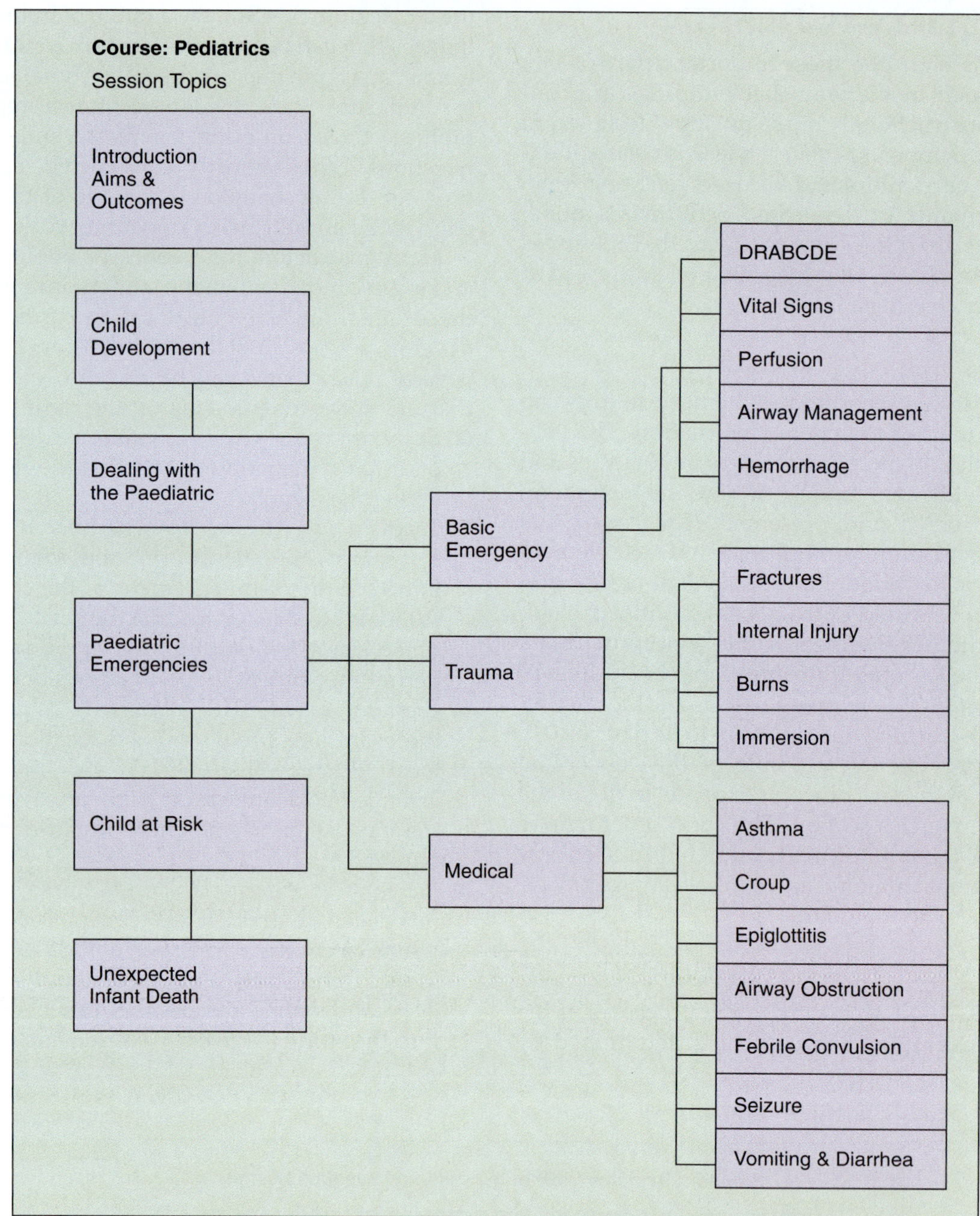

FIGURE 17-3 Conceptual model of a course map. (From O'Donnell M. Work in progress, unpublished. South Australia: Flinders University; 2003.)

FACULTY ADMINISTRATION MATTERS

Although an educational organization's student registrar is responsible for general student administration, some administrative matters must be dealt with at the local level. Some examples follow here:

- *Student enrollments must be entered into the LMS.* Student-related policies should mirror the protocol approach used for face-to-face courses. It is prudent for administrators to check the organization's handbook to ensure this has been addressed. If the DE course is about to be set up, the handbook may have to be amended to reflect the change in delivery mode
- *Student participation.* When an online program expects student participatory activities, instructors may be concerned about what constitutes a reasonable level of student participation or nonparticipation in the course. Before course commencement, a decision must be made and clearly communicated to students about how the course instructors will grade student participation. A participation policy

may need to be developed and a corresponding entry added to the student handbook
- *Grading collaborative work.* Students enrolled in the course must know how collaborative work will be graded. Without a clear statement on this, disputes can arise between students and faculty. A statement within the course instructions that defines how collaborative work will be graded significantly reduces the potential for problems

INSTRUCTOR SKILLS FOR ONLINE TEACHING AND LEARNING

Many enthusiastic instructors wish to develop their courses into DE format and are unsure how to go about it. If DE is already established at the instructor's educational facility, then the local staff development department may be able to offer workshops to provide the skills that instructors need to get started. An LMS will provide a comprehensive guide to assist the instructor in learning the technology, and the *Help* function within the LMS assists instructors during its use. When purchasing an LMS, the program director should make sure that the vendor includes training as part of the contract. Learning the technology to upload electronic files is not difficult; the challenge lies in learning the pedagogical framework and the different teaching methods available.

The instructor's experiences from classroom teaching provide a range of teaching skills that are readily adaptable to online teaching. Successful online teaching strategies include the following:

- Posing real-life scenarios—Students are able to relate learning to clinical practice. Real life scenarios provide sound foundations from which participants can explore a range of "what-if's" on the discussion board
- Asking students for their opinion—Students bring varied life experiences to the classroom; many will have encountered issues of social and health matters. Students learn from each other
- Acknowledging good progress—Feedback given to students through personal e-mail or the discussion board provides encouragement and allows students to gauge their progress
- Maintaining student self-esteem—Sometimes, the spoken word and the written word are in conflict when nonverbal cues are absent; instructors are encouraged to proofread e-mails sent to students to ensure that students' self-esteem is sustained
- Engaging students—Although students may be many miles away, online tasks and activities that require them to reflect on their learning create an environment that is meaningful to them
- Creating and maintaining a learning environment—this is the tenet of teaching principles

TEACHING TIP: Instructors must consider the way students process information; the learning environment that an instructor creates directly affects student learning. Instructors should do the following:

- Provide opportunities for students to share ideas
- Provide opportunities for students to feel supported and be challenged
- Empower students toward learning on their own by making course objectives clearly defined and accessible
- Establish relationships with students—relationships are essential if students are to be successful
- Instructors should design teaching to reflect high expectations for the success of all students

Because online learning does not provide the benefit of classroom visual cues, many instructors may be anxious to know if students are learning through the DE process. Additionally, very little research is described in the literature about DE from within the profession of EMS. One study wanted to find out whether two different distance learning techniques were as effective as classroom teaching for training EMT students at a rural location.[17] This study explored a range of technologies, including two-way audio and computers, and it employed synchronous teaching techniques. Study investigators concluded that, "No difference was found" between the two types of study, and they promoted distance learning techniques as an effective way to provide educational opportunities to rural EMS providers. Although it is imperative that EMS researchers undertake their own research into DE, research from general education and allied health disciplines confirms that learning does occur through DE courses.

ISSUES OF STUDENT LEARNING

Before a student embarks on an online program, several significant concerns must be considered. Basic computer skills are essential; although keyboard speed may present some limitations, skills for site navigation and basic software applications are required. Many local libraries or community centers offer short courses that teach computer basics. Therefore, it is prudent for instructors to provide potential students with a list of required computer skills needed to adequately participate in the course.

Potential students may find it helpful to be informed about course expectations and about how undertaking an online course can affect the home environment. Information packages that contain helpful hints about how to create a home study center and how to plan and attend to learning provide useful information for supporting and optimizing student learning.

Instructors may need to advise students that online learning requires self-regulated discipline because it is easy to defer course tasks in favor of personal commitments. To overcome this, it is recommended that students schedule specific times during the week to be dedicated to course activities and learning so that the benefits associated with accessing the online course can be balanced with personal endeavors (Figure 17-4).

Traditional classroom instruction is usually instructor centered, that is, the instructor is the center of attention, activities revolve around the demands and expectation of the instructor, and students are required to follow the instructor's lead. Online learning offers a different mode; the student is the center of attention, and the student is expected to lead topic activities and learning.

Many students are concerned about and question the equivalence of online learning and face-to-face learning. Although this is a valid query, evidence confirms that the learning that results is equivalent.[18] Instructors can help to alleviate student concerns by creating an active, vibrant online community that encourages participation.

CHALLENGES FOR DISTANCE EDUCATION IN EMS

EMS is a profession in its own right. As a profession, it is responsible for developing its own body of knowledge, as well as its own practices and paradigms.

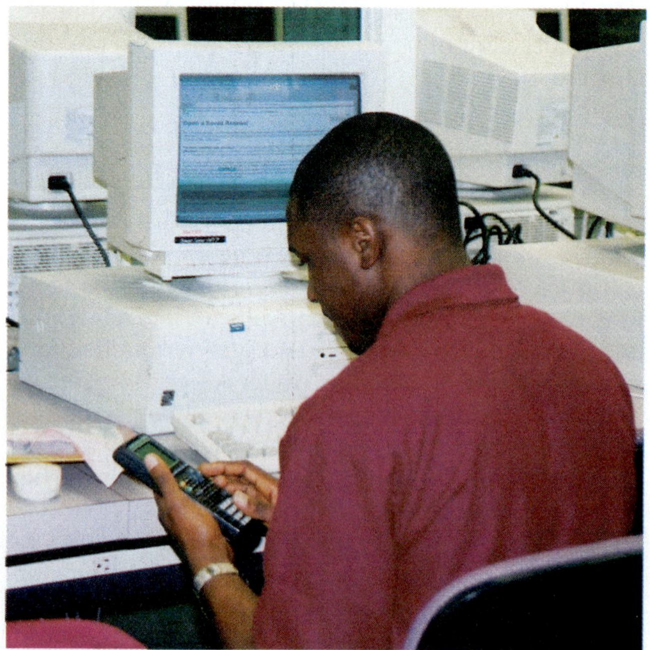

FIGURE 17-4 Students enrolled in distance learning courses are able to structure their class time around work time.

Internet-based DE offers many advantages for EMS; although it has been relatively slow to emerge as a teaching and learning option, EMS educators are encouraged to take advantage of this delivery method before other disciplines do it for them. The EMS environment of rural providers and shift-work rotations, as well as the range of educational programs to be delivered, makes DE a viable option.

EMS has an ongoing need for face-to-face practical skills labs—either on-site at the educational facility or at a central location that accommodates the needs of rural providers.

For online delivery of education, a system must be put into place that will retain a strong liaison between educational faculty and field instructors. Field instructors must be encouraged to participate in DE programs so that education and industry cohesiveness can be maintained. This results in the best outcomes for students.

Vocational and higher education institutions have policies that include access and equity. DE complements these policies by making education available to people who are unable to attend the classroom. Additionally, accrediting bodies have the expectation that educational programs will reflect contemporary methods by addressing access and equity.[19] The Continuing Education Coordinating Board for Emergency Medical Services is the body mandated to accredit courses offered via DL format within the United States. This organization can be found at http://www.cecbems.org; the Web site provides contact details and information about the process required for newly created DL programs to gain accreditation approval.

SUMMARY

Technology has paved the way for change in education delivery. A large percentage of students are enrolling in DE options, and DE programs appeal to many EMS professionals for various reasons. DE is a proven method of delivering education, with most educational institutions in the Western world and beyond taking advantage of the technological tools available to take education to those who have previously been unable to access such programs. The convenience and flexibility provided by courses that are free of the constraints of place and time are highly beneficial for learners.

REFERENCES

1. Newberger E. Home computers and Internet use in the United States. *Current Population Reports.* US Census Bureau, September 2001. Available at: http://usgovinfo.about.com
2. Gallagher S. The future of online learning: key trends and issues. The Distance Education and Training Council (DETC) 77th Annual Conference Summary, 2003.

3. Ashby CM. Distance education: growth in distance education programs and implications for federal education policy, 2002. US General Accounting Office Report GAO-02-1125T.
4. Redding TR. Comparative analysis of online learning versus classroom learning. *Journal of Interactive Instruction Development*. 2001;13:3-12.
5. Smeaton A, Keogh G. An analysis of the use of virtual delivery of undergraduate lectures. *Computers and Education*. 1999;32:83-94.
6. Wade W. Assessment in distance learning. *The Journal*. 1999;27:94-100.
7. Sener J, Stover M. Intergrating ALN into an independent study distance education program: NVCC case studies. *Journal of Asynchronous Learning Networks*. 2000;4.
8. Fallah MH, Ubell R. Blind scores in a graduate test: conventional compared with Web-based outcomes. *Journal Asynchronous Learning Network*. 2000;4. Available at: http://www.sloan-c.org/publications/magazine/v2n2fallah.asp
9. Thompson MM. Distance learners in higher education. In: Gibson CC, ed. *Distance Learners in Higher Education: Institutional Responses for Quality Outcomes*. Wisconsin: Atwood Publishing; 1998.
10. Halsne AM, Gatta LA. Online versus traditionally-delivered instruction: a descriptive study of learner characteristics in a community college setting. *Online Journal of Distance Learning Administration*. 2002;5.
11. Smith SL. Student services: the key to distance education programs. National Association of Student Personnel Administrators, 2001. Available at: http://www.naspa.org/netresults/
12. O'Shaughnessy MM. Designing for the distance learner—The diploma in social integration and enterprise for community development workers. Centre for Co-operative Studies, University College, Cork, undated. Available at: http://www.ucc.ie/acad/foodecon/c_dp3?b.html. Accessed August 1, 2003.
13. McDonnell A, Edwards D. From the classroom by Cyberland: 21st century education for paramedics. *Australasian Journal of Emergency Care*. 2000;7:231-234.
14. Lord W: The development of a degree qualification for paramedics at Charles Sturt University. *Journal for Prehospital Primary Health Care*. 2003.
15. O'Donnell M. Flinders University of South Australia, unpublished, 2003.
16. Schiffman SS. Instructional systems design: five views of the field. In: Angin GJ, ed. *Instructional Technology: Past, Present and Future*. 2nd ed. Englewood: Libraries Unlimited; 1995.
17. Hobbs GD, Moshinskie JF, Roden SK, Jarvis JL. Education and practice. A comparison of classroom and distance learning techniques for rural EMT-I instruction. *Prehospital Emergency Care*. 1998;2:190-191.
18. Boston RL. Remote delivery of instruction via the PC and modem: what have we learned? *American Journal of Distance Education*. 1992;6:345-357.
19. Council for Higher Education Accreditation. Accreditation and assuring quality in distance education. CHEA Monograph Series No. 1, 2002.

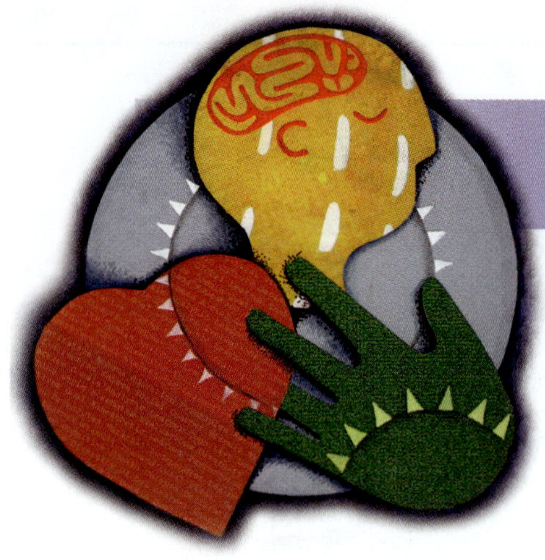

CHAPTER 18

Tools for Field and Clinical Learning

"Experience develops all our great flute players, but also unfortunately, all our worst players."

—*Plato*

The goals of an effective clinical educator are to demonstrate excellent clinical skills and behavior, recognize and take advantage of a student's teachable moments, and prepare students for the real world environment.

Both employers and patients expect graduates of healthcare programs to be competent healthcare providers. Theoretical knowledge and abstract skill performance, although important, are simply not sufficient to prepare someone to work in the hospital or field environment. All students of health care must experience real patient care if they are to gain a reasonable level of competency in their skills, as well as the appropriate level of confidence in their abilities. Clinical education is an essential component of emergency medical services (EMS) education, and the clinical educator may be the most influential teacher an EMS student will ever have.

The previous chapters of this text have focused on more traditional educational models and general instructional methods. These theories and strategies are applicable to all types of instruction, and the clinical educator should take time to become familiar with them. In this chapter, however, instructional theory and strategy focus specifically on clinical education, that is, education that is *experiential* and involves the student's observing, participating in, or leading patient care activities in an actual patient care setting.

CLINICAL EDUCATION

Clinical education in EMS is usually performed under the supervision of an experienced clinician who facilitates learning, teaches students, and acts as a patient advocate. The clinical educator is usually used by a healthcare facility or EMS responder agency but sometimes is employed by the educational institution. For the purposes of this chapter, the term *clinical educator* refers to all those persons who guide experiential learning, including mentors, preceptors, training officers, and instructors.

Clinical experience for the EMS student most often is acquired in a hospital emergency department (ED) or on an emergency ambulance. The term *field clinical* refers to prehospital or outdoor experiences; *hospital clinical* refers to experiences in a hospital, clinic, or other indoor setting.

The type and scope of clinical experience provided vary according to the level of education. Clinical education for entry level EMS providers, such as emergency medical technicians (EMTs) or First Responder students, is usually limited in scope, objective, and time. Basic clinical experience often involves observation in a hospital ED or a handful of ride-along shifts on an ambulance. At more advanced levels, such as EMT-Intermediate or Paramedic education, students may perform clinical rotations in a wide variety of hospital departments and healthcare settings. Specialized units within hospitals, such as operating rooms, cardiac units, catheterization labs, psychiatric crisis units, burn care units, obstetric departments, and intensive care units, are common at this level. Advanced field clinical rotations may also involve experiences with air ambulance services, critical care transport teams, law enforcement officers, fire or rescue personnel, and other EMS-related service providers. Some programs use innovative and nontraditional settings, such as homeless shelters, skilled nursing and geriatric care facilities, pediatric clinics, immunization outreach programs, and morgues, where students can gain a unique perspective (Figure 18-1).

Experiential Learning

Experiential learning is an educational philosophy that best describes the essence of clinical education. This philosophy is based largely on the original work of John Dewey, with later refinements by the German philosopher Kurt Hahn. At the core of this philosophy of education is the idea that learning begins with an experience. A particular circumstance may require an action on the part of the student, or it may simply be an observation of an action. Once it has been completed or the situation has been resolved, the student reflects on the experience, and with the assistance of a facilitator, draws meaningful lessons from his or her observations, actions, and reflections.

The goal of traditional didactic education in the classroom is for students to demonstrate a practical understanding of the knowledge imparted to them. In general, the student's role may be somewhat passive, although the student is encouraged to be attentive and to participate in class activities. In skills labs, the student is expected to practice and demonstrate the ability to perform step-by-step procedures after they have been properly demonstrated and rehearsed in a linear manner, usually under ideal conditions.[1-4] Less controlled and sometimes frenetic clinical experiences are often left until the final stages of the educational process. Because the quantity and quality of learning during the clinical phase can be unpredictable, clinical education is sometimes viewed as less valuable than other methods of instruction.[2]

Participation in clinical education in EMS, however, is one of the most important steps toward the development of confident and competent graduates.[5,6] Unlike the traditional classroom, the "real world" of clinical education requires that students be assertive, take initiative, and eventually even direct others to perform tasks.[3] He or she must be able to assess patients and circumstances, analyze conflicting information, apply acquired knowledge, perform technical skills, and exhibit professional attributes. This requires that the student perform at higher levels of intellectual functioning.[2] Therefore, the importance of an effective clinical education program for EMS students cannot be overstated.

In clinical education, experience is the catalyst for learning. In the course of treating patients, the student is actively engaging most, if not all, of his or her senses. The student is also immersed in a complex set of thoughts, actions, reactions, and evaluations. Reflecting on these experiences builds a library of knowledge that will help him or her identify similar patterns of disease and injury. This knowledge will aid EMS students in effectively assessing and treating future patients.[5]

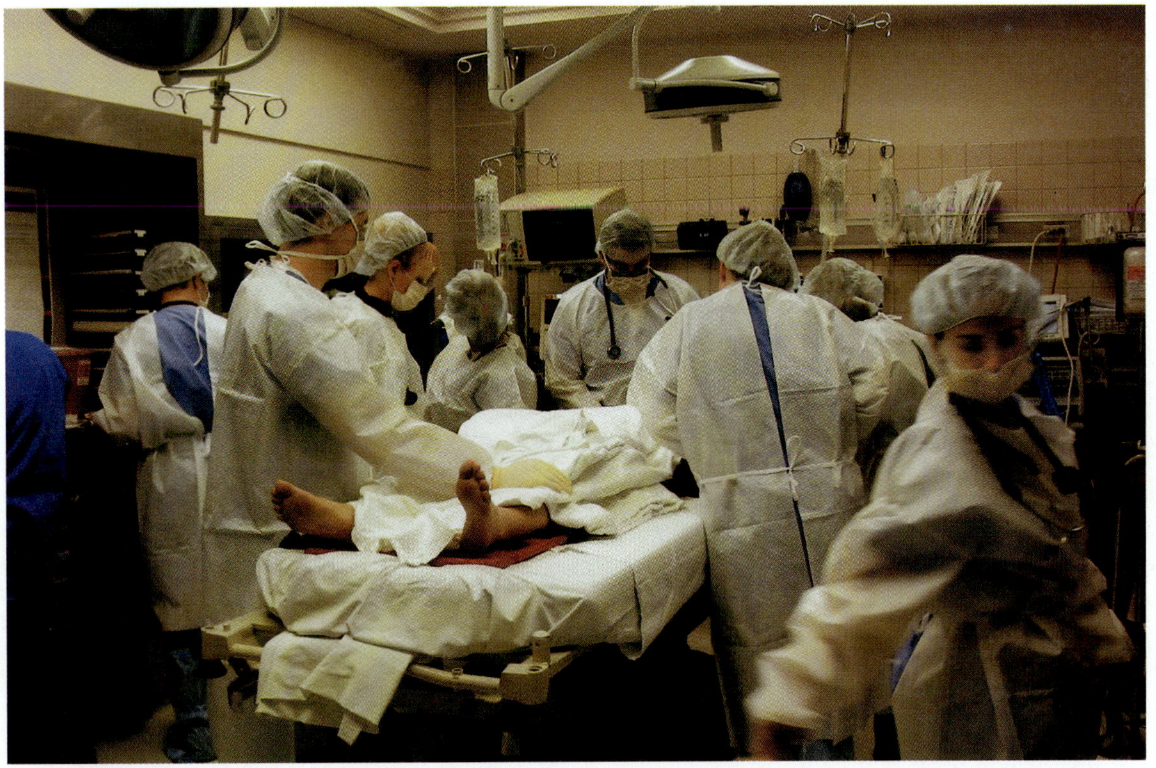

FIGURE 18-1 Airway management in the operating room is an important experience for paramedic students.

Experience alone, however, does not necessarily inspire learning. To be educationally sound, experiences should be carefully structured around specific learning goals and should include appropriate orientation, preparation, and critical evaluation.[7] It is the role of the clinical educator to provide background information, to ensure that experiences are put into context, to answer questions, and to direct further learning or review. A proper foundation, combined with timely communication, helps the student to organize learning and makes him or her aware of the fact that learning has just taken place.[3]

THE EFFECTIVE CLINICAL EDUCATOR

The clinical educator, beyond playing a central role during experience-based learning,[8,9] is a role model for students and is seen as an expert in the field. The characteristics of an effective clinical educator are discussed in Box 18-1.

Above all, clinical educators must create positive and professional interpersonal relationships with students (Figure 18-2). They must respect students, display confidence in them, show genuine interest in them, and encourage mutual respect. The personal attributes of an educator that promote learning include enthusiasm, patience, friendliness, a sense of humor, flexibility in the clinical setting, and a willingness to honestly admit limitations or mistakes.

TIPS FOR EFFECTIVE COMMUNICATION WITH STUDENTS IN THE CLINICAL SETTING

- Introduce yourself, and use your name
- Use your students' names
- Make and maintain eye contact
- Listen actively, providing verbal and nonverbal cues that you are following the conversation
- Clarify what is being said by paraphrasing key points and checking to make sure that you understand the communication
- Do not assume that you understand the student's words or actions until you have heard all of the facts or asked questions that confirm your understanding
- Watch for context: Most communication is paraverbal (tone, pitch, pace, and power) and nonverbal (behavior, gestures, and actions)
- Do not try to solve problems or give advice; instead, help students explore options to help themselves
- If you feel that your own feelings are clouding your ability to stay calm and communicate effectively, then take a break and return to the interaction when you are prepared to place students' needs above your own

BOX 18-1 Attributes of Effective Clinical Teachers[8,9]

Effective clinical teachers:

1. Create an environment that is conducive to learning with the following:
   - Knowledge of the practice area
   - Clinical competency
   - A desire to teach
2. Are supportive of learners; such support requires the following:
   - Knowledge of the learners
   - Knowledge of the practice area
   - Mutual respect
3. Possess teaching skills that maximize student learning; this requires an ability to:
   - Diagnose student needs
   - Learn about students as individuals, including their needs, personalities, and capabilities
4. Foster independence so that students learn how to learn
5. Encourage exploration and questions without penalty
6. Accept differences among students
7. Relate how clinical experiences facilitate the development of clinical competency
8. Practice effective communication and questioning skills
9. Serve as a role model with excellent clinical skills
10. Enjoy practice and teaching
11. Are friendly, approachable, understanding, enthusiastic, and confident about teaching
12. Are knowledgeable about the subject matter and able to convey that knowledge to students in their practice areas
13. Exhibit fairness and objectivity in evaluation
14. Provide frequent feedback and positive reinforcement

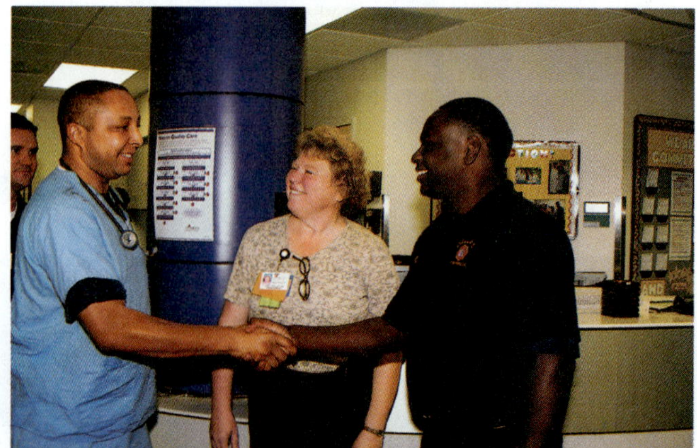

FIGURE 18-2 Clinical educators must create positive and professional interpersonal relationships with students.

Research shows that student learning is enhanced significantly when clinical educators are skilled at using teaching objectives, able to ask appropriate questions, and willing to provide specific and timely feedback. Additionally, formal preparation and instruction for clinical educators on how to teach in the clinical setting have proved to correlate with better student achievement.[9]

ROLE OF THE CLINICAL EDUCATOR

Through effective hospital and field clinical instruction, didactic knowledge and practical skills are reinforced by experience, which helps to prepare the student to be an entry level clinician.[5]

In general, the role of the clinical educator is to do the following:

- Size up the needs of the student
- Assist the student in creating a plan to facilitate learning
- Help the student put theoretical knowledge into practice
- Extend knowledge and learning by relating experience to general theory
- Promote skills development
- Promote professionalism
- Be responsive to the needs and concerns of other clinical staff
- Evaluate, document, and report student progress and achievement[2]

The clinical educator has a particularly challenging role in EMS education. In addition to regular patient care duties, either in the hospital or in the field, the clinical educator must balance the needs of the student with the needs of the patient, bystanders, family members, support staff, and coworkers (Figure 18-3).

By definition, students are not as skilled or competent as the clinical staff with whom they are working. The clinical educator must be willing to allow a student to attempt procedures and other patient care duties. This requires the ability to recognize any opportunity to do so and to perform a quick analysis of the risks to the patient versus the benefits to the student. An effective clinical educator can turn a nonemergent, superficial dog bite into a fascinating description of the importance of infection control, proper wound irrigation and dressing, the mechanism of healing, recognition of rabies or sepsis, and variations in animal and human bites.

CASE IN POINT

In the early stages of a clinical education, a student's performance may be unpredictable when he or she is attempting new skills. In this stage, the clinical educator should be authoritative and should ask the student to focus on specific objectives before the student encounters them in the next patient. For example, if a student is having difficulty obtaining a patient history, the instructor should try to have the student focus solely on creating a conversation with the next patient. An objective should be introduced for the student to simply introduce himself or herself, then to elicit the patient's name, chief complaint, and history. As the student successfully completes this task with the first patient, the instructor can add additional objectives for the next patient contact, such as getting a history from a family member or bystander. Giving feedback and building on small successes increases the student's level of confidence.

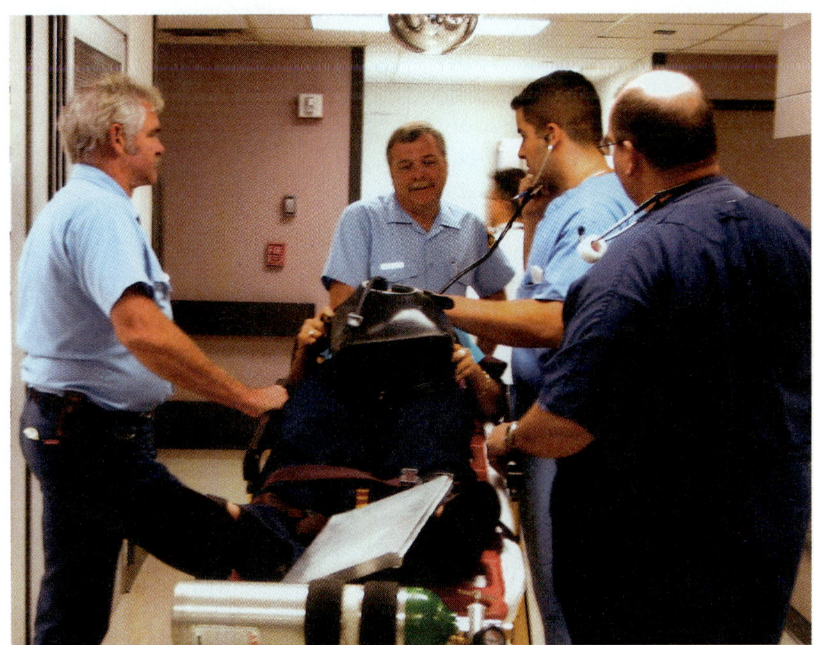

FIGURE 18-3 The clinical educator must balance the instructional needs of the student with the needs of the patient, bystanders, family members, support staff, and coworkers.

More importantly, clinical educators must have enough seniority and trust from coworkers to transfer patient care authority to the student. Eager and well-meaning staff members or First Responders wanting to perform rapid and efficient care can present an unintended barrier to student learning. Experienced clinical educators know to discuss the educational plan with other staff members, whenever possible, before a patient encounter. Students should be identified by a school badge, a distinctive uniform, or a patch reading "EMT Student" or "Paramedic Intern" so as to minimize confusion, particularly when advanced procedures are being performed.

The clinical educator should try to remain in the background as much as possible, seeming to carry on a casual social conversation, or quietly getting a private report from First Responders, family members, and other interested parties for the purpose of creating some space and time for the student to function. At the same time, a seasoned clinical educator should be able to keep an ear and a watchful eye on the student's performance. However, at times, education must be sacrificed in favor of patient care. Then, the role of the clinical educator is to help students reflect on events to find valuable learning points in their observations and in the actions of others.

The current EMT-Intermediate and EMT-Paramedic curricula recommend that students make the transition from the role of observer, to practitioner, and finally, to team leader.[5] Clinical educators must seek out opportunities for students to function at the level of their current abilities and to develop higher-level abilities. In some cases, students may be able to lead uncomplicated patient encounters, but they may function only as team members in situations that are more complex. The clinical educator must be keenly aware of students' strengths, weaknesses, current capabilities, previous successes, and ongoing challenges.

The clinical educator also plays a key role in reducing high levels of student stress. Evidence suggests that students experience significant stress and anxiety during clinical education.[2,9-11] Performance anxiety can be a serious barrier to achievement when students are unable to concentrate or receive and process information. Although stress and anxiety are common in emergency health care, the clinical educator should be able to recognize when a student's fear is actually preventing learning or inhibiting performance. Once this is recognized, the clinical educator should take steps to create a less threatening environment, and should focus the student on specific tasks that will serve to build self-confidence (Box 18-2).

BOX 18-2 Steps to Help Reduce Student Anxiety[10]

1. Establish a safe relationship
   - Be empathetic
   - Deal with mistakes calmly
   - Emphasize positives
   - Remember that a trusting relationship takes time to build
   - Be honest
2. Build self-esteem
3. Confront the problem (talk about the anxiety)
4. Draw from the student's past coping mechanisms
5. If the student appears blocked, give specific direction
6. Set strict limitations (insist that the student attempt or try to perform)
7. Divide tasks into smaller parts
8. Set realistic expectations

CASE IN POINT

A student is embarrassed about removing the shirt of a patient of the opposite sex. Each time this student is supposed to check the patient's breath sounds, he or she hesitates, then moves on to history-gathering questions. This is a case of anxiety masquerading as poor performance. Even though 5 minutes before the patient contact, the student perfectly described how to obtain breath sounds, the student is paralyzed at the instant of unbuttoning the patient's shirt.

The clinical educator is the best person to help the student get past the overwhelming feelings that are paralyzing him or her. The clinical educator should assist students by first identifying the fear, then rehearsing what he or she will say and do with a mock patient, such as a classmate or a patient that is not threatening. A good strategy is to take "baby steps." The student can be coached to listen to breath sounds through the shirt at first, then coached to raise the back of the shirt only; finally, once the student is more comfortable, he or she can begin removing the shirt altogether while taking steps to preserve the patient's modesty.

CLINICAL TEACHING STRATEGIES

Performance expectations of students at the end of their EMS clinical experiences are high. In a relatively short amount of time—as little as 3 to 6 months—students are expected to observe, practice, and direct emergency care. Entry level competency requires that the student master the building blocks of assessment, recognize pathophysiology in actual patients, demonstrate motor skills in adverse circumstances, and exhibit professional behavior in stressful situations. The clinical educator should help students move quickly through the learning process without overwhelming them. The following sections focus on strategies that are specific to clinical teaching and that complement previously discussed teaching techniques.

Do As I Do: Actions Speak Louder Than Words

One of the most effective clinical teching techniques is the consistent modeling of the behavior or skill that is being asked of the student.[2] When the instructor demonstrates the professionalism, technical aptitude, and leadership that are expected, a student learns by observing and emulating behavior. An educator should remember that a student is carefully observing his or her actions before, during, and after patient care activities.

Even if some clinical or operational steps seem redundant and unnecessary to the expert provider, clinical educators should practice all the good habits they would like to see in their students. For example, spending time at the beginning of a shift doing equipment checks and inventory may seem boring and routine to an expert, but it teaches the student that it is important to be thorough and prepared, and to have all equipment in working order. The instructor who arrives on time, well groomed, ready for duty, and wearing a smile teaches the student that he or she takes pride in the work.

When a choice exists between explaining and doing, the clinical educator should choose to *do*. Performing an action or exhibiting a behavior that demonstrates a point will make a more lasting impression on a student than will a simple explanation. The best teaching method is to involve the student in actively demonstrating, practicing, or researching the topic (Box 18-3).

BOX 18-3 Retention of Learning

Average retention rates from various instructional modes include the following:

- Lecture: 5%
- Reading: 10%
- Audiovisual: 20%
- Demonstration: 30%
- Discussion group: 50%
- Practice by doing: 75%
- Teaching others: 90%
- Immediate application of learning in a real situation: 90%

Of what we learn, we retain approximately the following:

- 10% of what we Read
- 20% of what we Hear
- 30% of what we See (We "see" what we read!)
- 50% of what we Hear and See
- 70% of what we Say
- 90% of what we Say as we Do

Modified from Erlendsson J. Learning retention rates. Available at: http://www.hi.is/~joner/eaps/cs_reten.htm.

CASE IN POINT

An EMT instructor is trying to teach professionalism. Upon discovering that the staff lounge is disastrously dirty, the instructor begins to clean up. With or without student participation, by emptying the trash and vacuuming, the educator sends a much stronger message than would be sent by verbally expressing disappointment in the situation.

Ask Questions

An instructor's effective questioning and answering of questions lead to improved student learning.[12] This reflection on observation and action is an essential element of learning by experience.[13] Clinical educators should encourage an atmosphere where it is safe to ask questions so that no detail is missed; also, the sophistication of the student's inquiries can be a good clue to the instructor about their level of progress. Simple or "dumb" questions can be especially important because hospital, EMS operations, protocols, and culture vary dramatically, and it is easy for misunderstanding to occur. Educators can also use questions to help students filter information and focus on the most important issues in patient care.[14]

Questions can be broadly categorized as convergent, where students are asked to analyze or synthesize information, or divergent, where students are asked to extrapolate on a concept. Convergent questions seek specific information, whereas divergent questions do not have a single right answer.[14]

Research shows that clinical educators have a tendency to pose low-level questions that ask the student to recall memorized facts.[9,14] The clinical educator should be careful not to fall into this common trap. More effective questioning revolves around asking the student to apply information, think critically, and make decisions. Higher-level questions improve reasoning and eventually lead to improved clinical performance[14] (Box 18-4).

The following are some tips on asking effective questions:

- *Slow down*. The slower the question and the longer the wait time for a response, the more time the student has to carefully consider possible answers, thus higher cognitive levels can be expected
- *Have students compare their actual experience with general theoretical expectations*. This helps bridge the conflict between the classroom (general didactic expectations) and the reality of actual practice. (*Examples:* Was the patient exhibiting classic signs and symptoms? Is it possible for a patient to have pulmonary edema and bronchospasm at the same time?)
- *Have students provide alternative solutions*. Encouraging students to think creatively about situations will improve their problem-solving abilities. These situ-

BOX 18-4 Examples of Questions Used to Evaluate the Cognitive Domain[8]

Knowledge (lower-level cognition)

Define ______.
List the five principles for ______.
Based on your assignment, what do you recall about ______?

Comprehension

Explain the meaning of ______.
Tell me in your own words what is meant by ______.
Which of the examples demonstrates ______?

Application

What is a new example of ______?
How could ______ be used to ______?
Show how this information could be graphed ______.

Analysis

What are the implications of ______?
What is the meaning of ______?
What are the key components of ______?

Synthesis of Ideas

What are some possible solutions to the problem of ______?
From this information, create your own model of ______.
Suppose you could ______. How would you approach ______?

Evaluation

Explain the effectiveness of this approach.
Which solution would you choose? ______. Justify your opinion.
What are the consequences of ______?

ations may involve real difficulties that they have encountered or hypothetical scenarios, but they should always be realistic[1]

- *Have students predict and anticipate changes in patient condition or reaction to treatment.* In addition, have the student propose possible plans to address these changes. (*Example:* What symptoms would you expect of this patient if her condition worsens? Improves? What will you do if there is no improvement after the first medication administration?)
- *Avoid yes/no questions.* These types of questions do not give you information about how the student is thinking or arriving at decisions[15]
- Limit each question to one main thought, and make sure that the question is understandable. Vague questions force students to guess what the teacher is asking

TEACHING TIP: Clinical educators should create an environment that welcomes questions and encourages curiosity. This does not mean that educators must know the answers to all questions. It is best to teach students to "fish for themselves" by showing them where and how to look up reference information. Modeling this continued quest for knowledge encourages lifelong learning that will serve the student well past the day of certification.

FIELD PRECEPTOR JOB REQUIREMENTS AND TRAINING

For the purposes of this section, the preceptor is the clinical educator in the field setting who is working directly with EMS students. Although all levels of EMS students can benefit from clinical and field preceptors, most of the emphasis in EMS clinical education is placed on the EMT-Intermediate or Paramedic level provider. In fact, the presumption is that if a preceptor can train paramedic students, he or she is also qualified to train basic level students. This may seem logical, but it remains one of the enduring myths of EMS. Providers such as First Responders and EMT-Basics have needs and expectations different from those of advanced level providers. Paramedic preceptors who provide training to entry level students may not be aware of the needs of basic providers. This phenomenon diminishes the advanced provider's oversight value, unless the preceptor is first tutored in the training needs and protocols of basic caregivers in the area.

Many EMS programs are measured by the capabilities of their preceptors. Just as with any other educational setting, high standards in both clinical skills and teaching strategies are to be expected. Programs should regularly evaluate past performance and should develop the skills of clinical educators. Pairing a student with the right preceptor can be challenging. Teaching and learning styles must be compatible. Care should be given to maintaining impartiality by pairing students with clinical educators who can be objective and fair, even if they have had previous working relationships with the student. Cases in which personal relationships between a student and his or her preceptor are already present should be avoided at all cost.

Preceptor Job Requirements

A clinical educator for any type of EMS student acts as a role model, and a preceptor's clinical knowledge and patient care skills—including the ability to establish patient rapport—should be carefully screened and evaluated. A preceptor candidate who will be overseeing interns new to advanced life support (ALS), should probably have at least 1 to 2 years of concentrated field experience. Preceptor candidates who will be evaluating interns with previous ALS field experience should probably have at least 3 to 4 years of concentrated field experience. It should not be assumed that an expert in ALS or the best-liked employee would make a good clinical educator. The candidate must be able to develop the capability to deal constructively with adult learners. He or she needs to view interns as active learners with whom the instructor will collaborate to solve problems; they must be seen as students who will require guidance regarding actions of human beings during a crisis, and who will need help to understand how to apply ALS protocols to specific situations.

The following is a list of qualifications exhibited by strong candidates for preceptor training programs:

- Significant field experience (measured by numbers of patients seen, as well as time spent at the provider level)
- Demonstrated ability to work with people (not the same skill as caring for patients)
- Experience with planning training events
- Supervisory or critical incident stress management training
- Experience or training in conflict management, negotiations, quality improvement, and similar subjects
- Awareness of current EMS research literature and of the value of clinical and educational research (candidate reads current journals and literature, participates in an EMS journal club, attends regional or national conferences, values continuing education)

If preceptor candidates do not possess any of these qualifications, then a different approach should be used for evaluation. For example, a teaching demonstration in front of a select panel or an appropriate audience might prove to be a useful evaluation tool. The candidate should also be observed while providing patient care and interacting with other responders and the public. Potential preceptors should be evaluated on calls rather than by talking with them about responses. Informal and formal interviews should focus on the candidate's attitudes toward and expectations regarding the role of clinical educator.

Preceptor Training

A combination of innate skills and proper training helps ensure success for preceptor candidates and prepares them for the challenges of teaching adults under stressful circumstances. The following is a suggested outline of topics that should be included in a preceptor training program:

- Preceptor roles and responsibilities
- Legal and ethical issues—confidentiality, harassment, and discrimination
- Principles of adult learning
- Effective learning environments
- Teaching methods—communication skills, teaching aids, and questioning techniques
- Purposes of evaluation
- Evaluation criteria and forms, and appropriate use
- Problem resolution and points of contact

Evaluation System

In addition to a preceptor training module, the field education program must have a well-defined written evaluation system for documenting the clinical progress of students. A rating system that removes as much ambiguity as possible from subjective evaluations is valuable. Understanding how one is to be graded can provide a great boost in confidence for the student and can provide a frame of reference for use as he or she moves through the educational process. Having a defendable evaluation tool also makes it easier for students who are seeking a change of preceptor, or who challenge the fairness of their evaluation (see Chapter 20, Using Written Evaluation Tools, for additional information).

Preceptors benefit from receiving program reference materials, such as a job description that includes reasonable expectations, limits on the numbers of interns (depending on the system, usually one to three per year with a break in between), and the supervisor and school representative to whom they will report.

Feedback and continuing education for the preceptor are highly desirable and should be based on the actual experiences of the preceptor, so as to fine-tune his or her skills and provide information on which the preceptor can base improvements. If possible, the preceptor program and other clinical education opportunities should be integrated into the provider organization's career ladder (Box 18-5). A well-defined training, education, and feedback system will improve the retention rate of quality clinical educators and will increase the educator's level of job satisfaction.

WRITTEN WORK

Both students and clinical educators must document learning activities thoroughly and must complete a standard patient care report for every patient contact. All records must be maintained in a manner consistent with the privacy practices of every public agency, corporation, and/or educational institution involved. At a minimum, the student should complete a summary of the complaints and field impressions of the patients he or she has encountered, skills that have been both observed and performed, and attempts at team leadership. Doing so is vitally important to the field education process as it actively reinforces learning and teaches the student the importance of keeping detailed records in future practice.

Clinical educators should confirm the accuracy of the student's documentation and should provide a written review of learning activities and performance. The process of reviewing the student's documentation allows the educator to identify patterns in student

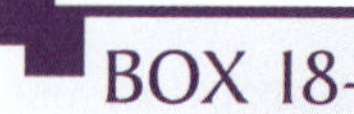

BOX 18-5 Cultivating Preceptors: Developing a Culture of Preceptorship

by Dean Vokey, BEd EMT-P

Introduction

Paramedic education has placed an emphasis on experiential, competency-based learning during the field internship. This emphasis provides students the opportunity to apply classroom theory and skill lab sessions in the real world classroom of the back of an ambulance under the watchful eye of a preceptor. Key to the success of this learning affirmation is the importance of the preceptor's role. Preceptors are tasked not only with the responsibility for patient care but also the role of clinical teachers, motivators, professional role models, and evaluators of student performance. With this in mind, it should be no surprise that there is a supply and demand problem with preceptors. This is due in part to paramedic programs steadily increasing their numbers of accepted students while the availability of preceptors is decreasing, causing paramedics to feel the effects of increased workloads and added responsibilities. To maintain the value of field internships and overall high standards of paramedic education, educators need to consider potential shortfalls in the preceptorship model and develop strategies that emphasize the development and sustainability of preceptorship programs focusing on establishing a culture of preceptorship.

The six R's of Developing a Culture of Preceptorship identify the key areas that focus on recognition of professional responsibilities, finding the right people for the job, providing them with essential skills, avoid burning them out, providing ongoing support, and recognizing their contribution.

The six R's of Establishing a Culture of Preceptorship:

- **R**esponsibility
- **R**ecruitment
- **R**eadiness
- **R**etention
- **R**eassurance
- **R**ecognition

Responsibility

As with other health professionals, there is a professional responsibility to participate in clinical education of new practitioners. For paramedics, this provides an opportunity to "give back" to the profession. Experienced paramedics have so much to offer students, not just in terms of skill performance but sharing their experiences and clinical judgment. Educational programs should place heavy emphasis on this aspect of professional responsibility when discussing the roles and responsibilities of the paramedic and throughout the course.

Recruitment

The next step in establishing a culture of preceptorship is to increase the numbers of preceptors. Right now the most significant challenge facing the preceptorship model is preceptor availability and fatigue. Educational programs are often competing with other programs for preceptors, often this constant stream of students leads to "burn out" of preceptors. To avoid preceptor fatigue and to increase the numbers of available preceptors, programs should consider developing a Preceptor Recruitment Strategy in response to these challenges. The strategy would focus on attracting new preceptors who exemplify excellence in clinical and professional competency, along with an interest in clinical teaching. This strategy would also set standards for preceptor qualifications, i.e., establish minimum years of service and certification level; develop a role description that defines expectations; get the word out that preceptors are needed by posting notices in stations and hospitals and holding information sessions; and develop a selection process, where potential preceptors could be interviewed.

What Educators Are Looking for in a Preceptor :

- Willingness
- Experience
- Above average skills
- Knowledgeable
- Excellent communicator
- Professional deportment
- Responsible
- Caring/Empathetic
- Patience
- Commitment

Readiness

Once you go out and recruit the right people for the job, the next step is to prepare them for their new responsibilities. The goal here is to provide new preceptors with skills and knowledge to ensure they are confident and competent to precept students with a focus on roles and responsibilities, facilitating clinical learning and student evaluation. Most programs provide some sort of preceptor preparation, usually in the form of a workshop. These workshops provide an excellent opportunity for faculty to meet the preceptors and discuss preceptorship issues. The disadvantage of workshops is it is often a challenge to fill classrooms due to scheduling or getting people to give up a day off to attend unpaid training. Perhaps one solution to increasing participation would be to put preceptor training online, just as many medical schools have done.

Some topics covered in preceptor workshops:

- Roles and responsibilities
- Principles of adult learning
- Motivating students
- Providing feedback
- Conflict resolution

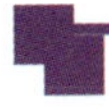

BOX 18-5 Cultivating Preceptors: Developing a Culture of Preceptorship—cont'd

by Dean Vokey, BEd EMT-P

- Evaluating student performance
- Practicum policies and procedures

Retention

Now that you have invested in a recruitment and training program and have established a highly trained and committed pool of preceptors, the biggest challenge is to keep them. To achieve this, programs must provide opportunities to keep preceptors involved and interested in the program, such as serving as adjunct faculty, guest lecturers, or participating on advisory committees. Programs must also be aware of the dangers of student overload and its effects on preceptors. If preceptors are constantly bombarded with students, they will steadily get tired of precepting. Some ways to avoid preceptor fatigue include rotating preceptors or limiting numbers of students going to a site. Consider expanding your preceptor pool by establishing new sites and having a recruitment drive.

Reassurance

One of the most common complaints from preceptors is that they feel that other than the occasional site visit or telephone conversation when a problem arises, they do not get the level of support they expect from program faculty. Remaining in constant contact and providing ongoing support is critical to keeping preceptors. Some ways to achieve this include increasing frequency of site visits; starting a preceptor newsletter or web site; establishing a faculty-preceptor committee; and developing a mentoring system where experienced preceptors can provide support to new preceptors.

Recognition

Most preceptors go above and beyond expectations when precepting students. While some preceptors are paid, most volunteer, receiving nothing more than a thank you. Whether they are paid or not, preceptors make a significant contribution to the development of their students, so it is important for programs to recognize their efforts and commitment. Programs would be wise to consider implementing Preceptor Recognition Programs to acknowledge the great work that preceptors do. A small token or gesture goes a long way in letting preceptors know that they are valued.

Preceptor recognition ideas:

- Thank you letters
- Preceptor time as CME
- Preceptor awards
- Prize draws
- Free CME courses
- Gift certificates
- Teaching opportunities
- Invitation to graduates
- Preceptor recognition socials
- Trinkets

Conclusion

The field internship is an essential component in the development of competent, "job ready" prehospital providers. The key ingredient to the success of this component is the availability of effective preceptors who are committed to clinical teaching. Paramedic programs need to be aware that, as the need for preceptors increases, so too does the demand placed on existing preceptor pools, and preceptor interest may drop due to the added demands. To avoid this scenario and to ensure sustainability of the preceptorship model, programs need to cultivate preceptors and look at ways to emphasize professional responsibility to new preceptors, attract new preceptors, train them, provide ongoing support, keep them interested, and recognize their contribution to paramedic education.

From NAEMSE, Domaine 3, Summer 2003.

performance, both good and bad, and to record the successful completion of learning objectives.

When possible, students and educators should go beyond the minimum data tracking and patient documentation requirements. Students can benefit greatly from a more detailed log of their activity and performance. By tracking detailed information over time, students can also identify patterns in their performance, or lack thereof. A review of the student's experiences will help the educator to anticipate needed learning opportunities or the need for more aggressive coaching.

Additional written work that is helpful in maximizing reflection and learning from experience includes the following activities for the student:

- Keeping a journal of learning activities, emotions, and specific milestones or accomplishments
- Creating a running log of prescription medications encountered. This log can include the indications for use, typical dosages and side effects, and a brief description of the diseases the medications are used to treat
- Documenting sources of references used to obtain additional information about a patient's disease, injury, or behavior
- Writing patient care reports in prose with the appropriate use of abbreviations. In some locations, patient care reports require only the completion of check boxes and short words. Students who must synthesize and compose full sentences on a relatively blank section of paper with the use of, for

CASE IN POINT

As an instructor, you have been assigned to evaluate a student who becomes quiet and withdrawn on select calls. After reviewing a report of the student's past clinical experiences, you note that when a psychiatric patient is encountered, the student steps back into the role of observer. Armed with this information, you investigate the cause of this particular problem and develop a plan to overcome it. The solution might be as simple as providing more time in a hospital psychiatric unit. Review of different types of psychiatric complaints and questions that would help the student assess these patients and defuse aggressive behavior might also be helpful.

You might discover that this student is shy and afraid, or has a family history of mental illness, which makes the student uncomfortable about talking with this patient. Working with the student one-on-one to discover this and to arrange for the student's personalized help with a counselor could be a life-changing strategy that will help the student grow as a caregiver and as a person.

instance, the Subjective Objective Assessment Plan (SOAP) method, will be intellectually stimulated

- After critical events, answering, in writing, a few questions regarding the nature of the experience. This exercise can spark critical thinking and pattern recognition

PREPARATION AND DEBRIEFING

Coming to a clinical experience properly prepared is as important for the educator as it is for the student. If the clinical educator is using a facility with a predictable pattern of patient complaints, volume, or population, much work can take place to maximize learning opportunities when students are present. Careful planning of goals, objectives, and specific activities can focus students, create a very productive learning environment, and make the experience more valuable. For example, a cardiac care unit with a predictable flow of patients with myocardial infarction or angiography is the ideal site for a student to practice cardiac assessments.

Preclinical and postclinical conferences have been found to be useful in the clinical setting.[16,17] In the preclinical conference, the educator can guide students through a goal-setting process that focuses student efforts for the day and sets the stage for later analysis of the experience. Focusing students' activities into concrete steps and assignments also helps to reduce anxiety, wasted time, and misdirection.[10] In the postclinical debriefing, students analyze their experiences, clarify relationships between theory and practice, and reflect on their actions and feelings, patients' conditions, and the learning process (Box 18-6).

MEASURING STUDENT PROGRESS AND COMPETENCY IN THE CLINICAL ENVIRONMENT

Currently, little research in EMS education definitively proves the value of clinical learning or explains the best way to track and measure it; however, it seems that something magical occurs when students get hands-on clinical experience. The transition from classroom theory to practical, lifesaving skills can quickly transform students into functional EMS practitioners. Field training is the setting in which some students and teachers discover that they may not be well suited for a career in EMS, and they look for an alternate pathway or an exit strategy. The educator's ability to manage and predict the quantity and quality of clinical experiences needed by the student directly correlates with the success of the clinical training program. But how does an educator manage and predict what will be needed? Once goals are created, how do educators track student achievement in the field?

The logistics of scheduling, creating documentation, evaluating progress, and keeping records during EMS clinical education can be overwhelming. Scheduling alone can become a logistical challenge depending on how many accommodations are made for clinical sites, preceptors, other classes, and student work commitments. More importantly, tracking the development of student learning and performance in a very unpredictable setting can be very time-consuming and too expensive to do with any accuracy or depth.

Terminal objectives, such as graduating competent entry level EMS practitioners, are often not easily measured, and patient census or run volume can vary greatly. Indeed, tracking student progress during clinical rotations is a challenging but essential task for the EMS educator. The educator must create a plan for student learning that is based on realistic expectations, focuses on developing competency, and includes measurable terminal goals and objectives. Students and preceptors should focus on the development of assessment, decision-making, and team leadership skills. Progress throughout the internship must be tracked and accomplishments rewarded in the areas of emphasis.

The Challenges

Measuring progress during EMS clinical experiences can often take the form of the easiest, most objective measurement available—time on task, also described as "seat-time" in more traditional educational settings. Hour-based clinical experiences from past EMS curric-

BOX 18-6 Guidelines for Clinical Educators

Before the Clinical Session Begins	During the Clinical Session	After the Clinical Session
■ Bring references Drug handbook Medical dictionary Pocket preferences Current SOPs Point-of-care resources ■ Set goals for the day Review and address students' past weakness List current successes that should continue If possible, visit the site or department, and determine patient census, patient and staff willingness to work with students, and potential learning opportunities ■ Come prepared with activities that can complement patient experiences or serve as guided tutorials when patient census or call volume is low. Examples of this include the following: Bringing real electrocardiogram (ECG) strips that you have collected over time to practice interpretation and verbalize treatment plans Going through the medication cart or ambulance drug box and randomly selecting medications and quizzing the student on indications, contraindications, dosage, route, mechanism of action, and antidotes or reversal agents Role playing past patient encounters and having the student ask interview questions and verbalize assessment impressions and treatment plans Practicing map reading by listening to other ambulance calls or selecting addresses out of a phone book Performing an ambulance inventory and having the student attempt to verbalize three uses for each piece of equipment	■ Do not be afraid to look up reference information and ask questions of experts in the presence of the student ■ Look for windows of opportunity (sometimes referred to as "teachable moments") to give the student a chance to practice skills and direct the team ■ Personal digital assistants (PDAs) may be used to carry everything from photographs of relatives to extensive reference material, such as the *Merck Manual*, standard operation procedures, and other useful point-of-care material.	■ Start by discussing positive aspects of the student's performance ■ Make the transition to areas that could be improved ■ Discuss whether the patient presented with typical signs and symptoms; ask about what could have been done sooner ■ Where possible, and without violating privacy, follow up on patient outcomes ■ Discuss some of the emotions noted in the patient and staff members, along with strategies to address those behaviors ■ Ask students to describe alternate methods for assessing and treating patients who were just encountered

ula were much simpler to schedule and track. Once the student completed a predetermined number of hours, the student's clinical experience was deemed completed, regardless of performance or ability. However, simply completing hour requirements does not necessarily translate to competency in EMS provider graduates.

Newer curricula now recommend that students perform multiple successful assessments and team leadership of patient contacts. Often, as is the case with the Paramedic curriculum, the students is required to perform more than a dozen assessments and treatments for a particular complaint before he or she is considered competent. Because patients often present with multiple complaints at the same time and must be simultaneously treated for several differential diagnoses, documentation of student learning may be very complex.

Performance rating criteria must be straightforward and easy to use because interrater reliability can also present a challenge. Many programs find that it can be logistically impossible to keep one student working with the same preceptor over time. As the student moves from preceptor to preceptor, coaching and evaluations may become inconsistent. Likewise, what constitutes a team leader or a patient at the ALS level may vary greatly from one clinical education site to another.

The Solutions

When tracking student progress during clinical training, educators should focus on the following areas:

- Confirming that the student attended the clinical, arriving on time, dressed in appropriate attire, and prepared to work (assess professionalism)
- Keeping accurate counts of the quantity of experiences the student has accumulated and has yet to finish, measured both in time and in number of patient encounters
- Identifying the nature of the illness or injury of patients with whom the student is coming in contact
- Identifying skills that the student has observed and performed during patient encounters
- Documenting instructor evaluation of the student and coaching the student on issues to address
- Continually assessing the student's progress toward completion of the goals stated in the clinical learning plan

Because so many variables are at play and so much information is managed simultaneously, a searchable computer database is one of the best ways of managing all the data being collected. Although these data have to be backed up and safeguarded, it is usually easier to do this than it is to store hard copy forms (paper and pen) in a secure location for a specified time. Although paper forms are necessary to confirm attendance and document preceptor evaluations, they are not so helpful in analyzing student clinical experiences. Using the power of the Internet to share and manage schedules has become much less cumbersome but may require expert advice to prevent data loss and to preserve patient and student privacy. An example of one student skill and experience tracking system is FISDAP. More information can be obtained on this product by visiting www.fisdap.net.

EVALUATION AND FEEDBACK

Educators must provide support and feedback throughout a student's clinical experience because this is a vital part of formative evaluation.[18] Students must have the opportunity to safely attempt, fail, regroup, and try again under the conscientious oversight of their instructor. Constructive criticism should lead to changes in style and habits and to experimentation by the student, all of which should be encouraged. Resultant positive achievements should be highlighted, no matter how minimal or small the progress might be. Educators may feel personally challenged and even frustrated when students are not progressing quickly or steadily. Discussions with peers and frequent breaks can alleviate some of the impatience and self-blame that an educator may feel.

Feedback can be given in many formats. One successful feedback tool that educators find helpful is called SMART. SMART provides educators with the following five guidelines for formatting feedback[19]:

S: *Specific*—Focus on behavior and performance. Give examples.

M: *Meaningful*—Focus on important issues and events. Avoid trivial events.

A: *Appropriate*—Provide balanced and fair review, keeping in mind that students respond best to positive feedback. Choose the right moment to praise improvement. The student must be receptive, and the educator has to stay professional.

R: *Reality based*—Give concrete examples that are based on actual behavior and performance.

T: *Time*—The closer to the event that feedback is given, the more helpful it is.

See Chapter 20, Using Written Evaluation Tools, for more information on evaluation of field and clinical experiences.

SUMMARY

Clinical education is effective when it meets predetermined objectives and provides opportunities for students to become competent and confident clinicians. The effective clinical educator uses actual patient care as the catalyst for learning and tracks students' experiences to plan a rounded clinical education. Many traditional teaching methods can be used in the clinical education environment. For example, the clinical educator should consistently model the behaviors and skills expected of the student. He or she should ask meaningful questions that enhance student learning and promote critical thinking. The clinical educator must prepare for clinical students just as in the traditional classroom environment. He or she must also evaluate a student's clinical performance. However, a clinical educator must plan for the unique challenges of educating a student in a busy patient care environment and must work hard to take advantage of a student's teachable moments. Being an effective clinical educator can be vastly rewarding and can make a difference in a student's readiness for a real work experience.

REFERENCES

1. Carpenito L, Duespohl TA. *A Guide for Effective Clinical Instruction.* 2nd ed. Rockville, Md: Aspen Systems Corporation; 1985.
2. Stengelhofen J. *Teaching Students in Clinical Settings* London: Chapman & Hall; 1996.
3. Hunt J. Dewey's philosophical method and its influence on his philosophy of education. In: *The Theory of Experi-*

ential Education. 2nd ed. Boulder, Colo: Association for Experiential Education.

4. Shuttenberg EM, Poppenhagen BW. Current theory and research in experiential learning for adults. In: *The Theory of Experiential Education.* 2nd ed. Boulder, Colo: Association for Experiential Education.
5. National Highway Traffic Safety Administration. EMT-Paramedic National Standard Curriculum. Washington, DC: NHTSA.
6. Cherry RA. *EMT Teaching: A Common Sense Approach.* Upper Saddle River: Prentice Hall; 1998:32.
7. Davis BG. *Tools for Teaching.* San Francisco, Calif: Jossey-Bass; 2001:167.
8. Billings DM, Halstead JA. *Teaching in Nursing: A Guide for Faculty.* Philadelphia, Pa: WB Saunders; 1998:286.
9. Oermann MH. *Research on Teaching in the Clinical Setting.*
10. Meisenhelder J. Anxiety: a block to clinical teaching. *Nurse Educator.* 1987;12:27-30.
11. Kleehammer K, Hart LA, Keck JF. Nursing students' perception of anxiety-producing situations in the clinical setting. *Journal of Nursing Education.* 1990;29:183-187.
12. Reese AC. Implications of results from cognitive science research for medical education. *Medical Education Online.* 1998;3. Available at: http://www.med-ed-online.org/f0000010.htm
13. Kolb D, et al. *Organizatonal Psychology: An Experiential Approach.* NJ: Prentice-Hall; 1971.
14. Wink DM. Using questioning as a teaching strategy. *Nurse Education.* 18(5).
15. Parvensky CA. *Teaching EMS: An Educator's Guide to Improved EMS Instruction.* St. Louis, Mo: MosbyLifeline; 1995.
16. Worlf ZR, O'Driscoll RW. How useful is the preclinical conference? *Nursing Outlook.* 1979;27:455-457.
17. Matheney RV. Pre- and post-conferences for students. *Americal Journal of Nursing.* 1969;69:286-289.
18. Joplin L. *On Defining Experiential Education. The Theory of Experiential Education.* 2nd ed. Boulder, Colo: Association for Experiential Education.
19. State of Georgia ASH. Quarry Products and State of Georgia Emergency Medical Services Paramedic Clinical Preceptor Program.

WORKS CONSULTED

Boney J, Baker J. Strategies for teaching clinical decision making. *Nurse Education Today.* 1997;17:16-21.

Bourn S, Smith M. Reliability of EMS instructors as evaluators of practical skills stations. Prehospital Care Research Forum. *Journal of Emergency Medical Services.* 1995;20:113.

Criss E. EMS research: obstacles of the past, opportunities in the present, models for the future. Prehospital Care Research Forum. Supplement to the *Journal of Emergency Medical Services.* March, 1998.

Dowd SB. Clock hours or competencies? *Radiology Technology.* 1994;65:325-326.

Duke M. Clinical evaluation—difficulties experienced by sessional clinical teachers of nursing: a qualitative study. *Journal of Advanced Nursing.* 1996;23:408-414.

Grubs K. Eureka: motor skills mastery. Paper presented at: EMS Conference Today; March 14, 1997.

Konrad C, Schupfer G, Wietlisbach M, Gerber H. Learning manual skills in anesthesiology: is there a recommended number of cases for anesthetic procedures? *Anesthesia and Analgesia.* 1998;86:635-639.

Kowlowitz V, Curtis P, Sloane P. The procedural skills of medical students: expectations and experiences. *Academic Medicine.* 1990;65:656-658.

Margolis G, Stoy W. (1997). Curricula update—How will it impact those who teach it. Keynote presentation at: Meeting of the National Association of EMS Educators, Second Annual Symposium; September 9, 1997; Atlanta, Ga.

Margolis G, Stoy W. The length of paramedic education programs in the United States. Prehospital Care Research Forum. Supplement to the *Journal of Emergency Medical Services.* March, 1998.

McGuire C, Babbott D. Simulation technique in the measurement of problem-solving skills. *Journal of Educational Measurement.* 1997;4.

Sloboda JA, Davidson JW, Howe MJA, Moore DG. The role of practice in the development of performing musicians. *British Journal of Psychology.* 1996;87:287-309.

Snyder W, Smit S. Evaluating the evaluators: inter-rater reliability on EMT licensing examinations. *Prehospital Emergency Care.* 1998;2:37-46.

Wilson ME. Assessing intravenous cannulation and tracheal intubation training. *Anesthesia.* 46:578-579.

US Congress. Emergency Medical Services System Act of 1973 (P.L. 93-154).

US Department of Transportation. National Standard Curriculum for the Emergency Medical Technician Paramedic, 1985.

PART V

Evaluation

In previous chapters, the emergency medical services (EMS) educator has been portrayed as a coach who works closely with students to bring out their best performance and help them achieve learning success. However, the instructor must play another key role—that of evaluator. Just as a coach assesses players at the end of the preseason, the EMS instructor must carefully evaluate whether the student is prepared to play in the "big league" of managing real world patients in real world environments.

This vital aspect of the teaching process is often overlooked or "thrown together" at the last minute. Evaluation is a challenging task that requires collaboration and sharing. Without a solid evaluation system that addresses students in all domains, instructors will fail at their goal to graduate competent providers in terms of knowledge, skills, and behaviors/attitudes. This part of the text is designed to jump start instructors in this area by describing general principles of evaluation, types of written and other evaluation tools, and ways for the instructor to implement the remediation process. The reader should return to these chapters when necessary for review of information.

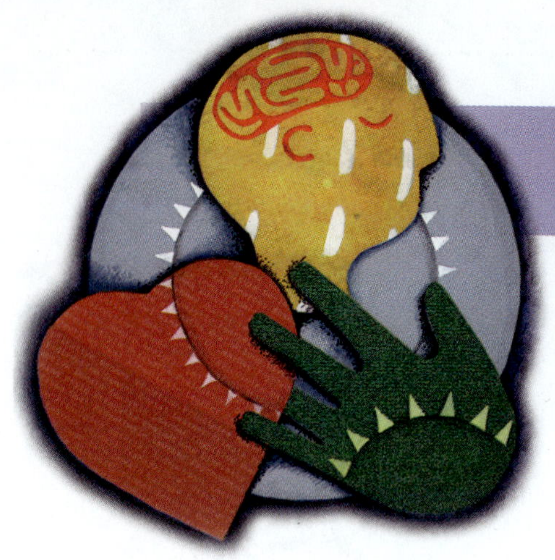

CHAPTER 19

Principles of Evaluation of Student Performance

"Good people are good because they've come to wisdom through failure. We get very little wisdom from success, you know."

—William Sarayan

Evaluating student performance is a task that can seem especially daunting. Creating appropriate tools for use in evaluating student performance requires knowledge of the core concepts of purpose, reliability, and validity. This chapter introduces these concepts and applies them to the development of an evaluation strategy.

EVALUATION

Definition

The act of teaching involves facilitating student acquisition of new knowledge, skills, and attitudes. The process of assessing whether the student has successfully acquired new capabilities is referred to as *evaluation*. To distinguish this process from evaluation of other aspects of a program, it is helpful for the instructor to consider student evaluation, or evaluation of student performance, as the process used to assess student understanding and ability to apply knowledge, skills, and attitudes. Appraisal of other aspects of the educational program, such as how the student rates the instructor, is discussed in other chapters. This chapter focuses on the principles involved in evaluating the student's knowledge and performance.

Multiple Messages of Evaluation

The results of any evaluation contain information that enables the instructor to make judgments. To make appropriate judgments on the basis of an evaluation, the instructor must understand several core concepts. First and foremost, the instructor must be aware that all evaluations comprise a combination of an assessment of the student and an assessment of the effectiveness of teaching. Thus, two messages are contained within each evaluation: how well the student is performing, and how well the instructor is performing. The effective instructor carefully considers each evaluation to look for both messages. Barbara Davis writes in her book *Tools for Teaching*, "... tests are powerful educational tools that serve at least four functions. First, tests help you evaluate students and assess whether they are learning what you are expecting them to learn. Second, well-designed tests serve to motivate and help students structure their academic efforts. . . . Third, tests can help you understand how successfully you are presenting the material. Finally, tests can reinforce learning by providing students with indicators of what topics or skills they have not yet mastered."[1]

Importance of Different Tools

The effective instructor does not rely solely on any single evaluation tool. Instructors evaluate student knowledge through formal methods such as written examinations, research projects, practical examinations, and observational reports. Instructors also use informal methods, such as questions delivered in class and homework assignments, to evaluate student performance. Typically, formal evaluations are used to formulate a "grade" for each student, and informal evaluations may not be part of the grading system. Informal evaluation systems are particularly valuable for providing immediate feedback regarding instructional effectiveness. On the other hand, informal evaluations lack the rigor necessary for justifiable decisions regarding student competency or pass/fail status. Although formal systems provide sound judgment regarding the student's mastery of objectives, formal systems are not particularly useful in providing timely feedback for modifying the teaching strategy.

TEACHING TIP: The effective instructor uses more than one evaluation tool to evaluate students.

Importance of a System for Constructing Evaluation Tools

Properly constructing appropriate evaluation tools from scratch can be a challenging task that is generally beyond the scope of an entry level instructor. Indeed, constructing evaluation tools often requires systems and processes, and even a seasoned instructor is unable to complete the task alone. Many EMS educational courses are taught and coordinated by individual instructors; it must be emphasized that an informal network of instructors can accomplish the same tasks as institutional systems that design evaluation tools. Nothing in this textbook should be construed as implying that appropriate evaluation can be performed only by educational institutions. Individual instructors can and should work together for the improvement of each instructor's evaluation strategies and tools. Although tasks and processes described for design of evaluation strategy, creation of evaluation tools, and analysis of the effectiveness of these tools may be beyond the capability of a single instructor, they can be effectively implemented by networks of instructors who are working for the common good. Professional associations, such as the National Association of EMS Educators, have a responsibility to encourage such networks. Individual instructors have the responsibility for actively participating in these networks, whether they are formed within a single institution, in collaboration with multiple institutions, or in a cooperative effort between independent instructors.

Evaluation of student performance is a core competency for all those who have a role in instruction. For example, although preceptors are unlikely to write examinations, they definitely do conduct observational reports and make assessments of candidates' knowledge through techniques such as informal questioning. It is important that instructors in all types of settings, from the classroom, to the lab, to the clinical site, understand the core concepts of evaluation and appreciate the implications of these for their particular application. Although specific tools may vary, the core concepts of student evaluation are applicable to all instructor roles.

PURPOSES OF EVALUATION

The first step in designing an evaluation tool is to decide on the purpose of the assessment. As long as the judgment that will be made through a particular evaluation is considered, appropriate design is ensured. Significant differences can be found among evaluation instruments and tools used to provide feedback to the student—from assessments used to determine whether the student is prepared to graduate from an educational program, to those that reveal whether a person is competent in his or her job performance.

Formative Versus Summative Evaluation

Formative evaluation is the ongoing evaluation of student performance throughout a course. Formative evaluation is important for instructors to use so they can gain insight early in the course, while changes to instructional strategy can still be made. Examples of formative evaluation tools include oral questions asked in class, having students write out questions for the instructor's consideration during a break, frequent short quizzes, practical drills, and homework assignments. The intent of these strategies is to provide feedback to students and to the instructor regarding progress made toward student mastery of course objectives. By using formative evaluation, the instructor can modify course structure, adapt presentation strategies, or provide remediation during the course.

CASE IN POINT

An instructor in an EMT program is teaching the airway and ventilation module. During the early phases of the module, she wishes to gain an understanding of how well students are absorbing the information and skills. She decides to give a daily quiz and intends to use the information to adapt her teaching strategy for the next class period. Quiz results will provide feedback to students and to the instructor, so that she can modify her teaching strategy before the time of the module exam. This is a formative evaluation.

Summative evaluation is the evaluation given to students at the end of a course, or at the end of a module within a course. Summative evaluation is used to determine whether the terminal goals and objectives of the course or module were met. Examples of summative evaluation tools include final written examinations, major projects (conducted at or near the end of a course or module), final practical examinations, and end-of-course survey instruments. Summative tools provide valuable feedback on student performance, instructor and preceptor performance, and effectiveness of clinical and field rotations. One downside to summative evaluations is that this feedback can be used only in future courses.

CASE IN POINT

A First Responder instructor is approaching the conclusion of the course. Before sending students to sit for licensure examinations, he knows he must verify that each student has mastered the knowledge and skills of the curriculum. He administers a final written and skills exam that each student must pass to qualify for licensure. This is a summative evaluation.

Of course, most evaluation tools represent a mix of formative and summative evaluations. An example of a mixed tool includes the module examination. A module exam is summative in the sense that it is used to assess a student's mastery of a complete block of instructional material with little to no time allowed for remediation; it is formative in the sense that students will complete several modules before they have successfully completed an entire program. Evaluation of the first module gives students feedback on the effectiveness of their strategies for study, while fulfilling the summative role of evaluating student mastery of that particular block of content.

High-Stakes Evaluations

Instructors should consider the stakes of the evaluation before they actually design the instrument (Figure 19-1). A high-stakes evaluation is one in which the student's continuation in the program depends on successful completion of (passing) the examination. An example of a high-stakes evaluation is a module or final exam that the student must pass if he or she is to pass the overall course. High-stakes examinations are primarily summative in nature, with little possibility that feedback can be used to modify learning strategies. Students taking high-stakes examinations often experience significant stress. Also, a high-stakes examination typically raises questions as to how well the examination was designed and the analysis conducted. With higher stakes come higher standards for defensibility of the examination. In EMS, the highest-stakes evaluation is a licensure examination. Thus, licensure examinations are subjected to the highest levels of scrutiny.

TEACHING TIP: High-stakes examinations must be created and analyzed with rigor so that they can withstand scrutiny.

CASE IN POINT

A clinical coordinator is concerned with *interrater reliability* among a group of preceptors. The coordinator reviews the forms used to evaluate intern performance to assure that clear behavioral descriptions are provided for each rating. The coordinator uses a spreadsheet to compare the scores of each preceptor. The average score of each preceptor is consistent, thus demonstrating *interrater reliability.*

CASE IN POINT

An EMS service training officer is asked by administration to prepare a written examination to be used as part of the screening process for candidates for employment. If a candidate scores poorly on the examination, he or she will not be hired, and no opportunity for retest will be provided. The training officer knows that the exam is a high-stakes evaluation; therefore, it will need careful analysis and construction.

Low-Stakes Evaluations

A low-stakes evaluation has relatively little effect on whether a student passes a particular course (Figure 19-1). Typically, low-stakes evaluations are used as a formative evaluation strategy. Examples include classroom quizzes and homework assignments. Although each individual evaluation may carry relatively low stakes, a number of these evaluations may collectively have a significant impact on the final grade. Low-stakes examinations are typically subjected to little scrutiny. If the instructor is using evaluation instruments of questionable quality, the safest strategy is to reduce the stakes associated with those instruments, while their quality is tested and improved as necessary. However, instructors should not consider low-stakes evaluations unimportant. Low-stakes formative evaluations serve the critical purpose of preparing students for higher-stakes summative evaluations. If an instructor uses only poorly constructed items for low-stakes formative evaluations, poor student performance on high-stakes evaluations related to properly

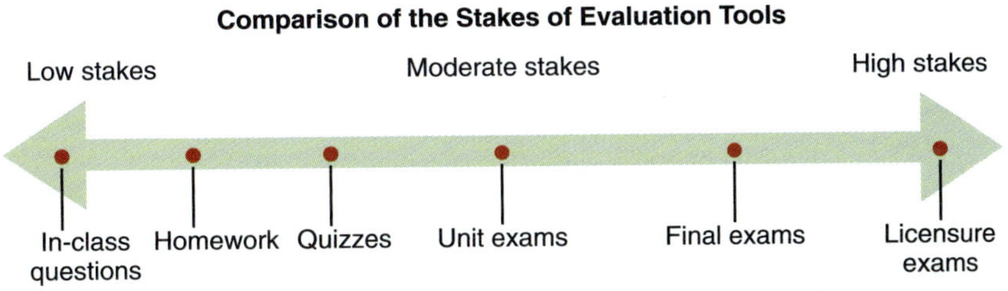

Comparison of the Stakes of Evaluation Tools

Low stakes — Moderate stakes — High stakes

In-class questions | Homework | Quizzes | Unit exams | Final exams | Licensure exams

FIGURE 19-1 Comparison of the stakes of evaluation tools.

constructed items is to be expected. The instructor should exercise care when selecting items for low-stakes formative evaluations, so that these evaluations will adequately prepare students for final summative evaluations.

CASE IN POINT

An instructor at a community college is using daily quizzes for formative evaluation. All quizzes in the course together count for 10% of the final grade. This is an example of low-stakes evaluation. The instructor uses these low-stakes evaluations to pilot test items for future use. If an item is shown to be reliable and valid, then the item is used for unit examinations.

Basis for Evaluation

The basis for the evaluation relates to consideration of purpose. A curriculum-based assessment is built on the objectives of the educational program. Performance agreement is the matching of the terminal goals for the course with lesson objectives, presentation of material, and evaluation tools used. In a well-designed and well-conducted course, the evaluation tools match the presented material, which is derived from the lesson objectives; in this way, the evaluation helps students to attain terminal course goals. Mismatch between goals, objectives, presentation, and evaluation often leads to difficulties. One symptom of lack of performance agreement is general complaints from students about the examinations. When a performance agreement exists, the examination is a natural and readily accepted component of the learning process.

Evaluations designed to verify the competency of the EMS provider, such as examinations issued by the National Registry of Emergency Medical Technicians (NREMT), are designed in a slightly different manner from those based on a prepared curriculum. Competency evaluations result from practice analysis. The practice analysis is a formal assessment of specific competencies that are needed for acceptable entry into the role of a provider. The distinction between an evaluation designed to verify competency, based on a practice analysis, and a curriculum-based evaluation is especially important for those instructors who serve as training officers for an EMS provider organization. Training officers are occasionally called upon to design an evaluation strategy that accurately verifies or reverifies the competency of EMS providers. The specific competencies needed within that particular EMS organization may or may not accurately match course objectives, particularly if the training was conducted by a different organization. In a perfect world, there would be agreement between curriculum objectives and practice analysis; however, perfect agreement rarely exists for nationally standardized curricula. For example, a delay is typically noted between the implementation of new treatment modalities and the inclusion of new treatment modalities in initial training programs for EMS providers. Another example involves competencies related to local navigation; these are critical to the success of the provider, yet they are unlikely to be included in a general EMS initial training program. This makes it essential that the instructor be prepared and willing to modify National Standard Curricula to meet local needs.

These concepts form the basis of decisions regarding the purpose of an evaluation tool. Consideration of summative versus formative evaluations is aided by information on what will be done with the results. Formative evaluations, which are used primarily to modify teaching and learning strategies, are associated with lower stakes. Summative evaluations, which are used to assess students' mastery of the material, are associated with higher stakes. High-stakes summative evaluations require item piloting and more careful construction than do low-stakes formative evaluations. Summative evaluations may be based on course objectives and used to determine whether students have learned the material covered in the course. Summative evaluations used to verify the competency of students as field providers should be based on formal practice analysis in the expected area of application.

RELIABILITY OF AN EVALUATION PROCESS

For an examination to be an appropriate assessment tool, it must measure consistently (Box 19-1). This property is referred to as *reliability*. In other words, an

BOX 19-1 Testing Exam Reliability

In the ideal world, the instructor could test reliability by administering the same exam to the same students at a later time. Exams that produce consistent results are said to exhibit temporal stability. This test of reliability is called *test-retest reliability*. Although temporal stability is important, this approach to testing reliability has a number of drawbacks. Test-retest is expensive and time-consuming. If the time interval between tests is short, students will remember some questions and their responses. If the time interval is longer, students will have learned more in the intervening time, in a sense representing a different group of students.

A different and probably better method of testing the reliability of an examination is to assess the same content using different forms of the test, then comparing the results. Exams that demonstrate consistent results according to this method have demonstrated form equivalence, or alternate form reliability. A drawback to this method of testing reliability is that there will invariably be some remaining differences in content or difficulty between forms of the exam, making apples-to-apples comparison difficult.

For example, after a new unit exam has been developed for a specific topic such as pediatrics, the instructor can compare the new examination scores with the scores of quizzes that were previously administered. The quizzes contained items different from those in the examination. If scores on the examination roughly match scores on the quizzes, alternate form reliability is demonstrated.

A different method of assessing reliability is to look for internal consistency among examination items. If a survey containing multiple questions is administered, respondents who agree with the statement, "I am comfortable dealing with pediatric patients," should also agree with the statement, "I am comfortable taking care of kids." Examinations can be assessed according to the same principle.

The split-half method of testing internal consistency consists of dividing the exam into halves (commonly odd and even questions), then comparing the percentages of correct answers between the two groups of items. The response pattern should be consistent. Of course, the instructor must exercise care to ensure that the two groups of items are comparable in terms of content and difficulty. One drawback of the split-half method is that results of the analysis will change according to how the data are grouped. To correct this weakness, more complex methods of assessing internal consistency, such as *Cronbach Alpha* and the *Kuder Richardson* formulas (KR20 and KR21), can be used. These statistical measures compare results for a particular item with all possible combinations of similar items, to assess internal consistency. The Cronbach and KR methods are typically completed with the use of specialized statistical software.

For example, an instructor in a certification course is using an examination of 40 items without access to statistical software. She assesses the reliability of the examination by comparing scores on the even-numbered items with scores on the odd-numbered items. The scores are roughly equivalent. This is an assessment of reliability performed by the split-half method.

exam with high reliability would produce a consistent result if repeated. If a person weighs in at 150 pounds, a highly reliable scale would produce the same result when the same person is weighed again. Similarly, a reliable exam produces similar results if it is re-taken by the same student later. A reliable exam would produce similar results in different students with the same degree of mastery of the material. Another example can be drawn from target shooting, in that reliability measures the grouping of shots on the target. A tight grouping is said to have high reliability. When an instructor gives an exam, he or she is aiming to measure the degree to which the student has mastered the material (aiming at the same point on the target). The reliability of the exam is dependent on the variation in results caused by extraneous factors not related to the student's mastery of course information (Figure 19-2).

One area of reliability that is particularly troublesome for EMS instructors is interrater reliability. This is the consistency in evaluation scores that different people assign in grading a particular exam. Concern for interrater reliability is especially high when the instructor is considering the use of practical examinations and other exams that consist of some degree of subjective evaluation, such as those made up of essay questions. Instructors must exercise special care to ensure consistency between evaluators when they use these types of exams. Interrater reliability is assessed through comparison of scores from different evaluators who are scoring the same examination. Several techniques can be employed to ensure interrater reliability. Clearly worded behavioral descriptors (anchors) can enhance consistency among items that are scored according to a rating scale. Interrater reliability can generally be improved by the use of a greater number of evaluators, although without behavioral anchors, these improvements may be obscured by measurement error. (A behavioral anchor is a description of observable behaviors that is linked to specific ratings in an evaluation.) This can be done by having a panel of evaluators grade the same student performance, or by having student performance repeated for multiple evaluators. Some instructors average scores among

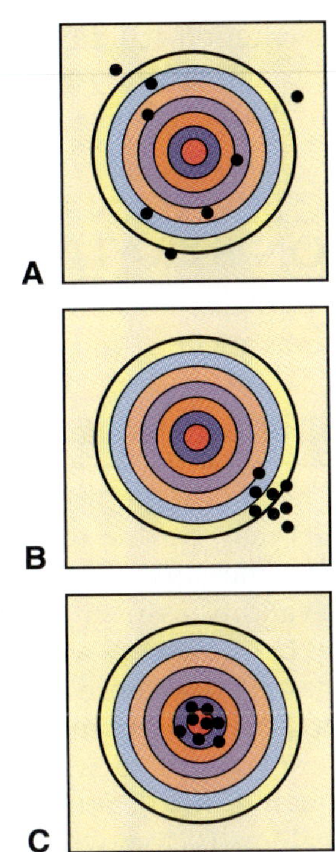

FIGURE 19-2 **A,** An example using the target shooting analogy of a low reliability exam. The examination results are not consistent; therefore, comparison with the objectives (the target) is meaningless. **B,** An example of an examination with high reliability and low validity. Although preferable to a low reliability examination, this exam is consistently measuring the wrong stuff. **C,** An example of an examination with high reliability and high validity. This tool is measuring knowledge consistently and appropriately.

evaluators; others eliminate outlying (highest and lowest) scores.

TEACHING TIP: Instructors must exercise special care to ensure consistency between evaluators when practical exams that consist of some degree of subjectivity are used.

CASE IN POINT

A clinical coordinator is concerned with interrater reliability among a group of preceptors. The coordinator reviews the forms used to evaluate intern performance to ensure that clear behavioral descriptions are provided for each rating. The coordinator uses a spreadsheet to compare the scores of each preceptor. The average scores for each preceptor are consistent, thus demonstrating interrater reliability.

VALIDITY OF EVALUATION PROCESS

Reliability of the examination tool is critical, but it is not sufficient by itself. An exam must also measure the knowledge or skills that it is intended to evaluate. This property is referred to as *validity*. Students with more knowledge of a particular subject area would score better on a valid exam than would students without the requisite knowledge. To return to the analogy of the scale, consistent performance of the scale is necessary for that scale to be accurate, but consistency is not enough. A scale can deliver results that are consistently 10 pounds too low and not be accurate. Returning to the analogy of target shooting, a tight grouping is necessary for a consistent bull's-eye, and once the shooter can produce reliable groups of shots, the aim is adjusted relative to the target. A tight grouping centered on the bull's-eye would be considered both reliable and valid. Consideration of reliability is the appropriate first step, but direct consideration of validity is also important.

The simplest aspect of validity is sometimes referred to as *face validity*, or commonsense validity. Although the concept is now considered to be a simplistic assessment of content validity (explained in the next paragraph), it may be useful for the EMS instructor. The practice of review of an examination by one's colleagues, with their agreement that the test items make sense, establishes face validity. Assessment of face validity is useful in the initial stages of examination analysis.

CASE IN POINT

An EMT instructor is building a new exam for use in the trauma section of his course. After drafting a number of questions, the instructor contacts a colleague, who is also an EMT instructor, to review the drafts. Of 40 draft items, the colleague identifies 5 that do not seem to match the objectives for the trauma section. The remaining items would be said to have face validity.

Content validity refers to the extent to which examination items accurately represent the wider body of knowledge that is being tested. Examination items should collectively form a reasonably representative sample of the body of knowledge. The depth of material covered in the course should be equal to the depth of items on the exam. For instance, testing advanced life support (ALS) knowledge by including only items related to basic life support (BLS) procedures would not provide sufficient depth. Also, the breadth of material on the exam should match the breadth covered in that portion of the class. For example, a test with a medical emergencies section that includes only questions related to cardiology would not provide sufficient breadth. According to Bloom's taxonomy, the level of thinking that is required by examination items should match the level of thinking required for the practice. High-level critical thinking

BOX 19-2 Criterion Validity

Criterion validity (sometimes known as predictive validity) refers to the ability of an examination to predict performance under other conditions. For example, a module exam is administered, and results match the results of observational reports in the clinical setting. This examination would have high criterion validity for performance in this particular clinical setting. In other words, a high score on the exam predicts high scores on observational reports. The measurement of this can be achieved through use of regression analysis. In the example cited previously, the score on the module exam would be the predictor variable, and the score on the observational reports would be the criterion variable. The calculated correlation coefficient would describe the strength of the predictive relationship.

cannot be effectively assessed through recall level items; the correct answer must be supported by course content, expert opinion, or science. In other words, examination items must be technically correct. Basic assurance of content validity can be achieved when performance agreement between course objectives and evaluation instruments is ensured.

CASE IN POINT

An Emergency Medical Technician-Basic Course (EMT-B) instructor is tasked with building a summative evaluation for the operations module. To ensure appropriate breadth, the instructor constructs an examination blueprint based on the objectives of the program (more on blueprints in Chapter 20). To assure appropriate depth, the instructor also includes criteria for each level of cognitive objectives in the blueprint. These efforts help to ensure content validity.

Many have argued that validity actually is a description of one's interpretation of examination results, rather than a description of characteristics of the test itself. All examination items test something. The important question is, What conclusions can be drawn from the results? To assess validity appropriately, the instructor must have defined the purpose of the evaluation at the start of the evaluation creation process. Without a clear statement of purpose, the assessment of validity becomes needlessly complex. For instance, in constructing a low-stakes, formative evaluation, assurance of face validity is usually sufficient. If the instructor is constructing a curriculum-based evaluation, checking content validity by comparing it with learning objectives is important. Consideration of criterion validity is key when one is constructing examinations designed to verify competency (Box 19-2).

CONSTRUCTING AN EVALUATION STRATEGY

The concepts of purpose, reliability, and validity are central to the construction and administration of appropriate evaluation instruments. Explicit discussion of purpose dramatically improves the chance that stated purpose will be achieved. Analysis and improvement of reliability are needed to reduce the chance that results may be due to error (rather than representing a true measure of knowledge). Careful consideration of validity assures that the evaluation matches the expected outcome, with clear linkage to learning objectives. Performance agreement among learning objectives, course presentation, and evaluation tools is a core concept to which all instructors must adhere if quality instruction is to be achieved. Even though not all instructors will be called upon to construct an evaluation strategy, the major steps required to construct one should be understood to maximize the quality of implementation.

Step One: Decide on a Purpose

The instructor must make a careful and explicit decision about the purpose of an evaluation. The key is to avoid leaving the purpose assumed, which can lead to confusion. Novice instructors sometimes assume that a test is an end in itself. Each test is nothing more (or less) than an assessment of students' knowledge and/or performance. Patient assessment can be considered as an example. Appropriate interpretation of an assessment finding requires that the EMT understand why the assessment is being conducted. If an EMT is unclear about the purpose of a particular step in patient assessment, it is unlikely that he or she will respond to patient need with the appropriate action. Just as with any research problem, the first step in constructing an evaluation tool is to have a clear question that the evaluation instrument is seeking to answer. Possibilities include the following:

- Does the student have the needed skills and knowledge to move into the clinical environment?
- Has the student mastered the objectives of a particular educational module?
- Does the student have more knowledge of the subject than when he or she started the course?
- Which students have the best mastery of the material in comparison with other students?
- Is the student competent to work independently as a provider?
- Is the student progressing toward mastery of the material?

The instructor must remember that each evaluation will carry messages regarding students' performance and the quality of instruction. Each of the purposes provided as examples earlier in this discussion will lead to dramatically different evaluation instruments, as well as to different ways of using the results. For example:

- *Does the student have the needed skills and knowledge to move into the clinical environment?* This purpose leads to a summative tool with high stakes. It includes aspects of competency verification, which results in the need for evaluation tools with high criterion (predictive) validity
- *Has the student mastered the objectives of a particular educational module?* This purpose also implies the use of a summative tool. Comparison with the stated objectives of the program is needed
- *Does the student have more knowledge of the subject than when he or she started the course?* This purpose can be accomplished with the use of a pretest and a posttest. Comparison of results before and after course administration will answer this question, without the need for grades or determination of a passing score
- *Which students have the best mastery of the material in comparison with other students?* This purpose leads to the use of a normative grading strategy (see the next chapter for explanation of normative grading). To answer this question, the instructor should grade on the curve, comparing each student's performance with that of each of the other students. This purpose leads the instructor away from establishing pass/fail criteria, or even issuing grades. A ranking of student performance is all that is required to meet this purpose
- *Is the student competent to work independently as a provider?* This purpose requires that the test be based on a practice analysis instead of on course objectives
- *Is the student progressing toward mastery of the material?* This question implies a formative strategy, with greater emphasis on providing feedback to the student than on grades

The purpose of each evaluation should be clearly communicated to students and to everyone involved in administration of the test. This helps to prevent misinterpretation of the results. Use of a tool designed for formative purposes to draw summative conclusions can lead to dramatic misinterpretation of test results.

Step Two: Specify What Will Be Done With the Results

After the purpose has been specified, the instructor must consider the meaning of the results. This follows naturally from a clearly stated purpose. To illustrate this, examples from earlier in the chapter are used here (the purpose is italicized):

- *Does the student have the needed skills and knowledge to move into the clinical environment?* Achieving a passing score on the examination is necessary before clinical rotations can begin
- *Has the student mastered the objectives of a particular educational module?* Achieving a passing score on the exam is necessary if the student is to move on to the next module
- *Does the student have more knowledge of the subject than when he or she started the course?* Comparison of knowledge before and after administration of the course is conducted
- *Which students have the best mastery of the material in comparison with other students?* (For example) Students with the top three scores on the examination qualify for preferential selection of their shift schedules
- *Is the student competent to work independently as a provider?* Achieving a passing score on the field evaluation is necessary for the employee to get off probation and work independently
- *Is the student progressing toward mastery of the material?* Graded quizzes will be returned to the student and collectively will count for 10% of the final grade. *Note:* Because some students will regard assignments without grade impact as unimportant, it is sometimes helpful for the instructor to assign small grade impact to formative assignments

Decisions regarding what will be done with results account for the potential stakes of an examination. The importance of these decisions determines the care with which the instructor must assure reliability and validity. The higher the stakes, the more diligent the instructor must be in constructing and using the exam.

Step Three: Select Evaluation Tools

Once the purpose and impact have been specified, evaluation tools are selected. In the ideal world, the instructor would simply select from a bank of valid and reliable tools. Unfortunately, this situation rarely exists. Test item banks and other tools available from publishers can provide valuable starting points, but these will generally need some modification before they can be used. The instructor should consider the objectives to be evaluated and should select tools that match the domain and level of performance specified by the objectives. For example, high-level psychomotor skills should be evaluated by simulation; however, cognitive objectives can be evaluated by a written examination.

Specific techniques for the construction, use, and analysis of different types of evaluation tools are contained in Chapters 20 and 21.

Step Four: Specify How Reliability Will Be Assured

After examination items have been selected, the instructor must next address the monitoring of reliability. The simplest method for assuring reliability is to reduce reliance on any single test. In essence, this is a form of assessing alternate form reliability. This approach to monitoring reliability is relatively easy and is almost always indicated. Assessment of internal reliability generally is indicated only for high-stakes examinations. For examinations that involve subjective evaluation by more than one grader, such as practical examinations, essay questions, and oral examinations, the instructor should have interrater reliability monitored.

Step Five: Specify How Validity Will Be Assured

Face validity and content validity should be checked throughout the item selection and editing processes. As examination items are selected, the instructor and at least one other colleague should review the items for face validity. Referencing the examination key to the stated course objectives can demonstrate content validity. Performance agreement and content validity are assured when each item is referenced to a specific course objective or reference.

TEACHING TIP: Some keys to validity include careful item review by one or more colleagues and referencing of each item according to a specific course objective.

Criterion (predictive) validity requires the piloting of examination items to test the predictive value of each. To test predictive value, the instructor must have access to good evaluations of actual performance data, as well as to examination item pilot results. Because most EMS instructors do not have ready access to actual performance data, the applicability of predictive testing is limited for most EMS programs.

Because examinations or examination items are commonly reused over multiple courses, it is important that their validity be tested periodically. A regular review process of the examination and key is essential for maintaining currency of the content validity. Testing students on outdated treatment modalities is useless.

CASE STUDIES IN CONSTRUCTION OF EVALUATION STRATEGY

Case I: A Preceptor Seeks to Confirm Progress

The instructor is a paramedic preceptor with a local ambulance service. She seeks to confirm that her intern is making progress throughout the internship and is incorporating lessons learned from previous shifts into development of patient assessment skills.

Purpose

The instructor believes she needs to confirm the student's knowledge of patient assessment and the lessons from previous shifts before beginning the next level of instruction. She decides to assess the intern's knowledge at the beginning of each shift to track the intern's development and guide that shift's activities. The instructor decides that the purpose of these evaluations is fundamentally formative, and that the assessments will not be graded.

Impact

The preceptor decides that providing feedback to the intern is the point of this evaluation. She will use this feedback to assess the effectiveness of the intern's work to date. She will provide the feedback to the intern to focus that shift's work and correct any misconceptions. After a short conversation with the program's clinical coordinator, the preceptor decides not to record the results, but to approach this as an informal evaluation.

Select tools

The preceptor elects to use an oral quiz of three to five questions at the beginning of each shift. At the end of each shift, she creates three to five questions, based on that day's calls, to ask the intern at the beginning of the next shift.

Reliability

Because the preceptor is the only grader, no problems will occur with interrater reliability. She talks with the clinical coordinator about reliability, and together, they decide to review the situation if the intern does poorly on 2 days of oral quizzes, then compare quiz results with the intern's evaluations in class (checking alternate form reliability).

Validity

The preceptor and clinical coordinator agree that if there are questions about a correct answer, the preceptor will check with the coordinator. The clinical coordinator gives the preceptor a copy of the program learning objectives to be used for reference purposes.

Case 2: A Primary Instructor Seeks to Confirm Mastery

The instructor is the lead instructor for an EMT course held at a community college. He is teaching at a remote satellite location and works with several part-time lab instructors to teach the program. He took over the program last year and does not have the tests used by previous instructors. He is preparing to begin the airway and ventilation module and is considering what to use as a module examination at the end of the section.

Purpose

In the course syllabus, the instructor told the students that there would be an exam for each module, and that successful completion of the module exam was necessary if students were to progress to the next module. The instructor decides that he is aiming for a summative strategy based on the course objectives.

Impact

The instructor has already decided that passing the exam will be required if students are to progress to the next module. This is a high-stakes examination, which requires increased vigilance. The exam will have a significant grade impact.

Select tools

The instructor decides to use a combination of a written exam and practical exams for each skill. He bases the examination on the airway and ventilation module objectives. Written exam items are drawn from a publisher's test bank, and practical examination check sheets are taken from the publisher's instructor resource kit. The instructor proceeds to construct the written examination, along with a key that references specific course objectives.

Reliability

The instructor divides the written exam into content sections so that he can use the split-half method to assess internal consistency. He has been using daily quizzes and expects to compare the results of the examination with those of the quizzes. He knows that he must monitor interrater reliability for the practical component, so he makes sure that students repeat each practical station so that different lab instructors can check for consistency. This allows him to assess the consistency of evaluation between practical stations. The instructor prepares lab examiners by meeting with them as a group before the time of the exam for a discussion regarding specific descriptions of acceptable, versus unacceptable, performance.

Validity

The instructor uses an examination blueprint (described in Chapter 20) to ensure that the breadth of the exam is representative of the entire module. The instructor edits each item, checking for face validity. He asks a colleague to review the exam for validity as well. He knows that this colleague will ask him to return the favor in the future. He then prepares the examination key, noting the objective and textbook reference that correlate with each item. After final preparation, he sends an e-mail to ask the medical director to review the exam for content validity.

Case 3: A Training Officer Seeks to Verify Competency

The instructor in this case is the training officer for an ambulance provider. The organization has just upgraded its monitor/defibrillators to include 12-lead capabilities. The medical director asks the training officer to verify the competency of all providers in 12-lead acquisitions before the new devices are implemented.

Purpose

The instructor is verifying competency in the acquisition of 12-lead electrocardiograms (ECGs). He realizes that although materials are available from the manufacturer, some aspects of the skill are probably not well covered by these materials. This is a summative evaluation that should be based on a practice analysis.

Impact

The medical director has made it clear that all providers must pass this test before the devices will be implemented. In a conversation with the service director, the training officer confirms that this will have no impact on performance appraisals, but that each provider must pass the test. Remediation and retest will be allowed until all have successfully completed the exam.

Select tools

The training officer starts by meeting with the medical director, an ECG tech from the local hospital, and a field paramedic. This group outlines the specific skills and knowledge necessary for acquisition of a 12-lead device. The training officer uses this rudimentary practice analysis to decide that a practical examination is needed. The training officer then has the ECG tech demonstrate the skill, while he identifies the steps required to complete the skill; from this, the practical check sheet will be constructed.

Reliability

The training officer decides to conduct each evaluation by himself, thereby minimizing problems with inter-rater reliability. To help assure temporal stability of the test, he uses the check sheet that he created, with critical criteria identified. He arranges for the medical director to monitor a random selection of the examinations to ensure reliability.

Validity

The training officer forwards the completed check sheet to participants in the practice analysis meeting to check for content validity. He and the medical director decide to review the first 25 real life applications of 12-lead ECGs to assess the criterion (predictive) validity of the practical examination.

SUMMARY

An understanding of the principles of student performance evaluation assists the instructor in the selection and development of evaluation tools. The effective instructor uses both formal and informal systems to assess student performance. Evaluation results provide information regarding student performance; they also help the instructor to assess the effectiveness of his teaching strategy. Formative evaluations provide feedback to the instructor and the student. Results of the formative evaluations lead to changes in instructional and learning strategies. Summative evaluations contain information regarding student mastery of the objectives; they do not allow modification of learning strategies.

Reliability and validity are characteristics of evaluation tools. Reliability refers to the ability of the exam to produce consistent results. A reliable exam maximizes the true measurement of knowledge and skills and minimizes the impact of measurement error due to irrelevant details. Validity refers to the applicability of the examination and confirms that the exam actually measures what it purports to measure. A valid examination is technically correct; contains content that is an accurate, representative sample of the wider body of knowledge; and, in some cases, can truly predict future performance. Validity and reliability are important characteristics of evaluation tools. The instructor must be prepared to monitor and improve examination reliability and validity.

As the instructor constructs an evaluation strategy and tools to support that strategy, the most important step is to explicitly identify the purpose of the evaluation. An explicit description of purpose is needed, so the instructor will select or create the appropriate tool, accurately interpret the results of the evaluation, and decide on best actions to take, as indicated by the results. Instructors who assume that everyone involved understands the intended purpose of an examination are likely to encounter problems. Explicit description of purpose is the foundation upon which successful evaluation is built.

REFERENCE

1. Davis BG. *Tools for Teaching*. San Francisco, Calif: Jossey-Bass; 2001.

WORKS CONSULTED

Davis BG. *Tools for Teaching*. San Francisco, Calif: Jossey-Bass; 2001.

Jacobs L, Chase C. *Developing and Using Tests Effectively: A Guide for Faculty*. San Francisco, Calif: Jossey-Bass; 1992.

Kittleson MJ. Evaluative approaches in health education. Southern Illinois University. Available at: http://www.kittle.siu.edu/course/hed526/default.htm

National Highway Traffic Safety Administration. National Guidelines for Educating EMS Instructors, 2002. Available at: http://www.nhtsa.dot.gov/people/injury/EMS

Rudner L. Questions to ask when evaluating tests. *Practical Assessment, Research & Evaluation*. 1994;4. Available at: http://edresearch.org/pare/getvn.asp?v= 4&n=2

Rudner L. Reliability. ERIC Digest. Educational Resources Information Center, April 2001. Available at: http://www.ericfacility.net/databases/ERIC_Digests/ed458213.html

Yu A (n.d.). Reliability and validity, educational assessment. Arizona State University. Available at: http://seamonkey.ed/asu.edu/~alex/teaching/assessment/alpha.html

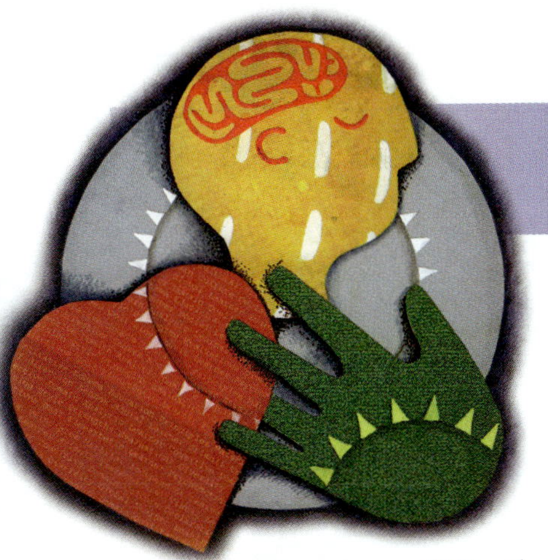

CHAPTER 20

Using Written Evaluation Tools

"To those of you who received honors, awards, and distinctions, I say well done. And to the "C" students, I say you too may one day become President of the United States."

—George W. Bush

One of the key tasks of instructors is to evaluate students' knowledge, usually through the use of written assignments and examinations. Each type of written evaluation has its strengths, weaknesses, and implications for use. This chapter presents information on the construction, use, and analysis of written evaluations.

THE WRITTEN EVALUATION

One of the most common formal evaluations of student performance is the written evaluation. By considering the purpose of the evaluation, the instructor can determine whether a written examination is the appropriate evaluation instrument. Written examinations can provide insight on student knowledge, but they provide little information about a student's ability to perform a skill or consistently demonstrate a given attitude. Thus, written examinations are most useful for evaluating the cognitive domain. Written exams have little usefulness in evaluating psychomotor objectives and can evaluate only lower levels within the affective domain. Grading, validating, and compiling results of written examinations is typically easier than is doing so with other types of evaluations. Because of this, written examinations can be easily used with large numbers of students in a single class setting or with multiple classes. Written examinations that rely largely on multiple-choice, true/false, and matching items are especially easy to grade; thus, they are very useful with large classes. Appropriate selection of an evaluation tool always depends on the proposed purpose of the evaluation. Written examinations are best suited to answer questions such as these:

- What does the student know about the subject?
- Which of the cognitive objectives has the student mastered?
- Does the student have the necessary knowledge to progress to more advanced material?
- Have the scheduled materials been presented adequately?

Properly constructed written exams can operate with high levels of reliability. Because each student is being asked the same questions in the same way during the exam, consistent administration of the test is ensured. Most written examinations provide for consistent scoring, although some types of short answer and essay questions can present challenges for ensuring reliability. Most written examination items can be easily checked and monitored for reliability. Of course, poorly constructed items can (and usually do) have low reliability. Monitoring and improving reliability promote the appropriate function of these easy-to-use tools.

Similarly, written examinations can operate at high levels of validity. The ability of the exam to measure what it purports to measure can be ensured by the use of carefully designed and written questions. Written exams generally encounter difficulties in this area. It is very easy to write examination items that assess low-level cognitive objectives, such as recall of key facts. Assessing higher-level thinking with written examinations is more difficult. Because of this, a common error for novice instructors is to assume that students have mastered higher-level objectives, simply because they scored well on an examination filled with recall items. Efforts to ensure validity should include consideration of (1) level of difficulty of required thinking (e.g., recall versus synthesis), (2) the breadth of the material covered, to ensure that the sampling of items is reasonable, and (3) the depth of the knowledge assessed by test items. This process is referred to as *blueprinting*.

Each type of written examination item has its strengths, weaknesses, and implications for use. Proper use of written examinations requires an understanding of these strengths and weaknesses. Just as the selection of an evaluation strategy is based on an understanding of the purpose of the evaluation, the construction of a written examination requires the instructor to apply knowledge of test item types to the objectives that the instructor is attempting to evaluate.

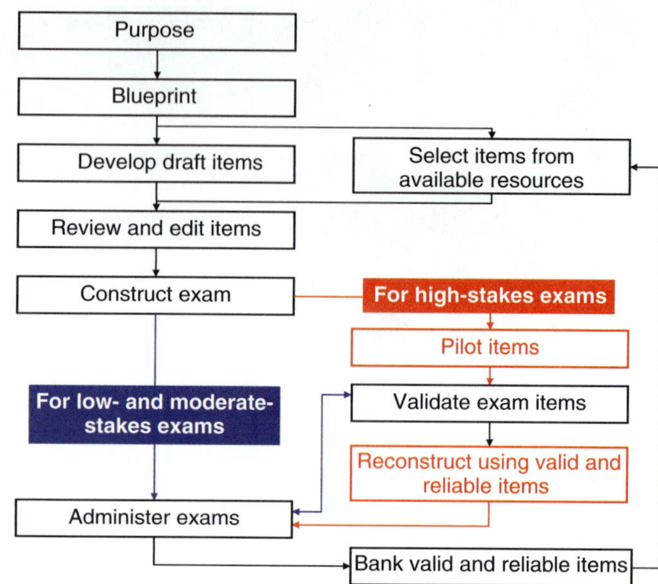

FIGURE 20-1 Reviewing exam items with other instructors or paramedics and with the program medical director is important for the instructor who wishes to verify the relationship of items to the objectives, to ensure their proper construction, to confirm the correct answer, and to discuss their relevance to practice.

CONSTRUCTION OF A WRITTEN EXAMINATION

Constructing good written examination items from scratch can be difficult and is beyond the expectation for most entry level instructors. Entry level instructors should focus their efforts on using and building on existing examination items from their educational institutions, other instructors, textbook publishers, and other available sources. However, the use of existing examination items presents challenges for the instructor. Just because examination items are available does not mean that those items are valid or reliable. The instructor still must review and edit examination items as needed.

Construction of a written examination consists of several key steps before the test can be put together. A flow chart of the examination construction process is shown in Figure 20-1. The first step is to carefully consider the purpose of the examination. The second step is to blueprint the examination, tying the breadth and depth of the examination to the stated objectives for the course. The third step is to develop or select draft examination items. Draft examination items are then reviewed by other instructors and are edited as needed (Figure 20-2). For high-stakes exams, test items should be piloted and validated.

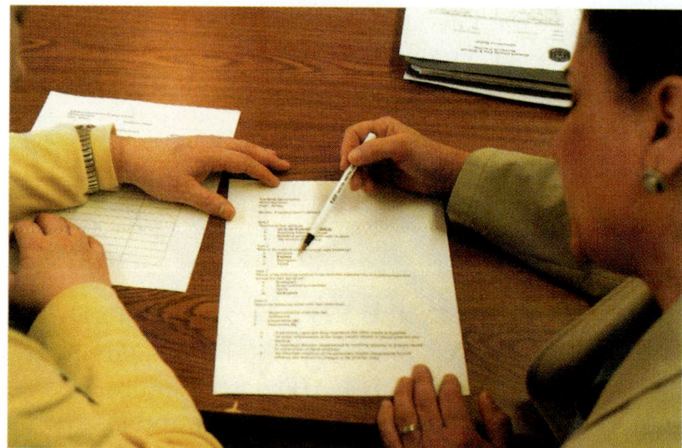

FIGURE 20-2 It is important that the instructor review exam items with knowledgeable sources (such as other instructors, paramedics, or the medical director) to verify that that they are constructed properly and are relevant to the objectives and the practice.

Carefully Consider the Purpose of the Written Examination

The types of written examination items and the content of those items depend on the purpose of the evaluation. Clear differences exist between the breadth of material used for formative exams and that used for summative exams. Elements to consider for purpose include the following:

- Are the subjects cumulative? In other words, is material from previous units to be included?
- What section(s) of the course curriculum is being evaluated? To which objectives will the exam be tied?
- Are there limiting factors within the course design that affect evaluation strategy? Examples include available class time, need for immediate grading, or a large number of students with only one instructor to grade exams

Blueprint the Examination

Once the purpose has been established, the next step is to blueprint the examination. The blueprinting process is conducted in the following steps:

1. The instructor lists the course objectives to be evaluated by the examination
2. The instructor assigns a percentage of total questions (or points, if varying numbers of points are to be assigned to each question) written to cover each objective. If necessary, objectives can be grouped together and percentages assigned to each group
3. The instructor selects exam length. In general, use of more questions increases reliability, but long tests (with more than 150 multiple-choice items) are much more difficult to develop and administer, and their use does not significantly improve reliability. Reliability is generally poor with less than 50 items, rises with additional questions up to about 150 items, and plateaus with more than 150 items
4. The instructor multiplies each section's percentage by the total exam length to determine the number of questions needed for each section

Using the same strategy, the instructor should also construct a blueprint of level of difficulty, based on the level of cognitive material that is being tested (i.e., recall versus synthesis).

CASE IN POINT

Blueprinting

An instructor is preparing a written examination to serve as a summative evaluation of the cognitive material for a medical emergencies unit that covers respiratory, cardiovascular, altered level of consciousness (LOC), and abdominal presentations. The instructor prepares a blueprint of the exam.

The first step performed by the instructor is to gather information on the emphasis to be placed on each content area. The instructor begins by consulting the National Registry of EMTs practice analysis, while using three parameters. He assesses each area for the risk of harm to the patient, assigning the greatest value to the riskiest, a lower value to the next riskiest, and so on. (Results are shown in Table A.) He then does the same for frequency and perceived difficulty. He follows by assessing the course objectives. The instructor notes that 35% of the module objectives are related to cardiovascular, 35% to respiratory, 25% to altered LOC, and 5% to abdominal complaints. Amount of class time spent on each content area is considered next, with the use of percentage allocation. The instructor also asks the medical director and the program coordinator to provide their opinions on the emphasis to be placed in each area, in terms of percentages. Results are averaged, and the totals are slightly adjusted by the instructor so the percentages add up to 100%. Table A shows the results.

TABLE A

	NREMT Practice Analysis			Curriculum Review		Expert Opinion		
Area	Risk of Harm	Frequency	Difficulty	Number of Objectives	Class Time Spent	Medical Director	Program Director	Adjusted Average
Respiratory	30	40	10	35	30	40	30	30
Cardiovascular	40	20	40	35	30	40	30	34
Altered LOC	20	30	20	25	30	15	25	25
Abdominal	10	10	30	5	10	5	15	11
Total	**100**	**100**	**100**	**100**	**100**	**100**	**100**	**100**

The instructor next considers the level of thinking required for the objectives. He assesses objectives written for the module and determines the percentage of objectives for each content area that are provided for each cognitive level. Table B shows the results.

TABLE B

Area	Recall (CI)	Application (C2)	Problem Solving (C3)
Respiratory	25%	30%	45%
Cardiovascular	30%	20%	50%
Altered LOC	20%	40%	40%
Abdominal	20%	30%	50%

Continued

CASE IN POINT—cont'd

The instructor next combines Tables A and B to determine the percentage of items that will be needed for each area and each level. This is calculated by multiplying the percentages assigned to each content area (Adjusted Average column from Table A) and the percentage of each level shown on Table B. The results are shown in Table C.

TABLE C

Area	Total	Recall (CI)	Application (C2)	Problem Solving (C3)
Respiratory	30%	7.5%	9%	13.5%
Cardiovascular	34%	10.2%	6.8%	17%
Altered LOC	25%	5%	10%	10%
Abdominal	11%	2.2%	3.3%	5.5%

The instructor previously decided that the examination would consist of 100 items of equal weight (each item worth 1 point). The number of questions required is determined by multiplying the percentage in each column by 100 (the total number of items on the examination). Table D shows the number of items needed for each level within each area.

TABLE D

Area	Recall Items	Application Items	Problem-Solving Items
Respiratory	8	9	13
Cardiovascular	10	7	17
Altered LOC	5	10	10
Abdominal	2	3	6

The instructor now knows how many questions of each level and content area are needed to for creation of a valid assessment of the student's knowledge of the content of this module of the course. The instructor can now select appropriate items from a test bank and proceed to the editing stage.

Develop or Select Draft Examination Items

From the blueprint, the process moves to the selection or drafting of items for use in the examination. The number of draft items collected should equal at least 2 times the number of items called for by the blueprint. This allows those involved in editing the selected examination items the option of selecting the best items. Some draft items will need extensive editing, and if substantially more draft items are included than needed, items that require considerable rework can be eliminated, if time becomes an issue.

Once an adequate number of draft items have been created or collected, the instructor can begin the review and editing stage. Only those examination items that have previously been validated can bypass this stage. During the editing phase, the instructor should have colleagues and the medical director review the items and assist in the editing process. Items taken from any commercially available test bank must also be reviewed and edited by the instructor before they are used. When possible, it is preferable for the instructor to employ unbiased editors who have not drafted the selected examination items or presented the material to students. These editors should consider the following questions for each exam item:

- Are any grammatical or spelling corrections needed?
- Is the item clearly related to a stated course objective? A common mistake is to base items on instructors' presentation materials instead of on the course curriculum. One method to help counter this tendency is to have those providing draft selections also provide an annotated key that references each item to a course objective
- Has the information/material been presented to the class in a lecture, reading assignment, or other means?
- Is the item constructed appropriately? (See the following sections of this chapter on technical considerations for specific types of items.)
- What is the correct answer that is being sought? If it is a multiple-choice item, is there only one correct (or clearly best) answer?
- Are there any inadvertent hints to the correct answer?
- Is the level of difficulty of the question appropriate?

TEACHING TIP: One possible strategy for facilitating item development and editing is for the instructor to work cooperatively with other educational providers. This could take the simple form of a test item exchange program between educators. A more complex approach would be for instructors to jointly host an item writing workshop, inviting participation from a number of educational programs, and allowing all participants to use the results of a day's worth of item writing and editing.

The Examination Construction Process

After items have been edited, the instructor can construct the examination. Instructors should consider the following guidelines regarding test construction:

- Be consistent in the use of punctuation and abbreviations
- Use a consistent strategy to draw attention to material in the test (underline, bold, italics, or a combination)
- Use capital and lower case formatting consistently for multiple-choice items and for the first word of each option
- If a separate answer sheet is to be used, ensure that the answer sheet and the test use consistent identification of options (e.g., 1, 2, 3, 4; A, B, C, D; or a, b, c, d)
- Provide clear and complete instructions for the examination—for example, whether the student can write on the test, time limits, whether breaks are allowed, and (specifically for multiple-choice items) whether there is only one correct answer versus whether students should select the *best* answer
- For short answer questions, students will commonly perceive the amount of space provided for response as a suggestion for length of the answer
- The exam should be organized in a logical manner, with items from a similar content area grouped together
- In general, the examination should begin with the easiest items, moving to harder items
- If several items are related to a single scenario, then those items should follow a logical sequence. Care should be taken to ensure that a single incorrect answer does not jeopardize students' ability to answer the next question correctly. In other words, although a single scenario can be used to set up a number of questions, each question should be capable of standing alone

Pilot use and validation should be conducted before an item is included in a high-stakes examination.[1] Items that demonstrate reliability and validity can then be included in future exams, and items that fail can be returned to the editing process for improvement. A common mistake made by instructors is to pilot examination items with the use of a single source that may not be representative of the intended audience. An example would be asking only other instructors their opinions on items for an entry level examination. Although this may be useful to check content validity, other instructors are clearly not the same population that will be evaluated by the examination items. It is more useful in this situation to pilot the items using a population of other entry level students.

For low- and moderate-stakes examinations, grading of the exams can be coupled with analysis. Two useful characteristics that can be identified in the analysis are difficulty level and item discrimination. Difficulty level is the percentage of students who answer each item correctly. Item discrimination is the degree to which a correct answer for a particular item is associated with high overall scores on the exam. Item discrimination is essentially a test of reliability. More on the analysis of written examinations is included on p. 247.

Well-constructed and validated examination items are extremely valuable to the instructor and to the evaluation process. This value is effectively destroyed if the security of items is compromised and items are distributed to students in advance of the test. At the very least, this would convert an item that potentially evaluated high-level cognitive thinking into a simple rote memorization question. As such, validated items should be secured in a test bank to preserve to the highest degree possible their usefulness.

Examination security can be breached in subtle ways. Letting students know which specific items are to be covered on a written examination is counterproductive in that students may then display false mastery of the material, which is not representative of their true abilities. A written evaluation typically comprises a sample or "biopsy" of the objectives included in the course content. For this reason, if the student knows which specific knowledge areas are contained within the sample from which a broader conclusion is drawn, then the validity of the conclusion is challenged. In this case, the conclusion that the student has mastered the necessary material can extend only to what is directly assessed, and the conclusion that the student has mastered the broader areas from which the sample is drawn cannot be made. Although it is unavoidable that the instructor should have previous knowledge of the test items, care must be exercised to not abnormally focus attention on specific content or items that will be covered in a future examination. An instructor need not know what specific items are covered on an examination, such as a licensure examination; he or she needs to know only the objectives on which the examination is based.

USING LIMITED RESPONSE ITEMS

The instructor may choose several different types of written examination items. Each offers its own advantages and disadvantages. Like other areas of evaluation of student performance, no single tool works for all situations. A combination of different types of examination items provides the strongest validity and reliability.

True/False Items

True/false items offer a complete statement with two possible choices: the statement is entirely true, or it is

BOX 20-1 Examples of True/False Items of Various Cognitive Levels

Recall (C1) Item

T/F Positive-pressure ventilation is used for patients with inadequate spontaneous ventilation.

Application (C2) Item

T/F A patient with cyanosis and a respiratory rate of 10 has adequate spontaneous ventilation.

Problem-Solving (C3) Item

T/F The head-tilt chin-lift is the preferred initial method of opening the airway for a child who is unconscious and is not breathing after being struck in the head by a baseball.

BOX 20-2 Examples of How to Edit True/False Items

Poor

T/F Effective splinting always immobilizes the joints above and below the injury.

Better

T/F Effective splinting of long bone fractures immobilizes the joints above and below the injury. *(Avoid absolutes.)*

Poor

T/F Oral airways are not used in conscious patients.

Better

T/F Oral airways are contraindicated in conscious patients. *(Use positive statements to avoid confusion.)*

entirely false. True/false questions can present complex ideas to be evaluated, and they can be easily scored. Additionally, because students can complete them quickly, much more content can be tested in the allotted examination time with true/false questions than with other types of questions. One difficulty is that with only true or false as options, the statement is either completely true or completely false. For example, if a statement is almost always true, the student is forced to guess whether the person writing the exam was thinking of the 99% of the time that the statement is true, or the 1% of the time that the statement is false. Another difficulty is that the chance of a random correct answer is 50%. In general, true/false questions tend to be very easy or very difficult. The result is that they do not always work well in discriminating between students of varying cognitive abilities (Box 20-1).

True/false items should be written in the positive voice, avoiding negatively worded statements such as "is not." It is also important to avoid absolute statements such as "always" or "never." Very few absolute statements are entirely true, and students know this (Box 20-2). The practice of taking statements directly out of the text should be avoided. To help eliminate problems in deciphering handwriting, instructors should have students indicate true or false by circling or otherwise marking among provided selections, rather than having students write "T" or "F."

Matching Items

Matching items typically present two columns of information with the intent that the test taker will select items from one column and match them to items in the second column to form correct statements or direct relationships. This strategy works best with terms and definitions, or with simple concepts and obvious relationships. However, this type of item can be confusing for the student unless very clear instructions are provided. This item does not work well when one is attempting to assess higher levels of cognitive learning, such as synthesis.

Items to be matched should bear some similarity to each other to avoid making the correct response obvious. In other words, the list of responses should be homogeneous (e.g., don't mix doses with administration routes) (Box 20-3). With matching items, it is important for the instructor to provide clear instructions such as, whether students will use each of the provided possible responses, whether one term can be used once or multiple times, or whether multiple answers are needed to complete a match. Poorly designed matching items are rather simple logic exercises, allowing students to use the process of elimination to greatly improve their chances of selecting the correct answer. The longer and more involved responses should be in the stem (the part of the item that is first offered, which may be written as a question or as an incomplete statement), keeping the responses short and simple. During construction, the instructor should take care to avoid giving grammatical cues to the correct answer. Matching sets should not exceed 15 items and should not break across pages.

Multiple-Choice Items

Multiple-choice items are commonly used in national and state certification examinations. Although multiple-choice items are extremely easy to grade

BOX 20-3 Examples of Matching Editing

Poor

1. Cyanosis	a. Used for unconscious patients
2. Nasal cannula	b. Used for airway control in conscious patients
3. Oral airway	c. Delivers low-flow oxygen
4. Bag-valve-mask	d. A sign of poor oxygenation
5. Nasopharyngeal airway	e. Used to assist ventilation

Better

1. Provides high-flow supplemental oxygen	a. Bag-valve-mask
2. Provides low-flow supplemental oxygen	b. Venturi mask
3. Provides precise concentrations of oxygen	c. Nonrebreather mask
	d. Nasal cannula

and demonstrate high interrater reliability (the reasons these items are used for certification exams), they are difficult to properly construct. Multiple-choice items consist of three main components: the stem, the distracters, and the key. The stem, as noted previously, is the part of the item that is first offered and can be written as a question or as an incomplete statement. The distracter is an incorrect answer designed to be a plausible alternative to the correct answer. The key is the correct (or best) answer to the stem.

Multiple-choice items can be used to test both low and high levels of cognitive thinking (Box 20-4), although constructing multiple-choice items that evaluate high-level thinking is challenging. Multiple-choice items are extremely easy to grade, and they allow for computer scoring of examinations. This makes it possible for a relatively large number of questions to be used, thus increasing the reliability of the evaluation instrument. On the other hand, because valid and reliable multiple-choice items are difficult to construct, the instructor is not able to rapidly develop these items. In other words, constructing the examination items the night before the evaluation is impossible. Because a limited number of responses is allowed with multiple-choice items, these items are unable to evaluate the thinking behind the selection of an answer. One variation on multiple-choice items designed to overcome this limitation is to provide space within which the student can explain a selection, if the student believes that the provided information is not sufficient for a clear choice.

Following are suggested strategies for the proper construction of multiple-choice items:

BOX 20-4 Examples of Multiple-Choice Items That Test Different Cognitive Levels

Recall (C1)

1. Which of the following parameters is included in the initial patient assessment?
   a. Blood pressure
   b. Level of consciousness
   c. Movement of distal extremities
   d. Bowel sounds

Application (C2)

2. Which of the following assessment findings is most helpful for determining the adequacy of ventilation?
   a. Skin color
   b. Heart rate
   c. Blood pressure
   d. Respiratory rate

Problem Solving (C3)

3. A patient from a motor vehicle accident presents with decreased level of consciousness, blood pressure of 170/100, heart rate of 60, and a respiratory rate of 10. The skin is pale, cool, and moist. Which of the following would be the most appropriate means of administering oxygen?
   a. Bag-valve-mask
   b. Nasal cannula
   c. Nonrebreather face mask
   d. Venturi mask

- Be on the watch for bias cueing (leading students to the correct answer by the way the stem is worded or from grammar choices) (Box 20-5)
- In general, negatively worded stems should be avoided. It is easy for students to misread negatively worded stems. Where negative stems are needed, the negative word, such as *not* or *except*, should be underlined or boldfaced so attention is drawn to it

In general, questions should not build on previous questions. Exceptions to this occur when the sequencing of steps is being evaluated, or when a number of multiple-choice items are related to a single provided scenario. When a single scenario is used as the basis for several multiple-choice items, the related items should be grouped together, should not break across pages, and may have a box drawn around the scenario and all related questions to ensure that students understand which questions belong to each scenario (Figure 20-3).

BOX 20-5 Example of Bias Cueing

Poor

A patient presents as unresponsive, with no spontaneous respirations, after being hit in the head with a baseball bat. Which of the following would be the most appropriate device to use to secure the airway?

a. Recovery position
b. Oral airway
c. Nasal airway
d. Head-tilt chin-lift

(The term "device" in this example immediately eliminates choices a and d.)

Better

A patient presents as unresponsive, with no spontaneous respirations, after being hit in the head with a baseball bat. Which of the following would be the most appropriate means of securing the airway?

a. Recovery position
b. Oral airway
c. Nasal airway
d. Head-tilt chin-lift

(Bias cueing is removed by rewording the stem to remove the clue.)

BOX 20-6 Example of Multiple-Choice With Fill-in-the-Blank

Poor

You have initiated CPR on a patient in cardiac arrest. As soon as the equipment arrives, connecting ______ would be the next appropriate step.

a. Oxygen
b. Automatic external defibrillator
c. Multilumen airway
d. Automatic transport ventilator

Better

You have initiated CPR on a patient in cardiac arrest. As soon as the equipment arrives, which of the following would be the next appropriate step?

a. Oxygen
b. Automatic external defibrillator
c. Multilumen airway
d. Automatic transport ventilator

(The blank in the middle of the statement can present unnecessary confusion, and is easily removed by rewording the stem.)

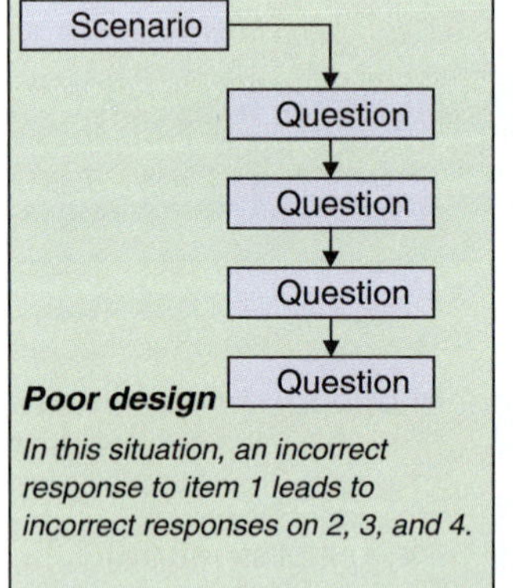

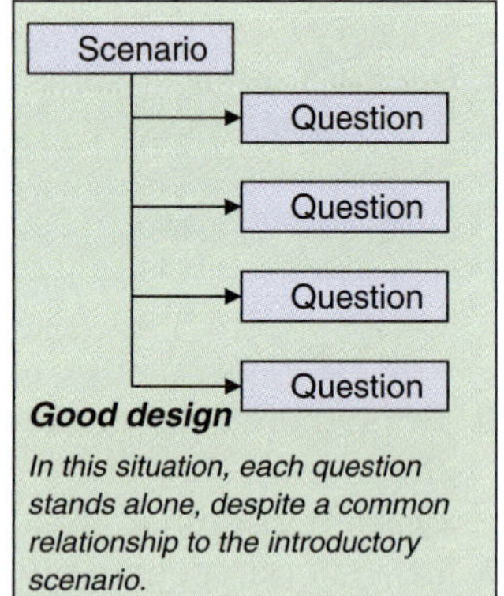

FIGURE 20-3 When a single scenario is used as the basis for several multiple-choice items, related items should be grouped together, should not break across pages, and may have a box drawn around them, along with the scenario, to ensure that students understand which questions relate to each scenario.

- Avoid questions written with a fill-in-the-blank segment in the middle of the stem; these are difficult to read (Box 20-6)
- Avoid the use of "all of the above" or "none of the above" as an option. Recognition of one incorrect distracter immediately eliminates "all of the above" as the key. Recognition of more than one distracter as correct immediately indicates "all of the above" as the correct answer. Although "none of the above" presents less of a problem, it still presents the student with the ability to use simple logic instead of content knowledge to derive the correct answer. Often, rewriting the stem can prevent the use of "all of the above" and "none of the above" as choices. Additionally, if the instructions for the examination are to select the "best" answer, then use of "none of the above" is inappropriate, as one of the choices will be the best of those provided (Box 20-7)
- Avoid the use of "multiple-multiple-choice" items, questions that provide a list of possible components to the answer, with distracters and keys containing different combinations of components. This type of item can be solved with basic knowledge, and these items are actually nothing more than a series of true/false questions. An exception occurs when this type of question is used to evaluate proper sequencing. Instructors can easily convert "multiple-multiple-choice" items to a series of true/false items, thus correcting the deficiency (Box 20-8)
- Overlapping responses present unnecessary difficulty to students. If the stem asks for a range and a distracter offers a single number, this can be immediately eliminated. Overlap of distracters into the correct range can be very confusing for the student (Box 20-9)
- Ensure that all distracters are approximately the same length (Box 20-10). Common wisdom is that

BOX 20-7 Example of Removing "All of the Above" as an Answer Choice

Poor

Which of the following would be appropriate care for the patient with a serious chest injury from a motor vehicle accident?

a. High-flow oxygen
b. Spinal motion restriction
c. Rapid transport
d. All of the above

Better

Which of the following would **NOT** be appropriate care for the patient with a serious chest injury from a motor vehicle accident?

a. High-flow oxygen
b. Spinal motion restriction
c. Rapid transport to the nearest trauma center
d. Application of sandbags to the chest

(The easiest way to remove the "all of the above" option is to convert the stem into a negative phrase. In this case, the negative "not" is in boldface and is capitalized to minimize confusion. Also, in the revised example, one of the distracters is lengthened, so the key is not the longest phrase among the choices.)

the longest option is usually the correct choice. This is because the writer of the item typically spends the most time with the wording of the correct option (to ensure that it is completely correct) and spends less time with the distracters

- Ensure that all distracters make grammatical sense. Frequent issues include problems with agreement of plural/singular and a/an. One method of avoiding grammatical cueing is to use complete sentences as the stem (Box 20-11)
- Ensure that the correct answer is randomly distributed. A general tendency is for instructors to predominantly use (b) and (c) as the key

TEACHING TIP: One method of ensuring random distribution of the correct answer involves the use of a deck of cards. With each item, a card is selected:

- If the suit is hearts, A is used as the key
- If the suit is clubs, B is used
- If the suit is spades, C is used
- If the suit is diamonds, D is used

One must be sure to shuffle the deck before cards are chosen.

BOX 20-8 Example of Removing Multiple-Multiples

Poor

Which of the following assessment findings is consistent with a patient who is suffering from hypoperfusion due to internal bleeding?

1. Warm and flushed skin 2. Rapid pulse rate
3. Low blood pressure 4. Anxiety

a. 1, 2, and 3
b. 1, 3, and 4
c. 1 and 3
d. 2, 3, and 4

Better

Which of the following assessment findings is **NOT** consistent with a patient who is suffering from hypoperfusion due to internal bleeding?

a. Warm and flushed skin
b. Rapid pulse rate
c. Low blood pressure
d. Anxiety

or, as another option,

Questions 12-15 refer to the following statement:

The following assessment findings are consistent with a patient who is suffering from hypoperfusion due to internal bleeding. Circle true or false for each assessment finding.

12. Warm and flushed skin	True	False
13. Rapid pulse rate	True	False
14. Low blood pressure	True	False
15. Anxiety	True	False

BOX 20-9 Example of Fixing Overlapping Ranges

Poor

Which of the following is a normal respiratory rate for a patient who is 4 years old?

a. 8-16
b. 12-20
c. 15-30
d. 20-40

Better

Which of the following is a normal respiratory rate for a patient who is 4 years old?

a. 10-15
b. 15-30
c. 30-50
d. 80-100

(The overlapping ranges present an unnecessary difficulty. The situation is best avoided, even with the addition of a distracter that is far outside the range.)

BOX 20-10 Example of Ensuring Comparable Length of Answer Choices

Poor

A patient with severe respiratory distress should be transported in which of the following positions?

a. Sitting, if the patient has a normal level of consciousness
b. Supine
c. Prone
d. Recovery position

Better

A conscious patient with severe respiratory distress should be transported in which of the following positions?

a. Sitting
b. Supine
c. Prone
d. Recovery position

(Any necessary conditions for the key to be correct are moved to the stem, removing the obvious clue to the correct answer.)

BOX 20-11 Example of Removing Grammar Cues

Poor

A patient has an injury to the leg with severe pain and bone fragments protruding from the site of injury. This patient has an

a. Closed fracture
b. Open fracture
c. Dislocation
d. Sprain

Better

A patient has an injury to the leg with severe pain and bone fragments protruding from the site of injury. This patient has

a. A closed fracture
b. An open fracture
c. A dislocation
d. A sprain

(Grammatical cueing, or grammar cueing, is easily avoided by using a complete sentence as the stem.)

- Be aware that in constructing a multiple-choice question, instructors tend to distribute the distracters so that two of the three are at the extreme positions, leaving the correct choice among the two middle answers (e.g., if the correct answer is 4, options would typically be 1, 3, 4, and 7) (Box 20-12). Students are aware of this tendency as well
- Place responses in a logical order. If the responses are assigned a numeric value, place the lowest numeric response as the first choice, the next highest as the second, and so forth
- Do not create words or abbreviations just to fill a response

USING OPEN RESPONSE ITEMS

Completion Items

Completion (also known as fill-in-the-blank) items are statements from which part of the information has been omitted, so students must complete the statement. Enough information must be included for students to glean the intent of the statement without being led to the answer. One issue with open response items arises when the meaning of the incomplete state-

BOX 20-12 Example of the Middle Value

Poor

Which of the following best expresses the range of respiratory rates considered normal for an infant?

a. 12-20
b. 15-30
c. 25-50
d. 50-70

Better

Which of the following best expresses the range of respiratory rates considered normal for an infant?

a. 8-12
b. 12-20
c. 15-30
d. 25-50

(Although all cases of the middle value being the correct choice do not need to be changed, the instructor should be aware of the tendency and take care to avoid patterns. Occasional use of an extreme value as the correct choice is appropriate. Although overlapping ranges are seen in this example, the student is being clearly asked to identify which range best describes normal, and the ranges in this case are taken directly from the NSC for EMT-B: 12-20 normal for adults, 15-30 normal for children, and 25-50 normal for infants. The overlap in this case is unavoidable.)

ment is unclear and several student responses emerge as correct, presenting a problem for the test grader. Items with unclear statements present a challenge for maintaining interrater reliability, if more than one person is grading the exam. Completion items are not capable of evaluating higher-order thinking such as with problem solving. These items are best used to evaluate recall, especially for key phrases that should be known verbatim or for definitions of key terms.

The provided answer space may present a problem for completion items. If one blank is used for each word of the correct response, the student is presented with a significant clue as to the answer. If only one blank is provided, students frequently assume that the answer consists of one word when multiple words are necessary.

Essay Items

Essay items pose a question or situation for which students are required to provide a relatively long, prose-style answer. Essay items are capable of evaluating higher levels of cognitive thinking, but they also require that the student be capable of expressing this knowledge in coherent written fashion. Essays can be used to effectively evaluate lower and middle levels within the affective domain. These questions also have the advantage of not being as easily susceptible to student guessing, although students may try to bluff. Because essay items are time-consuming for students to complete, it is seldom practical to include more than a couple of essay items during a classroom evaluation. Use of only essay questions on an examination presents a challenge to validity; this results from obvious problems with the breadth of material. Ensuring reliability during grading is difficult, as many factors other than knowledge can influence the assigned grade. In general, essay questions should be reserved for those objectives that cannot be effectively evaluated with limited response items.

The instructor should give his or her students advice for and practice with writing essays. This practice can be part of the formative evaluation strategies. The instructor should not give students a choice of questions to answer during examinations. It will be difficult to match the exam blueprint if different students answer different questions. Also, because some questions will be more difficult than others, the test could be unfair. When this choice is presented, each student is actually taking a different examination. Each essay question should be linked to a single objective; the student should avoid attempting to evaluate several objectives with one item.

Short Answer Items

Between the essay question and the completion item lies the short answer question. Short answer questions are very similar to essay questions, except that essay questions typically require multipage responses, and short answer questions rarely exceed a full page. Depending on the stated objectives, it may also be desirable to avoid requiring the use of full sentences to respond to short answer questions. Allowing students to use bulleted lists or outline forms may provide enough insight for the instructor to effectively evaluate knowledge, while not relying heavily on writing skills. Because they take less time and fewer writing skills for students to complete, more questions can be included. The strengths, weaknesses, and implications for short answer questions are otherwise the same as for essay questions. In most cases, essay questions have little usefulness in the EMS classroom compared with short answer questions.

TEACHING TIP: Both limited response items and short answer items can assess higher levels within the cognitive domain. A simple rule of thumb on which type the instructor should choose is that short answer or essay questions should be used when the time to prepare the examination is short and the time to grade the examination is long. When the time to prepare the examination is long and the time to grade the examination is short, limited response items (such as multiple-choice and true/false questions) are the preferred tool.

HOMEWORK AND RESEARCH PROJECTS

Homework

One tool that is especially valuable as a formative evaluation tool is the routine assignment of homework to be completed by students. Homework should be spread out relatively evenly across the course. Each assignment need not be graded, but many students will interpret the lack of grade impact as lack of importance. Assigning a minimal grade impact to a random selection of homework assignments is recommended to counter this tendency. The instructor should review homework assignments for level of difficulty and should include a mix of easy and difficult items. Encouraging students to collaborate on homework is a useful practice that helps to build teamwork and peer learning. Frequent assignments, which help to build regular study habits in students, provide the instructor with regular, formative feedback on student progress.

Examples of homework assignments for the emergency medical services (EMS) classroom include assignments from workbooks, completion and definition worksheets, short research projects, writing a summary of key points from lecture and description of care for a supplied scenario. Homework assignments also provide students with examples of what types of problems they will be expected to solve for summative evaluations. To be effective as formative evaluations, homework assignments must be graded and returned to students in a timely manner.

Research Project Assignments

Project assignments based on students' own research are another means of evaluating the ability of students to synthesize information. These assignments are a tool for assessing higher-level cognitive learning. Individual projects allow students to use their own specific learning preferences to complete the assignment. Research projects promote student autonomy, enhance student confidence, and encourage independent learning.

Assignment or choice of topic is an important, yet commonly overlooked, component of the project assignment. Allowing students to choose a topic that appeals to them is appropriate, but the instructor must be an active part of the topic selection and determination of project scope. Students should not waste valuable time on consideration of topics. One way of avoiding this scenario is to prepare a list of potential topics from which students can choose. Controlling the project scope is necessary to ensure that projects assigned to different students are roughly equivalent in terms of difficulty. Many instructors require that students get approval from them on project scope early in the process.

Another option is to prepare guidelines for determination of grades based on the amount of work that students complete. For example, "To get a C, the student will complete a written paper of at least 10 pages and a classroom presentation; to get a B, the student will also complete at least one optional activity; and to get an A, the student will complete at least two additional optional activities. Optional activities include reporting on an interview of a local medical director, creating a project-related Web site, completing a survey of at least 20 local EMS providers, and creating and demonstrating a working mechanical model related to a particular topic."

A measure of negotiation between the instructor and the student is appropriate in determining scope while still allowing students to express their own talents and learning preferences. It is also helpful for the instructor to reinforce relevance by creating realistic writing scenarios, such as, "Your medical director has asked you to submit a new protocol for the treatment of anaphylaxis. Please submit your protocol, which should include both assessment and treatment sections. Provide at least five sources from peer-reviewed medical journals that support the care you propose."

One problem with project assignments is the tendency of instructors to base the grade on product rather than on process. In most cases, the process used by students to prepare a project is just as important as the product itself. One way that instructors can avoid this trap is by requiring students to submit intermediary steps for consideration and possible impact on grade. An example is to have a "check-in" for the following steps: (1) description of title, purpose, and major points, (2) sources, data, and references, (3) outline, (4) first draft, and (5) final version.

The process of grading project assignments is essentially the same as that used to grade essay items on written exams. Recommendations provided in the "Grading Essays" section on p. 249 can be applied to written components of the project. Criteria for grading projects should be clearly communicated to students at the beginning on p. 249. The grade may contain components that measure the quality of the product, as well as the effectiveness of the process.

Project assignments are best viewed as a combination of a learning tool and an evaluation tool. As a learning tool, project assignments result in learning that is customized to the individual student's talents and preferences. Project assignments emphasize critical thinking, independent learning, and use of research skills. As an evaluation tool, project assignments permit assessment of high-level cognitive objectives and some affective objectives.

ADMINISTERING WRITTEN EXAMS

Environmental Considerations

The classroom setup for a written examination is essentially the same as that used for a lecture format (Figure 20-4). Students should be seated far enough apart to discourage them from looking at each other's papers. Exam proctors should be positioned so that they are able to see students' faces. Appropriate temperature and lighting should be ensured. Special attention should be given to providing a quiet environment. For examinations that last longer than an hour, the instructor should set clear rules for restroom breaks. It is helpful to have available extra copies of the examination and answer sheet, scratch paper, and pencils.

Proctoring

An instructor should supervise written examinations to discourage cheating and to address problems or process questions as they arise. Lead instructors communicate the importance of examinations by proctoring the examination themselves. Proctors should

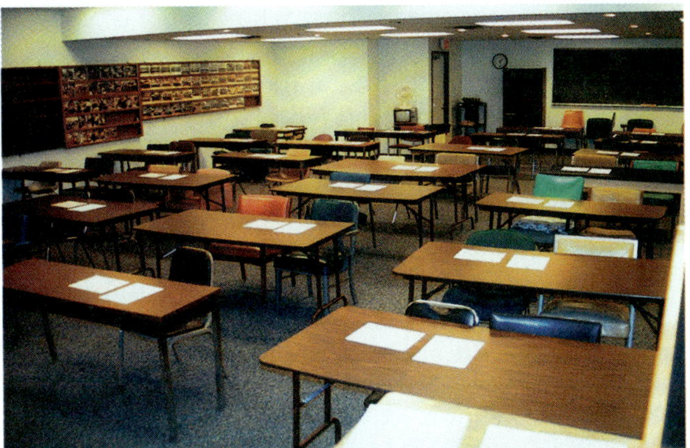

FIGURE 20-4 Answer sheets and test booklets (face down) can be placed at student seats before the examination. Student notebooks and backpacks should be placed at the back or side of the room.

arrive early and should be prepared to leave late. During the examination, the proctor should monitor the room without hovering over students. The proctor should have a strategy for addressing questions asked by students during the exam. One common strategy is to allow the proctor to answer only questions regarding examination process—not questions related to examination content. If multiple proctors are used, only one should be allowed to answer questions, thus maintaining consistency. The proctor should keep students apprised as to the time by having a clock in the room, writing (and updating) the time on a whiteboard, or periodically announcing the time remaining for the test.

Time Limits

Each student will take a different amount of time to complete the examination. To exert some measure of control over the time spent on the examination, the instructor must set some limits on time. Setting time limits for examinations is a legitimate strategy for (1) preparing students for certifying examinations, and (2) evaluating students' ability to think quickly. The drawback to setting time limits is that students should be able to complete the examination in the time allowed. In estimating the amount of time a student is given to complete an examination, the instructor can give students 4 times as long as it takes the instructor to complete the test. As an alternative, Barbara Gross Davis, in *Tools for Teaching*, suggests the following timing strategies:

1. Allow half a minute per true/false item
2. Allow 1 minute per multiple-choice item
3. Allow 2 minutes per short answer item
4. Allow 10 to 15 minutes per limited essay item
5. Allow 30 minutes per broader essay item
6. Allow 5 to 10 minutes for students to review their work
7. Factor in time to distribute and collect tests

ANALYSIS OF WRITTEN EXAMINATIONS

Posttest Review

A useful strategy after an examination has been administered is to allow class time for students to review the examination as a group with the instructor. This review highlights areas of weakness for individual students, as well as for the class as a whole. Review can also help the instructor to identify areas where the presentation of material did not adequately prepare students for mastery of the stated objectives. It can serve to alleviate concerns about bias when students see what items other students missed. A climate of fairness is promoted when students can discuss questions, answers, or the wording of a question. Some instructors allow students to retain the examination after classroom discussion. Allowing students to retain the examination provides a learning aid for future examinations; however, it greatly reduces the validity of test items that are reused. Conducting a classroom discussion breaches examination security, but the breach is less significant than when students are allowed to retain copies of the examination.

Pilot use and previous validation may not be possible for all examinations, but they should be conducted before an item is included in a high-stakes examination. One possible strategy for pilot use is to present pilot items for formative evaluations, such as quizzes. Another is to have an examination include several (not more than 10%) pilot items that do not count toward the exam score; these should be interspersed among regular items. Pilot items that demonstrate reliability and validity can then be included in future examinations. Pilot items that fail validation can be returned to the editing process for revision.

Difficulty Level and Discrimination Index

For low- or moderate-stakes examinations, grading of the examination is coupled with validation of test items. Validation is particularly applicable to limited response items such as true/false, multiple-choice, and matching questions. Although validation seems difficult, a simplified procedure can be performed by any instructor. The two characteristics of tests that are useful in validation are difficulty level and item discrimination. The difficulty level is the percentage of students who answer each item correctly (Box 20-13). The item discrimination index (Box 20-14) compares the performance of those who scored well on the exam

BOX 20-13 Calculation of Difficulty Index

The following procedure can be used to calculate the difficulty index and the discrimination index for limited response items, such as multiple-choice or true/false questions.

To calculate the item difficulty, the instructor should calculate the percentage of students who had correct responses. The formula for this is ID = (C/T)*100, where ID is the item difficulty, C is the number of correct responses, and T is the total number of students who took the examination. The goal is to use only a few items that more than 90% or less than 30% of students answer correctly.[2]

BOX 20-14 Calculating the Item Discrimination

The purpose of calculating the item discrimination is to compare the correct response with an item between the high and low scoring groups of students. If an item is constructed correctly, the instructor can expect more individuals in the highest scoring group to answer the question correctly compared with the lowest scoring group. This would be referred to as a *positive discrimination value.* If, for some reason, more individuals from the lowest scoring group than from the highest scoring group select the correct answer, the result would be a negative discrimination value. In general, items with a low (or negative) discrimination value would need to be reviewed and probably edited. As with calculating item difficulty, calculating item discrimination can be accomplished through the application of simple mathematical skills.

The item discrimination is calculated (in a simplified manner) by completing the following steps[2]:

1. Instructor identifies the exams with the 10 highest and the 10 lowest scores
2. For each question, the instructor records the number of students in the top group of 10 who answered correctly. He or she does the same for the bottom group of 10 students
3. The instructor then computes the discrimination ratio by subtracting the number of students in the bottom group who answered correctly from the number of students in the top group who answered correctly, and dividing by 10 (the number of students in each group). The discrimination ratio will fall between −1.0 and + 1.0. The closer the ratio is to +1.0, the more effectively the item distinguishes students who know the material (the top group) from those who don't (the bottom group)

with the performance of those who did not score well. Computerized programs will perform the necessary calculations (Figure 20-5), but the same measurements can be manually calculated when some simple mathematical skills are applied.

Students may find an item difficult for numerous reasons, including that the item may be poorly worded. Adding the discrimination index into the analysis for potential revision of items separates those items that have questionable reliability and validity from those that are appropriately constructed, yet challenging. Items that have extreme difficulty levels (either high or low) will not discriminate as well as those with a difficulty level near 50%. As a result, different thresholds are used to indicate the need for revision depending on the difficulty level of the item. When the difficulty level and the discrimination ratio are used, the process shown in Figure 20-6 can help identify items that need revision.

Negative discrimination indices indicate that students who scored well overall did worse on those particular questions than did students who did not score well overall. Items with a negative discrimination index should be reviewed for validity and revised before they are used again. A common cause of a

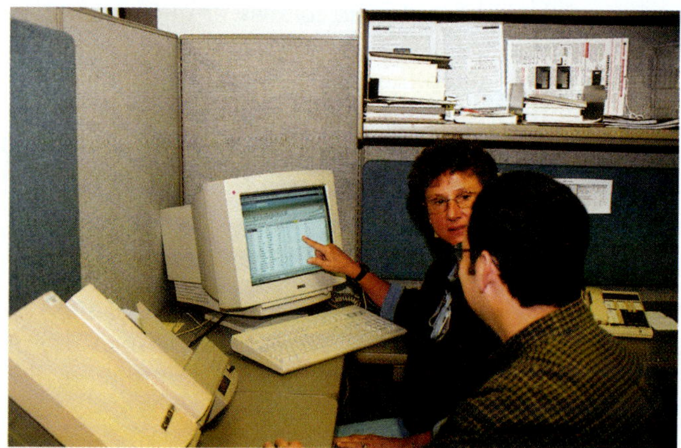

FIGURE 20-5 Scannable answer sheets and grading software can facilitate quick scoring of multiple-choice exams and provide a means of performing item analysis.

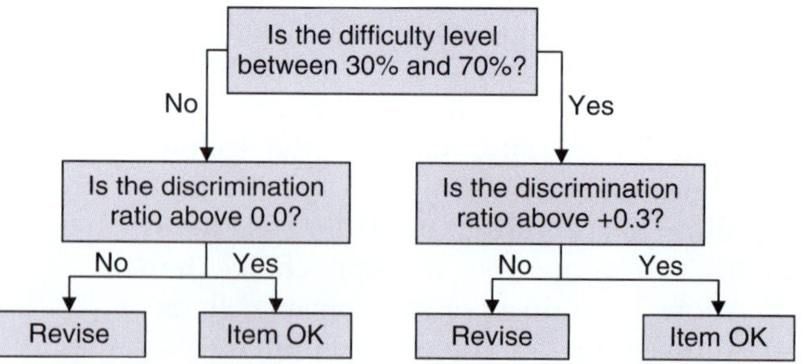

FIGURE 20-6 The difficulty level and the discrimination ratio can help the instructor identify test items that need revision.

strongly negative item discrimination index (near to –1.0) is an incorrectly keyed item. Editing of examination items should extend to a check of the answer key as well.

GRADING STRATEGIES

Grading Essays

Grading essays and written assignments can be particularly difficult. Because grading essays is inherently subjective, reliability is difficult to ensure. Some suggested strategies that help to improve reliability in the grading of essays follow:

- Skim all writing assignments quickly before grading them, to gain an overview of the general level of performance and the range of responses[3]
- Before the writing assignment is given or the test is administered, the instructor should decide on guidelines for full or partial credit. This is referred to as the *analytic method of grading*. The instructor assigns a number of points to each designated content area. The instructor decides on partial credit for each area, and totals the points for an easy grade calculation. It may be useful for the instructor to anchor these points to specific words, phrases, or concepts to help ensure reliability[4]
- Choose examples of student responses to serve as anchors for different levels of performance. The instructor chooses one student response as an example of a good essay, one as an example of middle performance, and one as a poor example. This approach is referred to as the *global method* of grading. It is generally helpful for instructors to also compare responses with those on an "ideal" paper prepared before the assignment[4]
- Grade essay items question-by-question rather than student-by-student. This allows more meaningful comparison of responses between students. Instructors should shuffle the exams between questions to avoid bias in grading caused by student performance on the previous question[3]
- Avoid judging assignments on the basis of extraneous factors such as illegible handwriting and the use of pen versus pencil. Judge essays on the intellectual quality of the response. Instructors must remember the purpose of the essay question when they are grading[2]
- If possible, repeat the grading process a couple of days later. Another option is to use multiple graders. Agreement in grades across independent grading sessions indicates reliability[4]

Norm-Referenced Grading

Normative (or norm-referenced) grading strategies are those that compare student performance with the performance of other students for assignment of a grade. This is commonly referred to as *grading on the curve*. The result of this strategy is that a set percentage of students receive A's, a second group gets B's, another group receives C's, and some are given D's and F's. Each student's grade is determined by the group's performance—not by comparison with objectives. This method of grading is commonly attacked because it is based on class performance rather than on comparison of performance with objectives. On the other hand, an advantage of normative grading strategies is that the grading strategy automatically compensates for poorly constructed examinations. If a test is very easy, the curve automatically shifts to require a higher passing score. If a test is very difficult, the passing score shifts lower to compensate. This occurs without additional calculation or analysis by the instructor. A number of variations of normative grading strategies include setting a percentage of students that will receive each grade, assigning grade levels based on natural breaks in the distribution, and assigning grade levels based on a normal statistical distribution. Although purely normative strategies are generally considered inappropriate for summative evaluation in EMS courses, normative strategies are useful for assigning grades to formative evaluations with minimal impact on final grade. Normative strategies are especially useful as an interim grading strategy when piloting evaluation tools are used during formative evaluations.

Criterion-Referenced Grading

Criterion-referenced grading strategies base grade assignment on mastery of course objectives. This approach requires the presence of relatively specific course objectives on which evaluation tools can be based. According to a criterion-referenced strategy, the evaluation is drawn from the blueprint, and setting grades is guided by the degree to which objectives are mastered. One example would be that 90% mastery is assigned an A, 80% is assigned a B, and so forth. This can be based on depth of mastery (90% knowledge of each objective) or breadth of mastery (complete knowledge of 90% of the objectives). A criterion-referenced strategy requires the use of valid and reliable items to ensure fairness in the evaluation process. Because the setting of grades does not automatically adjust for difficulty, the instructor must perform additional analysis to set an appropriate passing score.

Setting a Cut Score

In general, the instructor has two strategies from which to choose. In the first, the instructor can build the evaluations, analyze exam items, and set the passing score based on the difficulty of the exam (Box 20-15). In the

BOX 20-15 Setting a Cut Score

An instructor who is teaching a paramedic course at a community college is preparing a module examination for trauma. After collecting and editing a number of examination items, the instructor prepares to predict the difficulty by using the Angoff method. The instructor plans to use the information to set an appropriate passing score.

The instructor contacts four preceptors and three lab assistants who will serve as the expert panel. She starts the process by initiating a discussion on the concept of entry level competency. She describes the concept in this manner: ". . . the idea is to describe the provider who is barely competent. Not a great paramedic, or even a good paramedic, but instead, the paramedic who has just the amount of knowledge to be considered competent." She asks panel members to describe in their own words the depth of knowledge required for entry level competency related to trauma. The discussion continues for a short time until the instructor believes that the panel has reached consensus on the concept.

Next, the instructor distributes a set of examination items that have been used for past courses and for which the actual difficulty level is known. The instructor places the item, without the answer indicated, on an overhead projector and asks the panel, "What percentage of entry level providers would get this question correct?" After panel members have given their thoughts, she shares with the group the answer to the item. Panel members are then allowed to reconsider their rating. The instructor then shows the group how the item actually performed (the difficulty level of each item from previous administrations), and the results of each panel member are shown to the group. The panel has a short discussion on the difference between their estimates and the actual performance of the item. This exercise is repeated several times.

After reviewing these practice items, the instructor distributes the ones she will be using for the examination, without an answer key. Each panel member then rates each item as to the percentage of entry level providers who would answer the item correctly. The answer key is then provided, and panel members are allowed to reconsider their estimate. The instructor collects and averages the results, as the table below shows.

Item	Judge 1	Judge 2	Judge 3	Judge 4	Judge 5	Judge 6	Judge 7	Average
1	85%	80%	90%	90%	95%	90%	95%	89%
2	75%	65%	70%	85%	80%	70%	80%	75%
3	70%	80%	80%	75%	70%	80%	80%	76%
4	50%	60%	40%	50%	50%	55%	70%	54%
5	50%	45%	40%	50%	50%	50%	55%	49%
6	60%	60%	75%	65%	45%	55%	55%	59%
7	80%	90%	80%	85%	80%	85%	80%	83%
8	90%	85%	85%	90%	75%	80%	85%	84%
9	50%	55%	45%	50%	45%	50%	80%	54%
10	75%	75%	80%	70%	70%	70%	80%	74%
(etc.)								
Total	69%	70%	69%	71%	66%	69%	76%	**70%**

Note: The "total" row is the calculated average for that column.

The panel of experts has recommended a cut score (minimum passing score) of 70% for this examination. The instructor takes this into consideration as she determines the passing score for the examination. She takes into account that during the practice session, the panel consistently predicted rates of correct responses that were slightly higher than the actual values (in other words, during the practice session, the panel slightly underestimated the difficulty of items). She also considers the potential for error and decides to set the cut score for this examination at 60%.

(Note: In this case, had the instructor been in an institution that mandated by policy a set passing score, he or she could just as easily use this procedure to predict the item difficulty for each item, then could base item selection on the predicted difficulty to construct an examination of appropriate difficulty for the mandated minimum passing score.)

second, the instructor can first set a passing score, then analyze draft items and construct an examination with difficulty appropriate for the preset passing score. In other words, the instructor can either set the passing score to fit the exam or engineer the exam to fit the passing score. Either option is appropriate. It is inappropriate for students to consider a course with an 80% passing score "harder" than a course with a 60% passing score, without consideration of the relative difficulty of the examinations.

Many educational institutions set the grade levels and passing scores as part of institutional policy. This fits with a common expectation that 90% = A, 80% = B, 70% = C, 60% = D, and below 60% is failing. Another common expectation is that 70% is passing, with grades interspersed. If instructors are teaching with preset passing scores and grading levels, then they must construct examinations of appropriate difficulty to match this preset passing score. The instructor does this by predicting the difficulty level for each item and computing the average difficulty index for all items on the examination (Box 20-16). The instructor can then adjust the examination to match the computed difficulty with the preset passing score.

SUMMARY

Properly constructed written evaluations remain the most effective means of easily assessing cognitive objectives. Careful consideration of evaluation purpose ensures that the function of the assessment matches the use of written exam items. Different types of written exam tools have varying abilities to assess diverse types of knowledge. Items such as completion and matching are well suited to testing recall. Essay and short answer items are better for testing synthesis and evaluation. Multiple-choice and true/false items can test different levels of thinking, but construction of items that evaluate higher-order thinking is challenging. Homework can provide valuable formative evaluation. Research projects are another tool that can be used to evaluate higher levels in the cognitive domain. A combination of these different tools provides the instructor with a valid and reliable assessment of a student's mastery of knowledge.

Security of examination materials is important for limited response tools that prove to be valid and reliable assessments of higher levels within the cognitive domain. Security is not an issue for homework and project assignments, and it is less critical for essay items. Because of the extensive effort needed to properly construct and analyze limited response items, it is necessary that the security of these items be protected. If security is compromised, items that would otherwise test high-end knowledge become items that test only recall. In addition, compromises of examination security may dramatically change the difficulty level and discrimination index of the compromised items.

Limited response items are extremely valuable for the EMS instructor. Testing a large number of cognitive objectives with acceptable reliability and validity requires the use of many more limited response items than essay and short answer items. This also serves to prepare EMS students for licensure examinations, which use limited response items almost exclusively. Unfortunately, these items become nearly worthless if security is compromised.

BOX 20-16 Predicting Item Difficulty

In instructor can use a number of methods to predict item difficulty. The most common is the Angoff method. This method is commonly used for high-stakes examinations in educational, certification, and licensure settings. The procedure is to first establish a panel of experts. The panel considers the concept of the "minimally competent candidate," in other words, the minimum acceptable level of knowledge. This is not the ideal or average candidate, but the candidate who is barely acceptable. The experts are then asked to estimate the percentage of minimally competent candidates who would answer that item correctly. This is done first with practice items, where the experts' estimates can be compared with actual performance of the item. As the experts rate the items, the consensus that is reached by the experts' estimates forms the Angoff rating. By computing the mean of the Angoff ratings for all items to be included in the exam, the instructor can determine a cut score. Conversion of this predicted cut score into a passing score is a matter of professional judgment for the instructor.

REFERENCES

1. Hertz NR, Chinn RN. *Licensure Examinations.* Lexington, Ky: Council on Licensure, Enforcement and Regulation; 2000.
2. Davis BG. *Tools for Teaching.* San Francisco, Calif: Jossey-Bass; 2001.
3. Jacobs L, Chase C. *Developing and Using Tests Effectively: A Guide for Faculty.* San Francisco, Calif: Jossey-Bass; 1992.
4. Cashin W. *Improving Essay Tests.* IDEA paper, no. 17. Manhattan, Ks: Kansas State University Center for Faculty Evaluation and Development; 1987.
5. Johnson RR, Squires JR, Whitney D. *Setting the Standard for Passing Professional Certification Examinations.* Tampa, Fla: Financial Management Association International; 2002.

SUGGESTED READINGS

Case SM, Swanson DB. *Constructing Written Test Questions for the Basic and Clinical Sciences.* 3rd ed. Philadelphia, Pa: National Board of Medical Examiners; 2001.

Cashin W. *Improving Essay Tests.* IDEA paper, no. 17. Manhattan, Ks: Kansas State University Center for Faculty Evaluation and Development; 1987.

Clegg VL, Cashin WE. *Improving Multiple-Choice Tests.* IDEA paper, no. 16. Manhattan, Ks: Kansas State University Center for Faculty Evaluation and Development; 1986.

Davis BG. *Tools for Teaching.* San Francisco, Calif: Jossey-Bass; 2001.

Frary RB. *More Multiple Choice Item Writing Do's and Don'ts.* Washington, DC: ERIC Clearinghouse on Assessment and Evaluation; 1995.

Hertz NR, Chinn RN. *Licensure Examinations.* Lexington, Ky: Council on Licensure, Enforcement and Regulation; 2000.

Jacobs L, Chase C. *Developing and Using Tests Effectively: A Guide for Faculty.* San Francisco, Calif: Jossey-Bass; 1992.

Johnson RR, Squires JR, Whitney D. *Setting the Standard for Passing Professional Certification Examinations.* Tampa, Fla: Financial Management Association International; 2002.

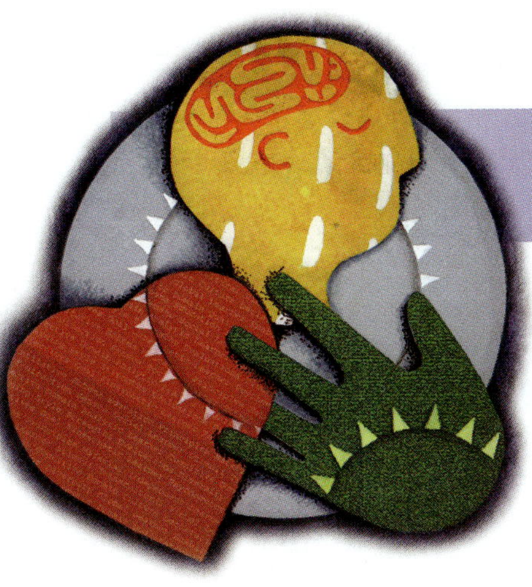

CHAPTER 21

Other Evaluation Tools

"There are no mistakes, save one: the failure to learn from a mistake."

—*Robert Fripp*

The practice of prehospital emergency medical care requires more than knowledge. Psychomotor skills and appropriate behaviors and attitudes are also essential if emergency medical services (EMS) students are to successfully perform. In addition to written examinations, other evaluations are needed to properly assess student performance. This chapter explores the use of oral examinations, practical examinations, attitudinal assessments, portfolios, and evaluations of student performance in the setting of actual patient care during clinical and field internships.

Bloom's taxonomy describes learning as divided into three domains: cognitive, psychomotor, and affective. Bloom's taxonomy is described in detail in Chapter 8. Most instructors are familiar with the methods used to evaluate the cognitive domain, or knowledge. As discussed in the previous chapter, knowledge is routinely evaluated through written examinations and writing assignments in a variety of educational settings, including the EMS classroom. The psychomotor domain, or practical skills, is better evaluated by observing the student's performance of skills in a controlled environment. Because attitudes and behaviors (contained within the affective domain) are heavily context dependent, evaluation of the affective domain is best done over time and in the applied setting. Attempts to evaluate the psychomotor domain through the use of a written examination seem patently ridiculous to the effective instructor. Selection of the appropriate evaluation tool can be guided by the domain of learning that is described by the objective. Written evaluations were discussed in the previous chapter; this chapter describes a number of other evaluation tools that are appropriate for the EMS instructor.

Different students exhibit preferences for different learning styles. Learning styles are described in detail in Chapter 4, Learning Styles. Howard Gardner takes this observation further when he asserts that different students actually have different levels of intelligence in various areas, a theory known as *multiple intelligences*.[1] He describes the areas of intelligence as verbal/linguistic, logical/mathematical, visual/spatial, body/kinesthetic, musical/rhythmic, and interpersonal/intrapersonal. It seems appropriate that evaluations can be administered in different ways to allow students to express their mastery of objectives in a manner that is comfortable for them according to their individual styles and talents. An awareness of learning styles and multiple intelligences can help the instructor distinguish between students who have not mastered objectives and those who have difficulty expressing knowledge or skills in a given format. As an example, Table 21-1[2] shows different evaluation methods that can be matched with Gardner's multiple intelligences.

It is recommended that the instructor use various methods of evaluation—not just the ones that play to a student's preferences. Some, and perhaps most, evaluation tools should be standardized and required for all students. However, the instructor must realize that learning preferences and multiple intelligences do have an impact on the evaluation process. For instance, written tests strongly favor those students with preferences and abilities in the verbal and logical areas. Similarly, kinesthetic learners may be favored by the use of practical examinations. Many instructors

TABLE 21-1 Evaluation Methods Matched With Multiple Intelligences

Intelligence Area	Evaluation of Knowledge of a Given Treatment Protocol
Verbal/linguistic	Essay
Logical/mathematical	Outline
Visual/spatial	Creation of treatment flow charts
Body/kinesthetic	Demonstration of procedure
Musical/rhythmic	Presentations of rhythmic mnemonic
Interpersonal	Classroom presentation; student leads a group discussion
Intrapersonal	Journaling, visualization

From Forte I, Schurr S. *Curriculum and Project Planner for Integrating Learning Styles, Thinking Skills and Authentic Instruction.* Nashville, Tenn: Incentive Publications; 1996.

describe situations in which the student who does poorly on written tests actually performs very well in the field. Allowing some evaluations to vary significantly in form of presentation according to student preference is desirable. This provides the effective instructor with another view of the student's acquisition of new knowledge, skills, and attitudes.[3]

Many of the tools described in this chapter require that multiple instructors be involved in performing evaluations. Effective evaluation of student performance across the domains of learning requires more than a single instructor—it requires a system. This does not mean that instructors who teach courses individually cannot perform meaningful evaluations, but individual class instructors must work together to create tools for evaluation. When the instructor works with the support of others to construct, use, and analyze evaluation instruments within a system, quality evaluation is possible.

ORAL EXAMINATIONS

Oral examinations are evaluations in which the questions and answers are given verbally in an exchange between a student and an instructor or group of instructors. Oral examinations are used to evaluate the cognitive domain and can extend to the affective domain. They may be used to evaluate the speed and confidence of response. The oral exam can evaluate the student's thought process and the thinking behind a particular answer. Oral examinations are similar in purpose to essay questions. Oral exams have the advantage of allowing evaluation by a group of instructors simultaneously. Another advantage is that different from essay questions, responding to oral questions does not require a high degree of compositional skills; consequently, oral examinations can more closely approximate the expectations of the entry level EMS professional in the job market.

For an oral exam to be fairly administered, a great deal of concentration is required by the student and the instructors. Any unexpected distractions can affect the test and may have a disparate impact on the student who is being examined when the distraction occurs. The instructor who is conducting an oral examination must exert strong control over the environment to minimize the potential for such distractions. This extends to ensuring that students and examiners minimize the potential for disturbance by having everyone turn off cell phones and pagers. The scheduling of examiners can present difficulties in that they may be expected to evaluate a large number of candidates with little opportunity for breaks. This can lead to uneven evaluation over time. Another potential problem is the identification of trends, leading to unfair emphasis on those who repeat mistakes made by previously examined students. For example, early in the day, the instructor who is testing may consider a mistake somewhat minor. However, as subsequent students repeat a seemingly minor mistake, it may take on greater significance as an error to the examiner, and expectations may change over the day.

Oral exam items should be blueprinted, drafted, and edited in a similar manner as written essay questions. Oral exam items should be scripted and clear instructions given to the examiners to minimize any variation from the script. Without scripting, oral examinations are very difficult to standardize. Examiners must be on the lookout for any clues they might inadvertently give to candidates, such as body language, comments, or gestures. By nature, grading of oral examinations is subjective. Ensuring reliability of scoring is also a challenge. One strategy for improving reliability is to use two or more examiners with independent scoring. These scores are later combined into a single composite grade.[4] Clear behavioral anchors are helpful in minimizing subjectivity.

Oral examinations are typically time-consuming and labor intensive. Efforts to address the disadvantages of being able to examine only one student at a time are countered by concerns about reliability. Running parallel stations with different examiners, although more efficient, would have a negative impact on exam reliability. Nonetheless, oral examination remains a valuable tool for use in a comprehensive evaluation strategy.

PRACTICAL EXAMINATIONS

Practical skill evaluation is conducted through the use of two major types of examination: the simple skill examination and the situational assessment (Figure 21-1).

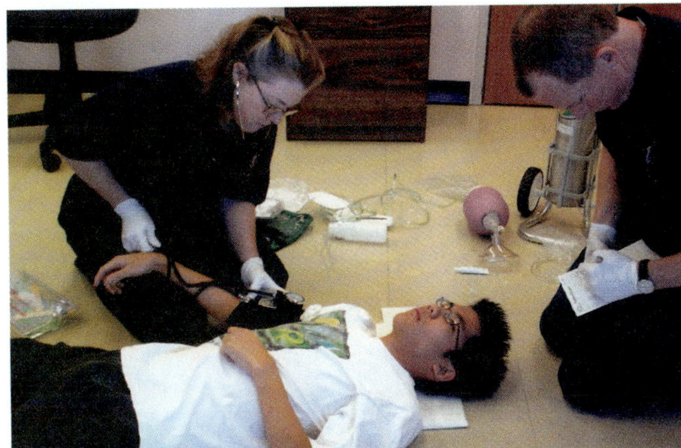

A

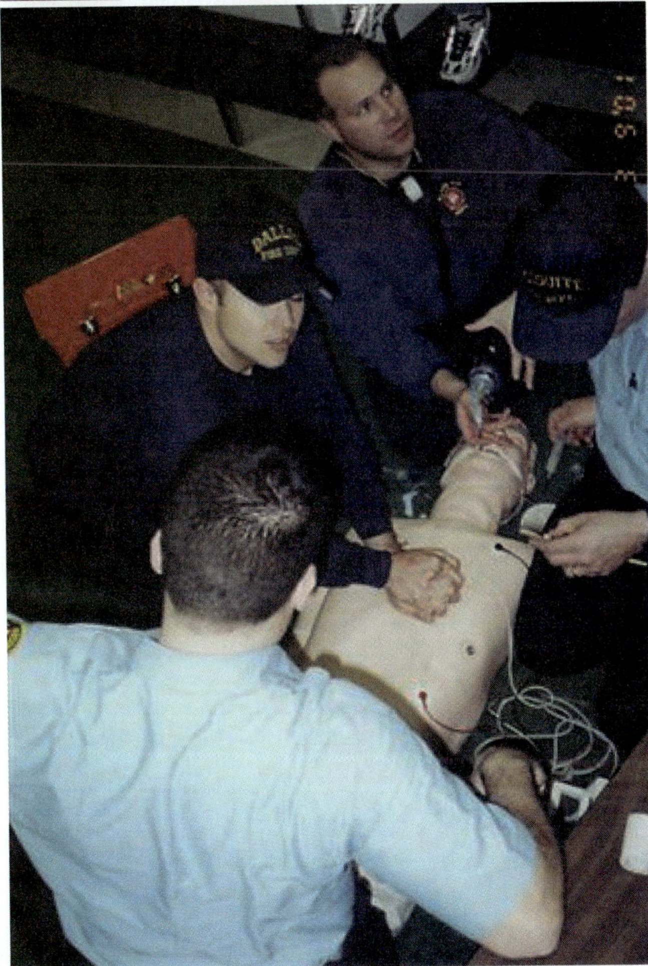

B

FIGURE 21-1 Practical skill evaluation includes the simple isolated skill exam **(A)** and the situational assessment that evaluates all three domains of learning **(B)**.

The evaluation of a rote mechanical skill is conducted through a simple task analysis. This is the easiest skill examination to administer. Simple skill examinations test at middle levels of the psychomotor domain, such as precision, and do not provide significant context for the skills. Situational assessment requires more elaborate simulation and is capable of assessing higher levels within the psychomotor domain, such as naturalization, as well as elements of the cognitive and affective domains.

Skill Evaluation

When a skill evaluation is conducted, the skill is first defined and the expected degree of proficiency is determined. Checklists are available for most skills, such as National Registry Practical Skills Examination Sheets and commercially available products (Figure 21-2). If checklists are not available, a performance checklist is developed from a task analysis, which provides a comprehensive list of the steps to be performed. Each step should include objective criteria, so that different examiners can agree on the criteria for successful completion of the step. It is usually best for instructors to keep the number of steps on the checklist to a minimum. This reduces errors in evaluation by allowing the examiner to observe the task as it is performed and complete the performance checklist afterward. The checklist should prioritize steps and list them in sequence. Critical steps should be identified, and important aspects should be weighted appropriately. Failure to properly perform any critical step results in failure of the exam. Whenever possible, the examiner should avoid qualifying or writing out the behavior; instead, the examiner should use the checklist to indicate whether a step was performed or not. The checklist should also provide any information that the examiner would need to give to the candidate. The more closely the examiner sticks to the script, the more reliable the evaluation is likely to be with various students and examiners.

To assess performance at the precision level of skill acquisition, context need not be provided and simple skill examinations can be used. Before the skill is tested in context, it is appropriate for the instructor to conduct simple skill evaluations to ensure that the student can perform the skill perfectly in isolation. Testing in context is done through the use of situational assessments. Situational assessments present the student with simulated scenarios; instructors evaluate the responses and judgments of the candidates in these specific situations. Situational assessments are more difficult to develop and deliver than are simple skill examinations. It is important that the situation and responses be simulated as accurately as possible.

The use of a programmed patient (also known as a *standardized patient*) is useful in conducting situational assessments. A programmed patient is an actor who plays the part of the patient. Programmed patients are provided with descriptions of what responses they should give to candidates when patient assessment is conducted. *Moulage* is the simulation of injuries with the use of make-up and special effects. Additional actors may be used to play the part of family members and bystanders. The environment of the situation

AIRWAY, OXYGEN, AND VENTILATION SKILLS
UPPER AIRWAY ADJUNCTS AND SUCTION

Start Time: ____________________

Stop Time: ____________________ Date: ____________________

Candidate's Name: ______________________________

Evaluator's Name: ______________________________

OROPHARYNGEAL AIRWAY	Points Possible	Points Awarded
Takes, or verbalizes, body substance isolation precautions	1	
Selects appropriately sized airway	1	
Measures airway	1	
Inserts airway without pushing the tongue posteriorly	1	
Note: The examiner must advise the candidate that the patient is gagging and becoming conscious		
Removes the oropharyngeal airway	1	
SUCTION		
Note: The examiner must advise the candidate to suction the patient's airway		
Turns on/prepares suction device	1	
Assures pressence of mechanical suction	1	
Inserts the suction tip without suction	1	
Applies suction to the oropharynx/nasopharynx	1	
NASOPHARYNGEAL AIRWAY		
Note: The examiner must advise the candidate to insert a nasopharyngeal airway		
Selects appropiately sized airway	1	
Measures airway	1	
Verbalizes lubrication of the nasal airway	1	
Fully inserts the airway with the bevel facing toward the septum	1	
Total:	13	

Critical Criteria

__________ Did not take, or verbalize, body substance isolation precautions

__________ Did not obtain a patent airway with the oropharyngeal airway

__________ Did not obtain a patent airway with the nasopharyngeal airway

__________ Did not demonstrate an acceptable suction technique

__________ Inserted any adjunct in a manner dangerous to the patient

FIGURE 21-2 The National Registry of Emergency Medical Technicians (NREMT) Airway, Oxygen, and Ventilation Skills testing sheet is a good example of a skill checklist.

should be as realistic as possible. This may require that simulations be conducted in office areas, restrooms, and outdoors rather than in the typical classroom.

A common problem with skill evaluations (both simple skill evaluations and situational assessments) is the tendency for examiners to allow candidates to verbalize elements of the skill. This can occur for a variety of reasons, including lack of appropriate equipment for the candidates to use. When candidates are allowed to verbalize components of a skill evaluation, validity is destroyed by the conversion of what would have been an evaluation of the psychomotor domain into a cognitive evaluation.

Another frequent issue is the consistency of administration of the examination. Unless carefully controlled, each scenario is likely to be presented in slightly different ways, leading to problems with reliability. This is countered by the careful attention of examiners in presenting information consistently. An instructor can ensure reliability by providing a script to examiners and insisting on compliance with the script.

Interrater Reliability

Interrater reliability can be a major problem with practical examinations. A well-constructed performance checklist can help reduce problems by not allowing examiners to qualify observations; instead, they must report and record whether a step was performed according to established criteria. Even with excellent checklists, reliability is a frequent problem when a single examiner observes the student's performance. A panel of examiners can help reduce reliability concerns. Another technique for improving reliability is the requirement of multiple iterations for a set type of skills being evaluated (e.g., successfully managing four of five trauma scenarios, each evaluated by a different examiner).[5]

High-Fidelity Simulations

Extremely realistic situational assessments (also known as *high-fidelity simulations*) have the capability of evaluating all three domains of learning in context. As such, these types of assessments are powerful tools for verifying mastery of objectives. These assessments present a rare opportunity for the instructor to evaluate the student's integration of needed knowledge, skills, and attitudes. Many courses use these assessments as a component of summative evaluations.

AFFECTIVE EVALUATIONS

Rubrics

Evaluation of the affective domain can be challenging for instructors. A useful tool for affective evaluations is the rubric. The rubric converts a list of characteristics into a graded set of observable criteria to be completed by the evaluator. Construction of the rubric consists of first identifying the characteristics to be evaluated. For instance, the following characteristics have been drawn from the 1994 Emergency Medical Technician (EMT)-Basic National Standard Curriculum: integrity, empathy, self-motivation, appearance/personal hygiene, self-confidence, communications, time management, teamwork/diplomacy, respect, patient advocacy, and careful delivery of service. A rating scale is then selected. A common rating system is 5 = excellent, 4 = above average, 3 = average, 2 = below average, and 1 = unacceptable.

TEACHING TIP: Another common rating system is 0 = unacceptable, 1 = acceptable, and 2 = excellent. Another alternative is to simply indicate that performance meets or does not meet the stated objective.

TEACHING TIP: To prevent clustering of scores at the middle value of a rating system, the instructor should use an even number of choices.

When the rubric is completed, observable behaviors are provided for each level of performance. Box 21-1, developed from Appendix 6 of the 2002 National Guidelines for Educating EMS Instructors,[6] provides a rubric for the characteristic of appearance/personal hygiene.

BOX 21-1 Sample Rubric

Point Value	Criteria
1	Inappropriate uniform or clothing worn to class or clinical settings. Poor hygiene or grooming.
2	Appropriate clothing or uniform selected most of the time, but the uniform may be unkempt (wrinkled), mildly soiled, or in need of minor repairs; appropriate personal hygiene is common, but occasionally, the individual is unkempt or disheveled.
3	Clothing and uniform are appropriate, neat, clean, and well maintained; good personal hygiene and grooming.
4	Clothing and uniform are above average. Uniform is pressed, and business casual is chosen when uniform is not worn. Grooming and hygiene are good or above average.
5	Uniform is always above average. Nonuniform clothing is business-like. Grooming and hygiene are impeccable. Hair is worn in an appropriate manner for the environment, and student is free of excessive jewelry. Make-up and perfume or cologne usage are discrete and tasteful.

From *National Guidelines for Educating EMS Instructors*, Appendix 6, 2002. Available at: http://www.nhtsa.dot.gov/people/injury/EMS

CASE IN POINT

A training officer at an EMS agency is tasked with designing an affective evaluation for new employees. The list of characteristics is drawn from the National Standard Curricula for the Emergency Medical Technician-Basic Course (EMT-B) and EMT-P. She has decided to use a 3-point rating system, with categories of unacceptable, average, and exemplary. She then collects a group of senior EMT-Bs and paramedics together to anchor the rating system with observable behaviors.

She begins the meeting by leading a discussion of the list of characteristics so as to develop consensus on the specific affective objectives to be evaluated. She follows with a discussion of the rating levels. She describes "unacceptable" as needing improvement before a student is released from probation. She describes "average" as the minimum level required for entry level competency. She describes "exemplary" as performance that makes the student a role model for that affective characteristic. Working at a whiteboard, she asks the group to describe behaviors that would be exhibited by a role model in the area of "integrity" (one characteristic from her list). She works with the group to describe each behavior in observable terms. After the group has reached consensus on a few observable behaviors to be linked with "exemplary," she leads the same process for "average." After this, the process is repeated for "unacceptable." The group then moves on to the next characteristic on the list and repeats the previous steps.

The rubric can be completed by a number of evaluators. By providing relatively detailed descriptions of affective characteristics, different evaluators can conduct assessments with some degree of interrater reliability. These tools should be provided to the student at or near the beginning of the course. Rubrics can be used for formative evaluation, and they provide valuable feedback to the student. Concrete examples of unacceptable conduct, including as much context as possible, should be provided to the student. When the discussion is framed in terms of observable behaviors rather than vaguely worded attitudes, student resistance to feedback is minimized. The more concrete and objective the feedback, the better received it will be. In some cases, the instructor may wish to have students fill out rubrics on each other, a technique known as *360-degree evaluation.* This is particularly valuable when group projects are assigned to class members. Group members can provide valuable feedback to each other regarding teamwork skills. Of course, summative evaluations of affective characteristics should also be conducted. The same rubrics can serve as summative tools.

Rubrics can fairly easily be converted to surveys that the student can use for self-assessment. Self-assessment is a useful formative strategy. Affective evaluations should be completed by the primary instructor and can also be completed by secondary and lab instructors who spend appreciable amounts of time with the student. The instructor who uses these affective rubrics in the clinical setting and internship can assess the degree to which a particular behavior is consistently exhibited in the applied care setting.

Impact on Grades

Converting rubric scores to grades is relatively easy. The degree of grade impact of affective evaluations is a matter of professional judgment for the instructor to decide. This excerpt from the 1994 EMT-Basic National Standard Curriculum provides recommendations on this issue[7]:

> Each student, therefore, must demonstrate attainment of knowledge, attitude, and skills in each area taught in the course. It is the responsibility of the course coordinator, medical director, primary instructor, and educational institution to assure that students obtain proficiency in each module of instruction before they proceed to the next area. If after counseling and remediation, a student fails to demonstrate the ability to learn specific knowledge, attitudes, and skills, the program director should not hesitate to dismiss the student.

Taken literally, this statement would indicate that evaluation of the affective domain should definitely yield a required minimum acceptable grade, as would assessment of the three domains. The implication is that the affective evaluation should account for a major portion of the grade and decision to pass the student, in that entry level competency in each of the domains is needed for a student to pass the course. The use of rubrics ensures a criterion-referenced strategy. Averaging scores from multiple evaluators can help ensure reliability. Content validity can be assessed through expert review, in a similar manner to written evaluations. Use of rubrics helps the instructor convert a subjective evaluation of the affective domain, with poor reliability, to a more reliable, more objective assessment.

Surveys

Another tool that is used to evaluate the affective domain is the completion of surveys by students. This tool is especially useful if the course is relatively short, and the purpose of the evaluation is to look for a change in behavior from pre-course evaluation to post-course evaluation. Surveys can be constructed as a series of statements for which students indicate the degree to which they agree with the statement. It is useful to use a Likert rating scale to indicate varying levels of agreement, for example, 5 = strongly agree, 4 = agree, 3 = neutral, 2 = disagree, and 1 = strongly disagree. By assessing the same objective with a number of different statements, the reliability of each statement can be assessed through a variety of statistical tests, such as split-half or Cronbach alpha (see Chapter 19, Principles of Evaluation of Student Performance, for further explanation of reliability tests). Surveys can also be used to assess the mastery of affective objectives related to the comfort level of the provider, such as "I am comfortable providing care for pediatric patients." Surveys are better than behavior-based rubrics for evaluating objectives that relate to confidence and comfort level because abstract characteristics like confidence are not easily assessed by observation of behavior. Thus, for affective objectives that are easily translated into observable behaviors, the rubric is the preferred tool; student surveys are more accurate for assessing internal characteristics.

PORTFOLIO PROJECTS

Research projects were discussed in the previous chapter. A variation on the traditional research paper is the use of a portfolio project. Portfolios are discussed in greater detail in Chapter 14, Tools for Individual Learning. The grading strategies used for portfolios vary considerably, depending on the specific forms of presentation used. Grading intermediate steps provides important feedback and an opportunity for formative evaluation. It is recommended that a portion of the grade be based on the results of the intermediate assessments. Guidelines for grading the written components are provided in the previous chapter. Other formats for presentation of information should have separate grading criteria. In grading written work, it is important to look past the handwriting and style to evaluate the content. Similarly, in evaluating other formats, it is important to look past the stylistic elements to evaluate the content of the presentation. It is helpful to use rubrics to assess alternative presentation formats. Instead of trying to create brand new rubrics, the instructor can modify rubrics through commonly available sources such as Rubistar.[8] Building the rubric with the student or group during the intermediate check-ins ensures that the grading criteria are well known to the student. The student can then use the rubrics as a self-assessment tool when working through the final stages of the project. If students are working together in a group to complete the project, the instructor should evaluate the interpersonal skills used. This can be done with the use of rubrics constructed for this purpose. The instructor who directly observes the group working together can assess teamwork, or a combination of self-assessment and 360-degree evaluation can be used to achieve this.

Portfolio projects can be used evaluate any of the domains of learning and appeal to different learning preferences. Portfolios take time for the student to develop; information is commonly collected over the duration of the course. This allows the project to serve both as a learning tool and as an evaluation tool. These projects can be a challenge for the instructor to grade, and rubrics may have to be created for each of the styles of presentation. Fortunately, generic rubrics are available. Typically, generic rubrics are designed for teachers in elementary and secondary schools; they may require some degree of modification by the EMS instructor.

APPLIED CARE EVALUATION

The primary goal of an EMS educational program is to prepare graduates to function competently as EMS providers. It is impossible for the instructor to fully simulate the environment and conditions of a medical emergency. Therefore, some degree of evaluation in the actual setting in which care is being provided is necessary. The instructor must supervise the experience because at this early stage, he or she may still be unsure about the competency of the student. Evaluating the student in the hospital and field environment is difficult. Among the challenges are maintaining appropriate patient care during the evaluation experience, ensuring reliability of the evaluations, and working with a team of preceptors. Appropriately conducting evaluation in the applied care environment requires well-constructed evaluation instruments that match the clinical experience to the objectives, a team of high-quality preceptors, and a systematic approach by the primary instructor.

Global Rating Scales

The most commonly used tool for evaluating student performance in the clinical setting is a set of global ratings of performance. When this tool is used, a set of characteristics are listed, along with a Likert scale for each. In some cases, a short description is provided for each rating. Box 21-2 provides an example.

BOX 21-2 Example of Global Rating

The student uses assistants well:

1	2	3	4	5
Consistently fails to direct assistants		Uses assistants well most of the time		Consistently makes best use of assistants

Global ratings are easy for the preceptor to complete. They can be constructed and completed very quickly. The major difficulty with global rating scales is that without extensive training and continuous reminders, interrater reliability is very difficult to achieve. Many instructors compensate for this lack of reliability by requiring that a large number of ratings be performed by multiple preceptors. Other instructors bolster reliability by providing detailed descriptions for each rating, effectively converting the global rating tool into a rubric.

Other Evaluation Tools

Neal Whitman, in *A Guide to Clinical Performance Testing*,[9] describes a model for using other tools to evaluate student performance in the clinical setting. Whitman draws distinctions between aspects of evaluated performance that are related to a specific objective in the course and aspects that are not well described by course objectives. This is discussed in terms of whether predescribed specific steps are to be performed (as in patient assessment), or the specifics are not predescribed (as in scene management). The matrix shown in Box 21-3 shows this relationship.

Checklists as Whitman describes them would be very similar to those checklists used in skill evaluations and simulations. Observable aspects would be listed in well-constructed checklists, generally in the order in which they should be performed (Figure 21-3). The preceptor indicates whether the student performed the step or not. Preceptors should be discouraged from making qualitative ratings. In some variations, the checklist includes categories for whether the step was performed correctly, performed incorrectly, or not performed (Figure 21-4). Affective

BOX 21-3 Objectives Matrix

	Specifics Pre-established	Specifics Not Pre-established
Objectives	Checklists	Observation logs
Other aspects	Critical incident forms	Anecdotal records

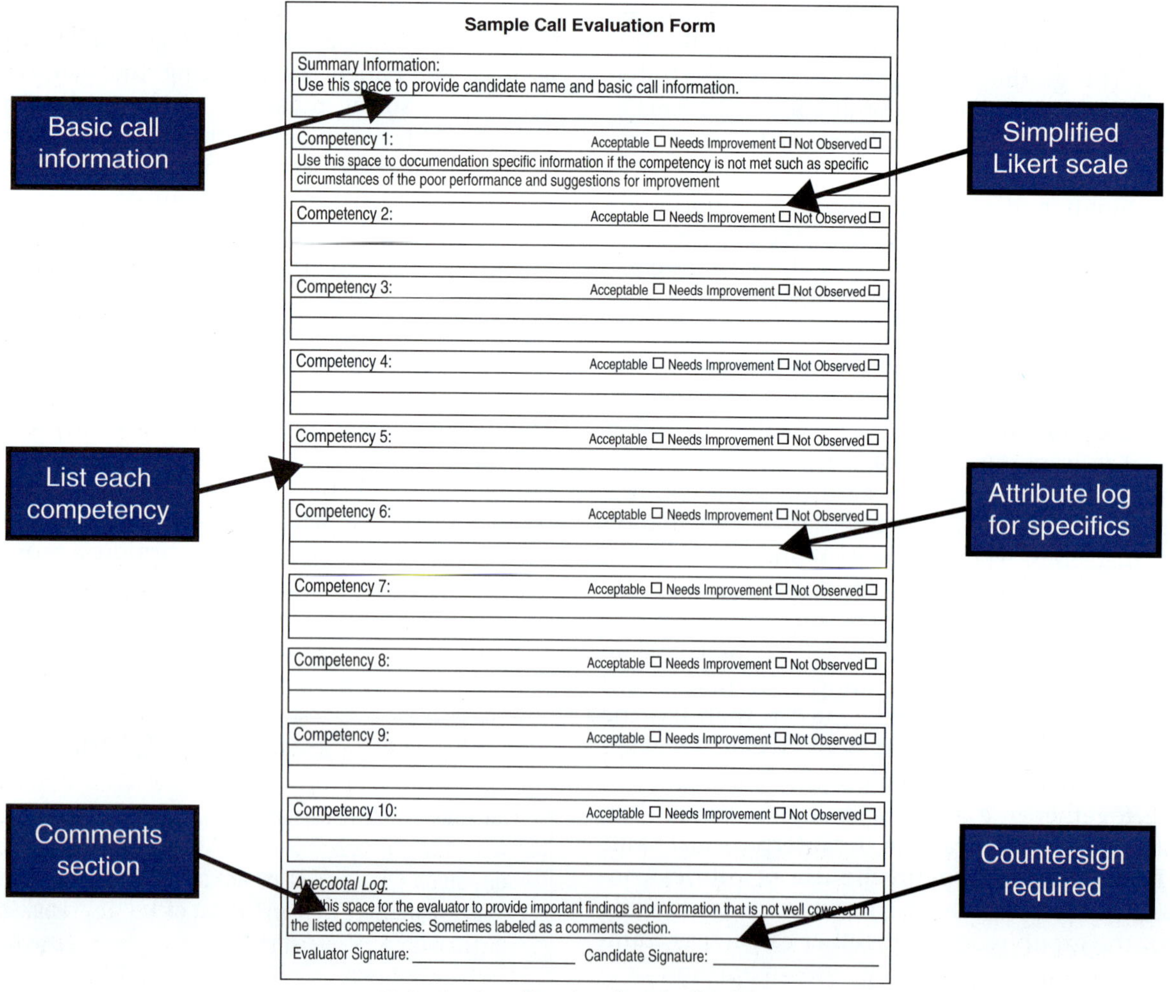

Sample Call Evaluation Form

Summary Information:
Use this space to provide candidate name and basic call information.

Competency 1: Acceptable ☐ Needs Improvement ☐ Not Observed ☐
Use this space to documendation specific information if the competency is not met such as specific circumstances of the poor performance and suggestions for improvement

Competency 2: Acceptable ☐ Needs Improvement ☐ Not Observed ☐

Competency 3: Acceptable ☐ Needs Improvement ☐ Not Observed ☐

Competency 4: Acceptable ☐ Needs Improvement ☐ Not Observed ☐

Competency 5: Acceptable ☐ Needs Improvement ☐ Not Observed ☐

Competency 6: Acceptable ☐ Needs Improvement ☐ Not Observed ☐

Competency 7: Acceptable ☐ Needs Improvement ☐ Not Observed ☐

Competency 8: Acceptable ☐ Needs Improvement ☐ Not Observed ☐

Competency 9: Acceptable ☐ Needs Improvement ☐ Not Observed ☐

Competency 10: Acceptable ☐ Needs Improvement ☐ Not Observed ☐

Anecdotal Log:
Use this space for the evaluator to provide important findings and information that is not well covered in the listed competencies. Sometimes labeled as a comments section.

Evaluator Signature: ______________ Candidate Signature: ______________

FIGURE 21-3 Sample call evaluation form.

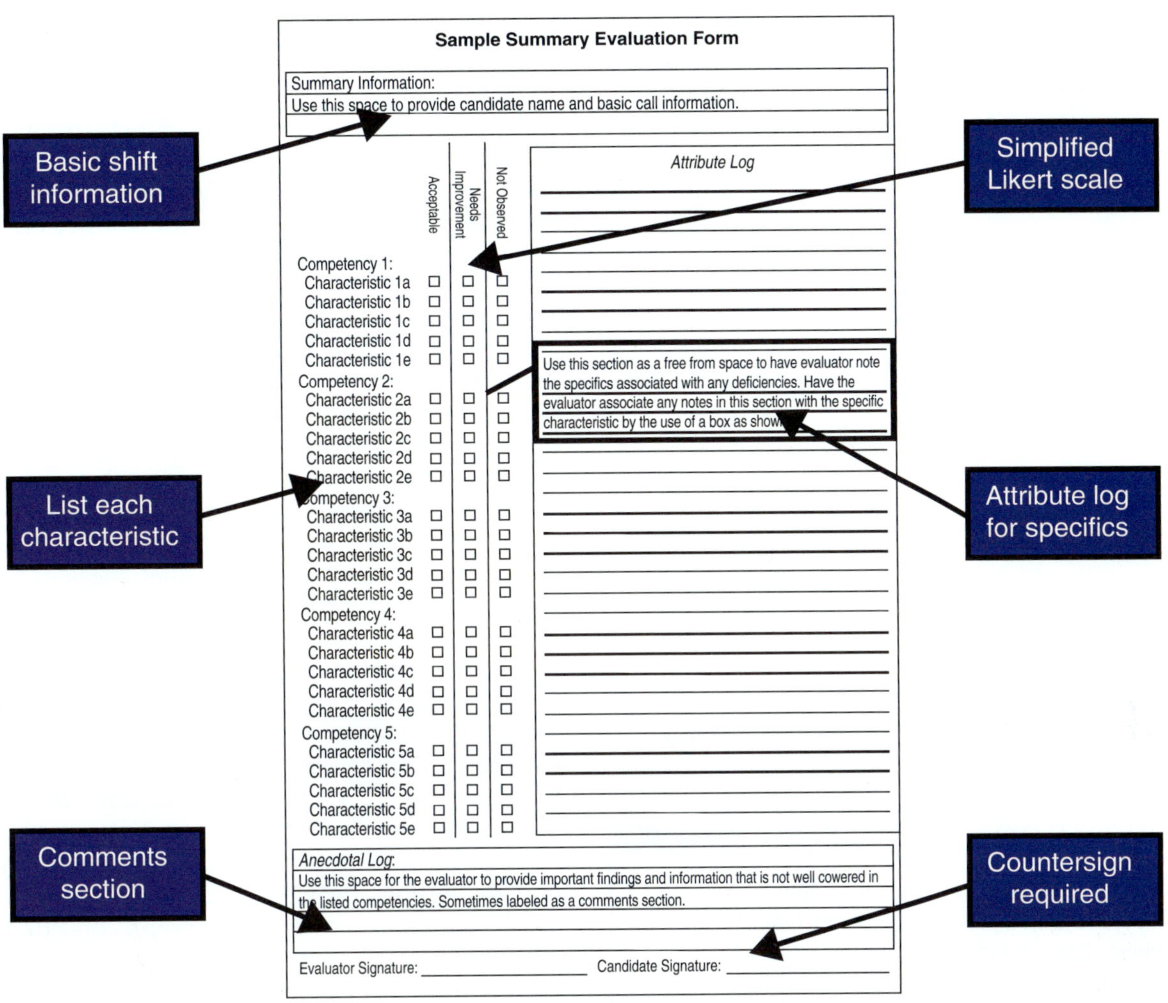

Sample Summary Evaluation Form

Summary Information:
Use this space to provide candidate name and basic call information.

	Acceptable	Needs Improvement	Not Observed
Competency 1:			
Characteristic 1a	☐	☐	☐
Characteristic 1b	☐	☐	☐
Characteristic 1c	☐	☐	☐
Characteristic 1d	☐	☐	☐
Characteristic 1e	☐	☐	☐
Competency 2:			
Characteristic 2a	☐	☐	☐
Characteristic 2b	☐	☐	☐
Characteristic 2c	☐	☐	☐
Characteristic 2d	☐	☐	☐
Characteristic 2e	☐	☐	☐
Competency 3:			
Characteristic 3a	☐	☐	☐
Characteristic 3b	☐	☐	☐
Characteristic 3c	☐	☐	☐
Characteristic 3d	☐	☐	☐
Characteristic 3e	☐	☐	☐
Competency 4:			
Characteristic 4a	☐	☐	☐
Characteristic 4b	☐	☐	☐
Characteristic 4c	☐	☐	☐
Characteristic 4d	☐	☐	☐
Characteristic 4e	☐	☐	☐
Competency 5:			
Characteristic 5a	☐	☐	☐
Characteristic 5b	☐	☐	☐
Characteristic 5c	☐	☐	☐
Characteristic 5d	☐	☐	☐
Characteristic 5e	☐	☐	☐

Attribute Log

Use this section as a free from space to have evaluator note the specifics associated with any deficiencies. Have the evaluator associate any notes in this section with the specific characteristic by the use of a box as show

Anecdotal Log:
Use this space for the evaluator to provide important findings and information that is not well cowered in the listed competencies. Sometimes labeled as a comments section.

Evaluator Signature: ____________ Candidate Signature: ____________

FIGURE 21-4 Sample skill evaluation form.

components can be evaluated with rubrics that contain observable behaviors associated with levels of performance, instead of checklists.

Observation logs list the various objectives, and open space is provided beside each in which the preceptor can note how that objective was met during the encounter. For example, an objective might be, "The student keeps the patient's family informed." Preceptors would make notes next to this objective when they observe that objective being performed. Although checklists work well for those skills and qualities that can be standardized for nearly all patient encounters, observation logs should be used when the specifics of skills and qualities are heavily dependent on the situation.

Critical incident forms are used to identify a specific aspect of performance, and the preceptor describes the situation when a positive or negative example is observed. As an example, the characteristic might be, "Promotes interagency cooperation." When the preceptor observes the student bringing a drink to the incident commander on a fire scene, the preceptor would make notes on the critical incident form to describe the positive example.

Anecdotal records are simply a means of describing any other behavior that the preceptor deems relevant. Room is often left on the evaluation form for anecdotal comments. Anecdotal records are valuable for capturing information that is not well described in advance by the other tools. Use of anecdotal records acknowledges that no evaluation system is perfect, and that all tools will invariably miss some important aspect of performance.

The effective instructor uses a combination of the previously described evaluation tools to form a system for observational reports to be completed by the preceptor of the experience. An effective strategy is to use a pyramid approach to the evaluation system. This consists of a report for each clinical encounter; these reports form the base of the pyramid. These encounter reports could include components of checklists, observation logs, critical incident forms, and anecdotal records. The preceptor would then complete a report for the entire shift (the next tier on the pyramid), combining information from encounter reports. This has the advantage of giving the student a degree of perspective on how the patient encounters combine to form a general impression for the shift. A number of shifts would be combined into a summative report for the entire rotation, forming the next higher tier on the pyramid. This builds from formative evaluation into a summative tool. An overall summary would be included at the end of the clinical cycle. Each tier builds on information obtained from the lower tier (Figure 21-5).

Selection of Experiences

The instructor should provide student experiences in relevant areas. For initial courses of instruction, guidelines for clinical experiences can be drawn from national standard curricula or state regulatory agency documents. The instructor should review such guidelines before beginning a course of instruction. Working from these guidelines, the instructor can plan for relevant clinical experiences. Early clinical experiences are typically used to evaluate student performance of skills on actual patients. The student is usually moved from less specialized areas of the hospital (such as labor and delivery) to more relevant areas (such as the emergency department) to the field environment. This model illustrates the concept of scaffolding experiences. The instructor should evaluate each clinical area according to two dimensions. The first dimension is one of educational experiences. In other words, what can the student learn in this environment? Educational experiences in the applied care environment should be clearly linked to educational experiences in the classroom and lab to build relevance. The second dimension is one of evaluation potential. In other words, what conclusions can the instructor draw from evaluations of the student performance in the given environment? For example, say a paramedic instructor requires venipuncture experiences with the hospital laboratory team. The student will learn the variation of vein locations and will learn techniques for finding a vein. The student can be evaluated on finding veins, and on hitting the veins accurately during a blood draw. This may be a necessary precondition before intravenous infusions on patients are initiated. However, the instructor should not draw the conclusion that the paramedic student can initiate intravenous lines after observing performance only in lab settings.

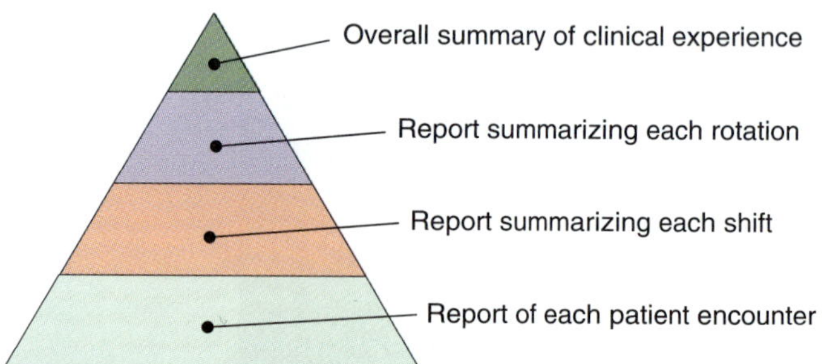

FIGURE 21-5 Pyramid approach to the evaluation system.

CASE IN POINT

A clinical coordinator is revising the documentation tools used for students in a paramedic program during their field internships. She decides that because different types of forms will be required for different elements, each student will be given a notebook with a set of forms to be completed by the preceptor. Each notebook contains the following, which are designed for up to 15 shifts with a preceptor:

- 40 call evaluations, each including an observation log that lists 10 objectives that can be demonstrated during any call
- 15 shift evaluations, each including an observation log that lists 10 objectives; these can act as a tool for the preceptor in summarizing the day's performance
- 20 performance checklists for patient assessment, to be completed by the preceptor after observing the intern's performance of an assessment
- 5 performance checklists for a variety of advanced life support (ALS) skills, to be completed by the preceptor after observing the intern's performance of each skill
- A knowledge checklist for each of several common protocols used by the service, to be completed by the preceptor after the student applies each protocol to an ambulance run
- 8 rubrics for affective objectives, to be completed by the preceptor on every other day of the internship
- 1 summary evaluation, along with a global rating for each objective, to be completed by the preceptor at the end of the internship

Preceptors

In most cases, the lead instructor will not be able to directly observe the performance of all students in the applied care setting. Preceptors must be used in the applied care setting. Preceptors should be proficient in the environment in which they perform. However, subject matter expertise is not enough. Preceptors also must serve as instructors for students in the clinical or field setting. In fact, many students take lessons from preceptors to heart much more than they do lessons from the classroom instructor (Figure 21-6). This can be effective if the lessons from the preceptor are aligned with those given in the classroom. If the lessons conflict, significant problems can arise. Thus, preceptors must be aware of the basic principles of adult education. They must also be aware of their role, and they must know what is being taught in the classroom. Regular communication between preceptors and classroom instructors is necessary. Preceptors should be trained in the use of the evaluation instruments they will be expected to use.

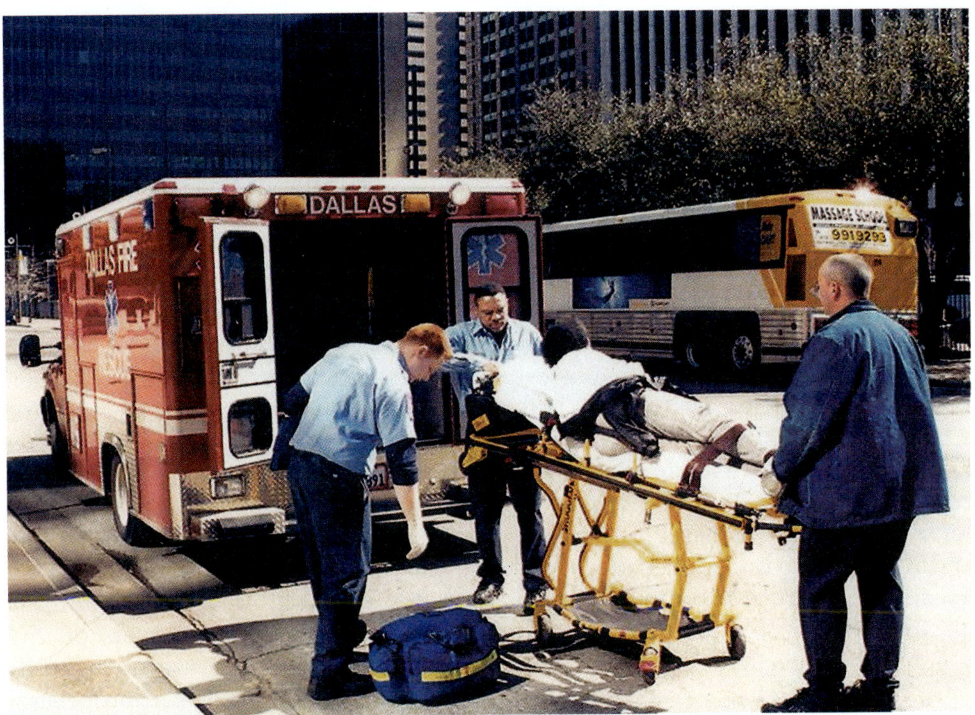

FIGURE 21-6 Feedback from preceptors is often instrumental in student learning. Feedback should be documented on the student evaluation tool.

Integration of Evaluation With Patient Care

A unique challenge to evaluating student performance in the applied care setting is the integration of educational goals, evaluation goals, and provision of excellent clinical care to the patient. It is essential that preceptors be prepared to meet this challenge. In terms of the educational goals of clinical experiences, the applied care setting is extremely effective in allowing students to experience the consequences of poor decisions. These lessons are extremely powerful and are likely to be retained by the student. However valuable these teachable moments may be, the educational value of having to deal with poor decisions must not be allowed to affect the patient. The preceptor must be prepared to intervene if it appears that the patient will suffer from a student's mistake. If the patient will not suffer, though, a valuable opportunity to drive a lesson home may be created. With regard to the goals of evaluating student performance, preceptor intervention can present difficulties. It is difficult for the preceptor to hold a student accountable for a mistake that was never allowed to occur. Intervention should occur just at the "point of no return," when it is apparent that the student will not realize and correct the mistake. If the preceptor frequently intervenes too early, the student may become hesitant and unwilling to commit to a decision. If the preceptor provides clues to the intervention, such as by asking, "Are you sure you want to do that?" on all critical steps, and not just when a poor decision is in progress, the evaluation has greater validity. Mastering this fine balance is an important skill for preceptors.

Even with extensive clinical and internship opportunities, it is unlikely that the student will be evaluated on all skills in the clinical environment. The instructor must be prepared to extrapolate from the results of evaluations that have been conducted. This extrapolation should be reasonable, based on the types of situations in which the student has demonstrated acceptable performance. For example, it is unlikely that all students will have the opportunity to manage a cardiac arrest in the applied care environment. The instructor may choose to extrapolate from the student's actual performance in caring for a critically ill patient and from simulations of cardiac arrest to conclude that the student can adequately manage a cardiac arrest in the field. This is a matter of professional judgment for the instructor, who combines personal opinion with input from the program director and the medical director. It is helpful to have guidelines regarding minimum exposure to different types of patients experiencing different types of emergencies. However, it is not feasible to require every student to see all types of calls. Reasonable extrapolations must be made.

TEACHING TIP: State regulations and program accreditation requirements typically have rules regarding minimum exposure for clinical environment (e.g., emergency department [ED] versus intensive care unit [ICU]), patients chosen from various age groups (e.g., adult versus pediatric), types of emergencies (e.g., cardiac versus respiratory), and procedures (e.g., initiating IV access versus performing endotracheal intubation).

SUMMARY

By combining written evaluations with other evaluation tools, an integrated strategy can be developed for assessing each of the domains of learning. Creating an effective evaluation strategy begins with careful consideration of the purpose of the evaluation. This purpose may be tied to a curriculum, in conjunction with established objectives that are used to anchor the evaluation tools used. The purpose may likewise be to verify competency with evaluations based on a practice analysis (that can be used to build objectives). It is sometimes helpful for the instructor to divide course objectives among the domains of learning, as the domain will be a significant consideration in the selection of evaluation tools. Based on the objectives, the instructor can decide on which tools will be used to evaluate student performance. Cognitive objectives can be effectively evaluated through the use of written examinations, oral examinations, and research projects. Psychomotor objectives can be assessed with practical examinations, simulations, and evaluations of student care of patients in a supervised clinical experience. Affective objectives can be evaluated through writing assignments, oral examinations, and surveys at lower levels; higher levels can be assessed through behavioral observations (with rubrics) that occur during class and during the clinical components of a course. Regardless of which domain area is to be evaluated, the student must be given previous knowledge of what objectives will be applied and to what degree they will be expected to perform.

When an integrated approach is used, a number of tools are required for effective assessment of the student. No one single tool will be capable of assessing the depth and breadth of objectives for the typical EMS course. The use of multiple tools also helps to ensure reliability of the evaluation process; consistency of results from different tools can be assessed. The grade assigned to a course should include elements from each of the formal evaluation tools. Each tool can be weighted according to the stated purpose of the evaluation strategy and the course objectives. Each tool will have strengths and weaknesses. By thoughtfully combining tools, the instructor can effectively minimize the weaknesses of each individual tool.

Based on the evaluation strategy chosen, specific tools and items can be selected and edited, and evaluation instruments constructed. The resourceful instructor collects tools and items from commonly available sources, instead of constructing each from scratch. Effective instructors also carefully edit each item and tool to ensure that the item has content validity for their particular course. Items are then analyzed to confirm reliability and validity. Over time, instructors can collect a powerful toolbox of evaluation instruments.[10,11] Although security is an issue for written examinations, other types of evaluation instruments are better shared with students. For example, students can use performance checklists and rubrics for meaningful self-assessment. Whether the student has prior knowledge of components to be assessed does not matter because knowledge is not being tested—performance evaluation is the object of these instruments.

Another point of view is to look at the evaluation of student performance as a set of progressive steps to be followed by the instructor. The use of formative evaluation is coupled with learning activities. Formative evaluation allows the student and the instructors to modify the learning strategy to ultimately master the course objectives. This mastery of course objectives is assessed through the use of curriculum-based summative evaluation tools. Appropriate instruments are combined after the instructor considers the appropriate domain of the objective drawn from the curriculum. The curriculum and the student together are tested through competency verification, which is a summative evaluation based on a practice analysis.

Evaluation of student performance can be complex. The results of each evaluation convey two intertwined messages that the instructor must decipher. The first of these messages is information regarding the performance of the student. The results of each evaluation can tell the instructor how well the student is performing. The effective instructor realizes though that the performance of the student is integrally tied to the performance of the instructor. This is the second message carried by the results. Poor results may reveal that the student is performing poorly, or they may indicate that the instructor has not provided adequate learning opportunities for the student to master the material. Of course, this assumes that the evaluation itself is giving accurate and meaningful results. To decipher these multiple messages requires an understanding of the fundamentals of student evaluation. Proper selection, construction, and analysis of evaluation instruments help to assure the instructor that evaluation is providing meaningful results. Proper formative evaluation provides feedback to the instructor about whether the learning activities have adequately prepared the student. With these fundamentals, the instructor can decode the results of tools that evaluate student performance.

REFERENCES

1. Gardner H. *Multiple Intelligences: The Theory in Practice.* New York: BasicBooks; 1993.

2. Forte I, Schurr S. *Curriculum and Project Planner for Integrating Learning Styles, Thinking Skills and Authentic Instruction*. Nashville, Tenn: Incentive Publications; 1996.
3. Sparks-Langer GM, Starko AJ, Pasch M, et al. *Teaching as Decision Making: Successful Practices for the Secondary Teacher*. 2nd ed. Philadelphia: Prentice Hall; 2003.
4. Jacobs LC, Chase CI. *Developing and Using Tests Effectively: A Guide for Faculty*. San Francisco, Calif: Jossey-Bass; 1992.
5. Davis BG. *Tools for Teaching*. San Francisco, Calif: Jossey-Bass; 2001.
6. National Highway Traffic Safety Administration. National guidelines for educating EMS instructors, 2002. Available at: http://www.nhtsa.dot.gov/people/injury/EMS
7. 1994 EMT-B National Standard Curriculum.
8. RubiStar. *Create Rubrics for Your Project Based Learning Activities*. Lawrence, Ks: Advanced Learning Technologies Center for Research on Learning at the University of Kansas; 2003. Available at: http://rubistar.4teachers.org
9. Whitman. (1982). *A guide to clinical performance testing*, IDEA paper No. 7. Manhattan, Kan: Kansas State University Center for Faculty Evaluation and Development. URL: http://www.idea.ksu.edu/papers/Idea_Paper_07.pdf
10. Accreditation Council of Graduate Medical Education and American Board of Medical Specialties. Toolbox of assessment methods, Version 1.1, 2002. Available at: http://www.acgme.org/Outcome/assess/Toolbox.pdf
11. Accreditation Council of Graduate Medical Education and American Board of Medical Specialties. Table of toolbox methods, 2000. Available at: http://www.acgme.org/Outcome/assess/ToolTable.pdf

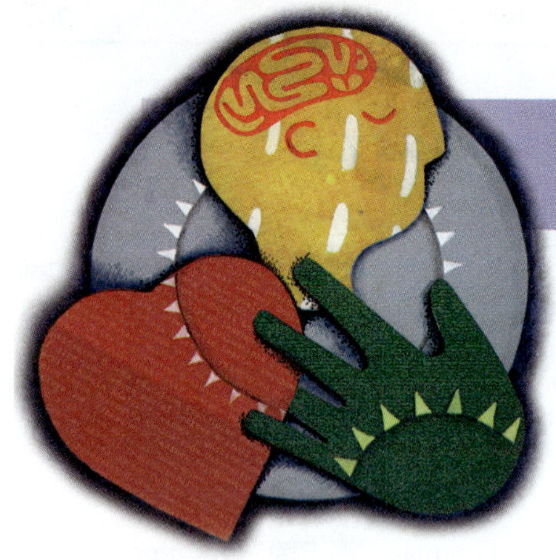

CHAPTER 22

Remediation

"You won't find a solution by saying there is no problem."

—*William Rotsler*

What should an educator do when a student doesn't meet the program's performance standards?

Performance standards are articulated at all levels of the Department of Transportation National Highway and Traffic Safety Administration National Standard Curricula (NSC) with terminology such as "entry level competency" when the educational goals for training are described.[1] Objectives included within each curriculum describe specific behaviors that are expected in accomplishing these goals; however, typically, curricula do not provide explicit guidance on how to measure goals or objectives, nor on how to conduct an effective remediation (retraining and retesting) process. Although this allows for a great deal of flexibility, it may not provide enough structure for the novice instructor.

In addition to the NSC, performance standards are found in state, regional, and local regulations for emergency medical services (EMS) education. Because regional guidelines are typically written to allow for flexibility in programs, they also may not contain specific evaluation or remediation processes. An instructor should use these references to provide the foundation on which to build an evaluation system for an educational program.

When a student does not meet the established performance standard, two options are available to the instructor: remediation, or removing the student from the educational process. When an evaluation system is in place for an educational program, a remediation process should also be included as a component of that system.[2] To be most effective, the remediation process must be clearly articulated and understood by all members of the education team and by students. The appropriate regulating bodies of the educational program should approve the remediation process.[3]

TEACHING TIP: You will have the greatest control of the remediation process if you have policies and procedures in place before remediation is ever needed.

REMEDIATION DEFINED

The term *remediation* is derived from the word root "remedial," which means to correct a deficiency.[4] The suffix "-ation" refers to an act or process. Therefore, the definition of remediation is the process of analysis and identification of deficits (or problems) and a plan for retraining or improving performance before retesting is undertaken.

The implication for evaluation is, "Here is the performance standard, and each student must meet this standard to pass."

Remediation is a critical component of the educational system because it provides solutions for situations in which students do not meet the performance standard. In these cases, the educational program must effectively respond with actions that go beyond the typical educational process (i.e., apply additional effort to help a student achieve competency). Research indicates that many, if not most, students need remediation at some point in their academic careers. In one study, 30% to 90% of all community college students needed remediation.[5] Given these statistics, if remediation is not an option because a program has not developed an effective process or cannot expend the necessary resources, a very high rate of failure may be noted in that program.

Still, other reasons besides the threat of low success rates must drive the need for remediation. The education process is a partnership between the student and the education team, and a successful student outcome is a reasonable expectation.[1] In this partnership, it is also reasonable to assume that the education team will be an advocate for student success. In this environment, a remediation process is a reasonable component designed to facilitate success.[6]

One component of the student-educator partnership that is difficult to design is a system that allows for remediation but does not compromise program integrity or fairness to the other students in the program. On the basis of student performance in a particular course, an instructor may feel one student "deserves" a second chance, and that another does not. Without a defined remediation system in place for guidance, the potential for bias is greater.

WHEN TO REMEDIATE

Remediation should follow a student's failure to meet an expected standard during an evaluation process. The remediation process should be initiated as soon as the failure is identified. Students should not be allowed to continue until remediation and reevaluation have taken place. Because of the schedule of some courses, this may mean that remediation must occur quickly.

CASE IN POINT

A student has just performed a series of skills associated with IV therapy and drug administration. During the student's demonstration, the instructor notes several times where the student repeats the same mistake; she sets an uncapped needle on the table as she prepares other steps of the process. When the instructor critiques her performance and provides feedback, the student tells the instructor that she knows she made the mistake and will "do better next time." Since the student repeated the mistake several times, the instructor is unsure whether the pupil actually does know the proper procedure, or if she was just being sloppy because it was a simulation versus a real patient encounter. A formal remediation cycle may be used to correct this mistake, then the student can be retested. In this case, the amount of time spent on the actual retraining may be minimal. In the remediation process, the student will be required to demonstrate proper skill performance and to provide evidence that she really does know the procedure.

Any type of evaluation, whether formal, informal, formative, or summative, can trigger the remediation process. Chapter 18 describes different evaluation types in detail.

The importance of remediation as an integral part of the evaluation process cannot be overemphasized. Student advocacy is a primary role for every EMS educator, just as patient advocacy is a primary role for every EMS provider.[1] In addition to discussing and describing student advocacy as a value, it is important that the instructor provide the necessary tools to accomplish this.

Although the range of students who may require remediation is not yet fully known, mounting evidence suggests that there is a need for it in every educational program (Box 22-1).[5] Given this need, educational programs must plan for remediation through establishment of deliberate steps and processes. A defined procedure allows classroom educators to focus on *how* to provide remediation for specific students, rather than getting bogged down in determining *whether* they should or can provide remediation. The administrative team for the program should create the remediation policies and procedures. The student handbook, syllabus, policies and procedure manual, and other program documents should contain policies and procedures that clearly outline the process. The remediation policy should also be provided to students during program orientation.[3]

STEPS IN THE REMEDIATION PROCESS

Once an evaluation reveals the failure of a student to meet an expected standard, the educator should initiate the remediation process. In some cases, the student may recognize this failure before the instructor does and will discuss concerns with the instructor; this discussion may result in initiation of the process.

The remediation process includes the following five steps:

1. Conduct an assessment of possible reasons for failure
2. Determine the cause for failure (attribution)
3. Develop a remediation plan
4. Implement the plan
5. Reevaluate

To ensure fairness in the remediation process and to maintain program integrity, a thorough assessment should occur before a remediation plan is developed. Information gathered during this step helps the instructor to determine whether remediation is allowable, possible, and appropriate. Information regarding the cause of a student's failure, from the student's perspective as well as from the instructor's, is needed for making this decision (Box 22-2).

The second step in the process, during which the root cause for the student's failure is identified, is known as attribution. Attribution helps identify the level of responsibility shared by the instructional process, educators, and the student. Attribution has a significant impact upon the remediation process.

BOX 22-1 An Update on Learning Disabilities

by Jeffrey T. Lindsey, M.Ed., EMT-P

Learning disabilities can be a complicated and confusing issue for an instructor. What are learning disabilities? How do you deal with learning disabilities in the classroom? What are the legal implications of identifying and accommodating a student with a learning disability? This article will address these issues regarding learning disabilities.

The National Center for Learning Disabilities defines the following words commonly associated with learning disabilities.

- Dyslexia—perhaps the most commonly known, is primarily used to describe difficulty with language processing and its impact on reading, writing, and spelling.
- Dyspraxia (Apraxia)—difficulty with motor planning, impacts upon a person's ability to coordinate appropriate body movements.
- Dysgraphia—involves difficulty with writing; problems might be seen in the actual motor patterns used in writing; also characteristic are difficulties with spelling and the formulation of written composition.
- Auditory Discrimination—is a key component of efficient language use, and is necessary to "break the code" for reading; it involves being able to perceive the differences between speech sounds, and to sequence these sounds into meaningful words.
- Visual Perception—is critical to the reading and writing processes as it addresses the ability to notice important details and assign meaning to what are seers.
- Attention Deficit (Hyperactivity) Disorder (ADD/ADHD)—may co-occur with learning disabilities (incidence estimates vary); features can include: marked over-activity, distractibility and/ or impulsivity which in turn can interfere with an individual's availability to benefit from instruction

In 1963, the term "learning disability" was introduced to describe the characteristics of a group of individuals of at least average intelligence who seemed less capable of school success, but who had unexplained difficulties in acquiring basic social and academic skills. There have been a variety of discussions among the experts as to developing a definition that is both clinically and educationally useful and also encompasses the wide range of characteristics found in those with learning disabilities. Professionals agree that individuals do not have a learning disability when the learning problems and/or school failures are due primarily to: impaired vision, mental retardation, emotional difficulties, hearing loss, environmental factors, or physical disabilities. Learning disabilities affect children and adults, and range from relatively mild to severe.

The criteria used to delineate whether an individual has a learning disability include the following:

- Has an average or above average intelligence
- Exhibits unexpected discrepancy between potential and actual achievement
- Performs poorly because of difficulty in one or more of the following areas: listening, reading, speaking, reasoning, writing, or mathematical skills.

  (National Center for Learning Disabilities)

Additional learning disabilities may also include difficulties in concentration and attention, memory and social skills.

There is no known exact correlation or cause of learning disabilities. A variety of factors may contribute to their occurrence. Learning disabilities may be due to:

- Heredity. Learning disabilities tend to run in families. Similar difficulties have been discovered in the same family.
- Problems during pregnancy and birth. Illness or injury during or before birth may cause learning disabilities. Learning disabilities may also be caused by the use of drugs and alcohol during pregnancy. Other factors may include: RH incompatibility with the mother (if untreated), premature or prolonged labor, lack of oxygen or low birth weight.
- Incidents after birth. Head injuries, nutritional deprivation, poisonous substances, (e.g., lead) and child abuse can contribute to learning disabilities.

Learning disabilities can have a significant impact on one's life. Learning disabilities are life-long. They can affect one's life including education, employment, daily activities, and interpersonal relationships.

The following are some of the more predominant characteristics of learning disabilities in adults:

- Reading or reading comprehension
- Math calculations, math language, and math concepts
- Social skills, or interpreting social cues
- Following a schedule, being on time, or meeting deadlines
- Reading or following maps
- Balancing a checkbook
- Following directions, especially on multi-step tasks
- Writing, sentence structure, spelling, and organizing written work
- Telling or understanding jokes

  (National Center for Learning Disabilities)

As an instructor you need to be aware that the individual may be able to learn information presented in one way, but not in others. The individual may be able to explain things verbally, but have difficulty writing ideas on paper. Other factors to consider include: misreading or miscopying, misinterpreting language, or have poor comprehension of what is said. These individuals may find it difficult to memorize information.

The Individuals with Disabilities Education Act is very clear as to which individuals should be included in the transition services available to children with learning disabilities. This act, has hopefully, identified the individual with a learning disability and directed them towards the proper path for their learning years. As an instructor, these individuals entering into

BOX 22-1 An Update on Learning Disabilities—cont'd

by Jeffrey T. Lindsey, M.Ed., EMT-P

our profession will have recognized their learning disability. We need to remember that; there are still a number of individuals in our society who have not had the luxury of these services available.

Section 504 of the Rehabilitation Act of 1973 and the Americans with Disabilities Act of 1990 (ADA) protect individuals with learning disabilities from discrimination. Students who have documented their learning disabilities are entitled to accommodations to support their educational success.

Students are responsible for making their learning disabilities known and for requesting adjustments in order to receive Section 504 accommodations.

The types of accommodations include:

- Extended time on tests
- Note-takers
- Assistance from the use of technology devices (tape recorders or laptop computers)
- Modified assignments
- Alternative assessments and test formats

(ADA)

The ADA is a federal anti-discriminatory statue designed to remove barriers, which prevent qualified individuals with disabilities from enjoying the same employment opportunities that are available to persons without disabilities.

Employers cannot discriminate against employees with disabilities. This prohibition covers all aspects of the employment process including:

- Application and promotion
- Testing and medical exams
- Hiring and layoff/recall
- Assignments and termination
- Evaluation and comprehension
- Disciplinary actions and leave
- Training and benefits

(ADA)

Employers are responsible and required to make reasonable accommodations to qualified applicants or employees with disabilities. Some examples of reasonable accommodations include:

- Job restructuring
- Modifying work schedules
- Reassignment to another position
- Acquiring or modifying equipment or devices
- Adjusting or modifying examinations, training materials, or policies
- Providing qualified readers or interpreters
- Making existing facilities used by employees readily accessible to, and usable by, individuals with disabilities.

(ADA)

Keep in mind, you are not required, nor are you expected to lower quality or quantity of standards to make an accommodation. Nor are you required to provide personal items, such as glasses or hearing aids, as accommodations.

Individuals with learning disabilities may have difficulty with social skills. These difficulties may spill over into the classroom. As instructor we need to be sensitive to these issues. Some social issues include:

- Self-esteem
- Interpersonal relationships
- Workplace functioning
- Community participation

(National Center for Learning Disabilities)

Additional considerations to take into account when dealing with learning disabilities, is the fact of the disability being overlooked as a hidden handicap. Learning disabilities are often not easily recognized, accepted, or considered serious once recognized. Attention deficits and hyperactivity sometimes co-occur with learning disabilities, but not always. Learning disabilities are NOT the same as the following handicaps: mental retardation, autism, deafness, blindness, or behavioral disorders.

As an instructor you need to be aware and sensitive to the students needs in your class. It is not your responsibility to identify those in your classes with a learning disability. It is your responsibility to reasonably accommodate those individuals with a learning disability.

For further information regarding this issue, there are a variety of resources.

- The National Center for Learning Disabilities is excellent resource to gain more information and knowledge on learning disabilities. You can contact them through the web at www.ncld.org or by phone at 1-888-575-7373.
- The U.S. Department of Justice, ADA Information line is 1-800-514-0301.

BIBLIOGRAPHY

National Center for Learning Disabilities www.ncld.org
American Disabilities Act www.ada.gov
VFIS Instructional Methodology (2001) York, PA

From NAEMSE: Domaine 3, Winter 2002.

BOX 22-2 Assessment Phase of Remediation

The assessment phase of the remediation process may reveal helpful information for the student on any of the following topics:

- Need for study skills enhancements
- Need for evaluation for learning disabilities
- Need for developmental or remedial classes
- Need to obtain additional clinical experience
- Need to work on motivation or attitude
- Understanding of the sacrifices necessary for the course
  - Contact for helpful resources
  - Schedule adjustments for work and family
  - Access to financial or other support

BOX 22-3 Remediation Algorithm

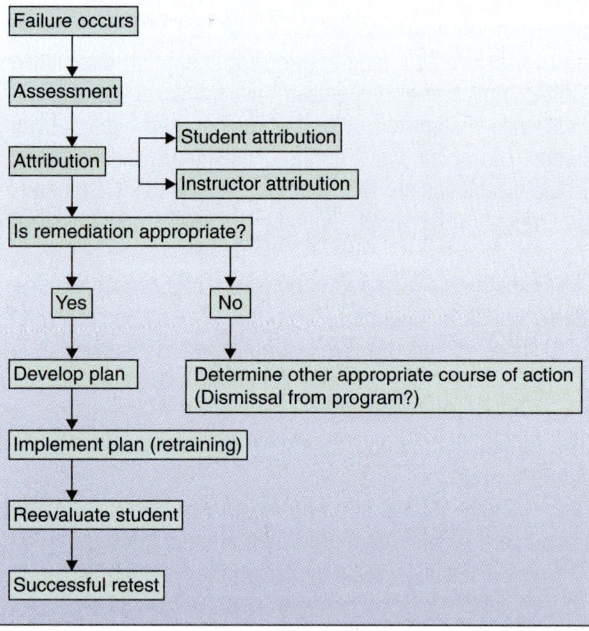

Failure occurs
↓
Assessment
↓
Attribution → Student attribution; → Instructor attribution
↓
Is remediation appropriate?
↓ Yes → Develop plan → Implement plan (retraining) → Reevaluate student → Successful retest
↓ No → Determine other appropriate course of action (Dismissal from program?)

TEACHING TIP: If you don't do a thorough front-end analysis to identify the problem, you may not get to the actual cause for the student's failure, and your remediation plan may not be successful.

Once the problem has been identified and retraining is found to be possible and appropriate, a remediation plan is developed. For the plan to be finalized, the student must agreed to the terms and conditions, including the consequences of repeated failure. Once the plan is in place, the retraining can begin. The progress of the student during the retraining process should be closely monitored. Once retraining has occurred, Step 5, reevaluation, can occur (Box 22-3).

CASE IN POINT

(Part 1 of 2)

An educator is teaching a First Responder course. The course is 40 hours long and adheres to the curriculum and syllabus developed and provided by the state EMS agency. The syllabus states that students are required to successfully pass three testing cycles during specified parts of the program to be eligible to take the state First Responder test for certification. Each test consists of two parts: 50 multiple choice questions and 3 psychomotor skill tests based on appropriate scenarios. The syllabus further states that students who fail the exam process are allowed to retake that part of the test one time. It also states that failure a second time results in dismissal (removal) from the program. One student just failed the practical examination portion for the first testing cycle. What should happen next?

A process allowing for remediation is included in the evaluation system for this course. The syllabus identifies three testing points that have relatively high stakes: (1) Students must successfully complete each examination to be able to continue in the course; (2) it further states that, in the event a student fails testing, one retesting opportunity is provided before dismissal; and (3) remediation should occur after failure of the first attempt, and before a retest is attempted.

Step I: Conduct an Assessment of Possible Reasons for Failure

Before ever setting foot in the classroom, the instructor should have read all program policies and procedures and should know where and how to access them. Once a failure occurs, the instructor should review the remediation policy and procedure early in the process to ensure compliance with program rules.

The following questions are useful in determining if a student is eligible for remediation, and in deciding whether remediation is possible and appropriate:

1. Is there a standard in place that indicates what level of student involvement is required for remediation to be provided?
   - Does the policy identify a score or range of scores required for remediation to occur?
   - Is there an attendance standard?
   - Are other criteria specified (e.g., limits on total number of attempts at remediation and retesting allowed in a program)?
2. Can remediation be accomplished in a timely manner to allow the student to continue in the program?
3. Are resources available for providing remediation?
4. How committed is the student to the remediation process and to improving his or her performance?

Time constraints are a critical factor to be analyzed. For example, if the course schedule does not allow enough time for remediation to occur, it may not be appropriate to proceed with retraining. If the time frame for retraining is not adequate, a second failure may result during the retesting phase. As the course continues to move forward, the student will face the additional burden of keeping up with new material at the same time that he or she is retraining.

Resource considerations are important also. Many programs have limitations on their equipment and supplies; some share resources among several simultaneous courses. Remediation requires careful scheduling and cooperation. The need to provide resources for remediation for one student can seriously disrupt programs that operate with tight resource constraints, adding additional importance to the need for incorporating remediation considerations into the evaluation process.

The final decision regarding eligibility for remediation usually requires an understanding of the reason for the failure. If the decision rests solely with one instructor, bias can enter into the decision-making process. Input from other members of the educational team can help reduce bias.

TEACHING TIP: Because of the commitment to student advocacy, when an educator is unsure whether a remediation attempt should proceed or is unclear of the standard in place, it is best to allow the student to attempt the remediation process.

Educational program strategies and educator knowledge and experience are important considerations in the assessment phase, but the student's role in the process is also critical. There is significant anecdotal evidence and action research (non-scientific or pseudo scientific evidence) on student attitudes and their impact on learning. Educational psychologists are placing greater emphasis on attitude, as noted by the increase of scientific papers on this subject. If the real cause of the failure is primarily attributed to the student and the student is unwilling to acknowledge that, then successful remediation may not be possible because the student may not be willing to correct their behavior.

Step 2: Determine the Cause for Failure (Attribution)

Some evidence suggests that attribution may be the single most important component affecting the remediation process.[7] To develop a meaningful remediation process, the educator must identify the root cause of the student's failure.

Intuitively, we know that incorrect problem identification can lead to implementation of the wrong or an ineffective solution. Therefore, seeking multiple points of input can help the instructor to identify the correct cause. In addition to reviewing the instructional process and evaluation instruments, the educator should interview the student and consider seeking input from instructors in all settings in which the student has participated, including the classroom, lab, clinical, and field settings. It may also be appropriate to seek input from the medical and program directors.

TEACHING TIP: The instructor must maintain the student's confidentiality during this process. Discussion of the issue of failure should be limited to appropriate members of the education team.

The educator should use active listening and clear communication skills, especially when interviewing the student. Considering that the student may have strong emotions during this time, it is important that professionalism and perspective be maintained.

It is not uncommon for the educator to assign a different attribution to the failure than what the student believes to be the cause, nor are multiple attributions uncommon. For example, a student believes that the reason for failure was inadequate time to prepare for the examination, but the instructor believes the root cause is that the student missed a practical skill development section. The impact of conflicting attributions on the solution is significant.

TEACHING TIP: Failure of a student, regardless of the cause, affects the instructor as well as the student. Input from members of the education team outside the situation should be considered to help limit bias and subjectivity.

Student attribution

The educator can identify the student's attribution of the cause for failure through an interview. The instructor should ask open-ended questions and should approach the interview in a nonjudgmental manner. It may be appropriate for the instructor to emphasize to the student that he or she is working on an educational solution to the problem. The instructor may find it helpful to tell the student that the goal of the remediation process is to determine what strategies will most likely result in the student's passing on the next attempt.

TEACHING TIP: Some students lack the maturity to accept responsibility for their action or inaction. The instructor should focus energies on developing a solid plan, with the hope that the student will eventually accept his or her responsibility in the failure.

As the educator conducts the interview, it is important that he or she assess the student's commitment to improving performance (Figure 22-1).[7] The instructor may find it necessary to make decisions regarding the student's abilities to succeed on future attempts. If the student does not possess the necessary tools (cognitive, affective, or psychomotor abilities), the resultant remediation plan may need to include strategies for developing these abilities. Inclusion of the program and medical directors in the decision process may be required.

As the instructor works through the process of attribution, it is important to ascertain whether the student ever successfully demonstrated the standard. This can reveal whether the student is capable of attaining the standard. If success was demonstrated previously, then the instructor should determine what has changed. Perhaps the progress of the student was not monitored appropriately, which allowed for uncorrected poor performance. If the instructor does not have evidence of successful attainment of the standards, corrective instruction should be provided to the student.

Program attribution

It is important for the instructor to examine what possible role the educational process played in the failure. It must be ensured that the faculty understood and articulated the performance standard clearly. Was the student informed of one standard, yet tested for another? The instructor must ensure that the goals and objectives of the course match the testing process.

The educator must analyze the evaluation process. Were the correct instruments used to evaluate students? Have these instruments been validated? And are they reliable? The evaluation section explains these processes in detail.

The educator also must analyze the learning plan. Was the plan appropriate and effective? Was adequate time allotted for students to learn the material? Were adequate teaching strategies used to appeal to the student's learning style or preference? Did the learning plan allow for reinforcement of concepts? And did it test for understanding? Were activities designed to facilitate the learning of metacognitive (critical thinking) processes?[8] Findings from the program attribution may indicate the need for changes and improvements in the course.

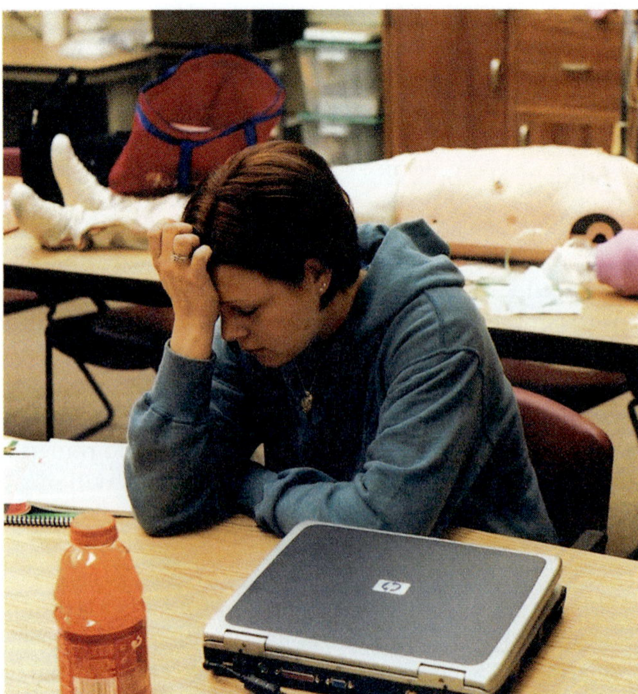

FIGURE 22-1 Student commitment to improving performance is imperative if the student is to succeed.

CASE IN POINT

(Part 2 of 2)

The policies and procedures indicate that remediation is allowed and encouraged for the student. During the problem assessment interview, the student is unclear about why he believes he failed, but he says he wishes he had had more time to practice the skill.

As the educator reviews the course syllabus and schedule, he notes that with the practical skill development session, many skills were listed on the sheet. Because of time constraints, the instructor ended up demonstrating all the skills, but students did not get much practice time. The instructor also notes that many of the students did not perform very well on the practical exam, even though only one failed. The educator immediately contacts the program coordinator to discuss rearranging the schedule to allow for additional practical skill time and permission to retest the entire class. A private skill session is also arranged for the student who failed.

On retest, all students pass.

Multiple attributions

Frequently, student failure is caused by multiple attributions. In many cases, the attributions identified by the student and the educational team do not match. The interrelationship between education, performance, environment, and student needs is complex. The instructor should consider the effect that each of these has on student performance.

CASE IN POINT

A program has an inadequate number of manikins for all students to remain active during class. A shy student feels the instructor is paying more attention to the other students and withdraws. The instructor is dividing his attention between too many students and does not notice that the student is withdrawing. When the student fails the examination, he blames the instructor for not providing appropriate instruction. The instructor counters that the student is not assertive and seems unwilling to practice skills. Consider the impact these multiple attributions have on development of a successful remediation plan.

This Case in Point highlighted two program problems: not enough manikins for students, and not enough instructors. One-on-one instruction may result in successful retesting of the student in this case, but unless the program can allot additional resources, the problem will likely reoccur.

A "teachable moment" is a concept employed at all levels of EMS curricula. It describes the opportune time to provide valuable information to people closely affected by traumatic emergency situations. For example, the fire department often visits households within weeks of a tragic fire to provide smoke detectors and fire safety information. Health professionals discuss healthy lifestyle choices with other family members after the near-death experience of a family member from cardiovascular disease. Often, people are willing to listen to advice and direction provided by professionals during these teachable moments. However, confronting a student while he or she is discussing attribution is usually NOT a teachable moment. Failure of an examination may be devastating to life plans and goals, and the student may be very emotional. It may not be helpful for the instructor to try to convince a student that his or her attribution is incorrect at this time.

Although students can benefit from understanding and accepting personal responsibility for failure, the student attribution interview may not be the time to approach the subject. Experience and strong interpersonal skills will help an educator to decide whether and when it is appropriate to confront a student about his or her perception of attribution. It is critical for the instructor to determine whether the remediation plan can account for the student's attribution.

Step 3: Develop a Remediation Plan

Input from the student and from the educational team is used to develop the remediation plan (see sample remediation plan document in Figure 22-2). The remediation plan should clearly describe the process and the expected outcomes for the student and instructional team. It should define any work (e.g., reading assignments, homework, or self-study) that should be completed independently by the student, and should describe the assistance to be provided by the instructor. A timeline for the remediation should be included that clearly identifies when the process will begin and end, including an estimated total number of hours that the retraining process should take. The plan should describe time the student and instructor may spend together and should suggest time the student should spend in independent work or study. If appropriate to the plan, the instructor can include the dates and times that progress reports will be issued. The plan should also identify the date and time of retesting, should specify what type of retesting will occur, and should tell about any observers (e.g., the medical director or other instructor) who will be present during retesting. The expected standard for successful completion should be reinforced, and the consequences of failure to comply with the terms specified in the remediation plan should be described. The consequences of failure of the retest should also be described.

The instructor should review the finished plan to ensure that it complies with the program remediation policy. The completed document, when signed by the student, instructor, program director, and medical director, becomes a learning contract. Copies of the document should be provided to all parties involved, and one should be maintained in the student's record.

TEACHING TIP: It may be helpful for another member of the education team to review the plan before it is finalized to ensure that it is reasonable and appropriate.

If the educational methods are not initially identified as the cause for the failure, they may become the basis for the retraining methods used in the remediation plan. For example, the teaching strategy can shift from a group approach to one targeted to the student's individual learning style and preference. If the educational method is attributed as the cause of failure, adjustments to the educational methods used should be made (an educator cannot continue to do the same thing and expect different results).

Step 4: Implement the Plan

The instructor must monitor the student's progress closely during remediation, ensuring that all involved parties are performing as described in the plan. The instructor should maintain progress reports and provide the student with corrective feedback. Students

Student Name: ______________________ Date: ________________

The above student has failed to attain a passing score on the following evaluation(s):

____.

A remediation plan has been approved for this student with the following conditions:

Describe all expectations and outcomes for each of the following. Include specific work required like reading assignments, independent study, skills development sessions etc. As appropriate include how many hours will be provided.

Student expectations and deliverables:

1.

2.

3.

Program expectations and deliverables:

1.

2.

3.

List each deliverable and the date required for completion:

Item: ____ Due date/time: __________________________________

Item: ____ Due date/time: __________________________________

Item: ____ Due date/time: __________________________________

A retest will follow the completion of remediation. List each evaluation tool to be utilized and required passing score.

Describe the consequences of non-completion of the remediation process or failure on the retest.

Signatures:

_____________________ _______________

Student Date

_____________________ _______________

Instructor Date

_____________________ _______________

Program Director Date

_____________________ _______________

Medical Director Date

The original document will be placed in the student's permanent record. Copies of this document will be provided for each member signing above.

FIGURE 22-2 **Remediation plan template.**

CASE IN POINT

An instructor's class meets for 4 hours on 1 evening each week. A student in the class fails a cognitive anatomy test on the circulatory system. During a problem assessment, the instructor determines that the student learns best through visual means. For the remediation plan, the educator provides the student with some pages from an anatomy coloring book and lends the student a heart model for the weekend. The instructor also furnishes the student with several Web addresses for sites with cardiac content. The student spends an hour with the instructor answering questions. On retesting during the next class session, the student attains a very high score. The instructor adds visual elements to all future class presentations.

should be held accountable for their responsibilities as outlined in the plan. Careful documentation is critical. In the event of legal challenge, the education team will be called upon to provide evidence to show how they advocated for the student.

Step 5: Reevaluate

Remediation plans require that both the student and the educator make sacrifices in time and resources, and often the stakes are high. The educator must carefully evaluate the tool that will be used to retest the student to ensure that it is fair and objective. All tools should undergo validity and reliability testing and should be approved by the program and medical directors. The instructor must decide whether the same evaluation tool will be used to retest the student. A psychomotor skill test will most likely use an identical tool, but the scenario used to prompt the student to perform the skill may be different. Using the same tool for a written exam will likely increase the score without necessarily resulting in an increase in the student's knowledge level. Having seen the exam and identifying what was missed may lead the student to correct only those specific item errors, with no increased knowledge or improved understanding in that area. Consequently, retesting a written exam with a different tool provides a more accurate measure for determining that true remediation has occurred. Educators should seek advice from other members of the educational team if they are not sure about reevaluation decisions.

If retesting involves an instrument with a high level of subjectivity, such as a psychomotor skill test, the instructor should consider using an independent evaluator who has limited knowledge of the student's previous failure.

An educator must ensure that the grading of the reevaluation tool complies with the policies for remediation. Depending on how the policy is written, it may be appropriate for the original grade to remain unchanged, with the grade book indicating that a "pass" occurred on retest, or it may be appropriate for the two grades to be averaged. Another process may be appropriate as well; this decision should be based on how the policy is written.

SUMMARY

Remediation is needed when a student fails to attain a passing score or an acceptable performance on an evaluation. The remediation process is an integral component of the evaluation system, and it is a reasonable expectation for a program that values advocating for students. Remediation helps maintain partnership within the education process.

Remediation is necessary for many students. It will not be appropriate in all situations, but it is important that clear guidelines and policies be established before the need arises. With deliberate design, the process can maintain program integrity and provide fair criteria for all students.

REFERENCES

1. Department of Transportation National Highway and Traffic Safety Administration National Standard Curricula.
2. Boylan HR, Bonham BS, Rodriguez LM. What are remedial courses and do they work: results of national and local studies. *Learning Assistance Review.* 2000;5:5-14.
3. CoAEMSP Guidelines and The Agenda for the Future.
4. *Riverside Webster's II Dictionary.* Revised Edition. New York: Berkley Books; 1996.
5. Spann MG Jr. Remediation: a must for the 21st century learning society, Policy Paper, 2000. Center for Community College Policy, Education Commission of the States, Denver, Colo. (Available from ESC Distribution Center, 707 17th St. Suite 2700, Denver, CO 80202-3427.)
6. Colby A, Opp R. Controversies surrounding developmental education in the community college. *ERIC Digest,* 1987.
7. Brenner P. From novice to expert. *American Journal of Nursing.* 1982;82:402-407.
8. Adult Education Resource Information Service. *Adult Learning. ARIS Information Sheet.* Melbourne, Australia: National Languages and Literacy Institute of Australia; September 1999.

PART VI

Administration

The topic of administration appears in this foundation level educator textbook for two major reasons. First, although many beginning instructors can focus on their craft without needing to deal with administrative issues, many others must tackle them because of the circumstances in which they operate, whether budgetary or resource dependent. Second, although great emergency medical services (EMS) providers often attribute their success to great instructors, great EMS educators depend on a well-administered, well-managed training program.

This part of the text provides information about the administrative issues that affect any EMS training program. Every educator need not be proficient in administrative issues; however, every educator should be familiar with them.

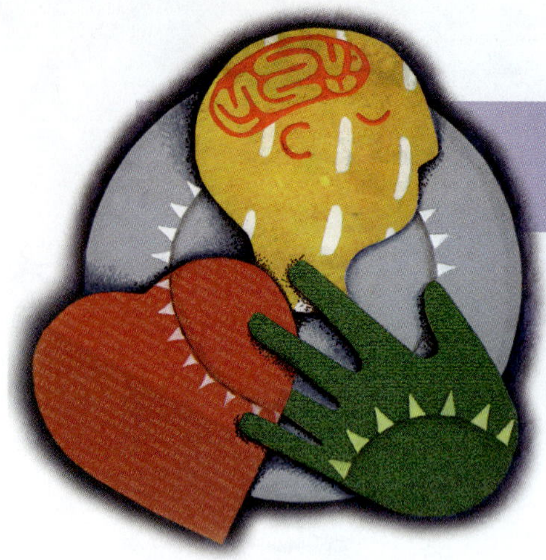

CHAPTER 23

Administrative Issues

"It is the mark of an educated mind to be able to entertain a thought without accepting it."

—*Aristotle*

It is no secret that most educators would rather be in the classroom with students than dealing with administrative "headaches." Although tending to administrative issues may be the primary responsibility of a course coordinator or program director, every educator has a role in administration of the course, from documenting attendance and enforcing conduct rules, to completing student evaluations. Additionally, every educator should have a basic understanding of, and appreciation for, all administrative tasks to maintain order and organization; to protect the institution, program, and faculty from liability; and to ensure fairness and consistency with students. Paying close attention to administrative policies and procedures can also promote the best possible educational experience for students and everyone else involved in the program. This chapter discusses both the general administrative matters common to most programs and issues about which the emergency medical services (EMS) instructor should be particularly aware.

FEDERAL LEVEL ADMINISTRATIVE ISSUES

The National Highway Traffic Safety Administration (NHTSA), a division of the US Department of Transportation (DOT), is currently recognized as the lead federal agency for the development of EMS. The Emergency Medical Services for Children (EMSC), a division of the Maternal and Child Health Bureau (MCHB) within the Department of Health Resources and Services Administration (HRSA), partners with NHTSA to support and promote many EMS activities.

Currently, the content of most EMS education programs in the United States is based on the National Standard Curriculum (NSC). The NSC has been developed for all nationally recognized levels of emergency medical technicians (EMTs) and consists of detailed objectives and course content outlines. Course curricula include First Responder, EMT-Basic, EMT-Intermediate, EMT-Paramedic, Emergency Medical Dispatcher (EMD), an Emergency Vehicle Operators Course (EVOC), and refresher programs for all previously mentioned EMT levels, as well as others. In addition, *Guidelines for Educating EMS Instructors* is a tool that has been developed by the National Association of Emergency Medical Services Educators (NAEMSE) with NHTSA and EMSC support. Other information regarding curricula and development of curricula is available to EMS instructors and program directors from NHTSA through its Web site at www.nhtsa.gov.

EMS Agenda for the Future was developed in 1995 and 1996 with funding from NHTSA and EMSC (Box 23-1, Box 23-2). The purpose of the document is to "predict the future by creating it."[1] This document is a strategic plan that needs assessment to be used as a blueprint for EMS in the 21st century. It serves as a guide for EMS providers, healthcare organizations and institutions, governmental agencies, and policy makers. Developed by a steering committee that represented a cross section of the EMS community, the *EMS Agenda* was extensively peer-reviewed by more than 500 organizations and individuals. A Blue Ribbon conference held in December of 1995 brought the EMS community together to finalize the vision for the future.

As a follow-up to the *EMS Agenda for the Future*, NHTSA and EMSC convened a task force in January

BOX 23-1 EMS Agenda for the Future: The Vision

The Vision

EMS in the future is envisioned as a community-based health management organization that is fully integrated into the larger healthcare system. It will have the ability to identify risk factors for the purposes of intervening and preventing illnesses and injuries, providing urgent or emergent episodic health care, providing transport and follow-up, and contributing to the management of chronic conditions and performance of community health monitoring. This new entity will be developed from redistribution of existing healthcare resources and will be integrated with other healthcare providers, public health entities, and public safety agencies. It will improve overall community health and will result in more appropriate and efficient use of healthcare resources. EMS will remain the public's emergency medical safety net but may have duties not traditionally associated with EMS.

To realize this vision, *EMS Agenda for the Future* proposed continued development of the following 14 EMS attributes:

- Integration of health services
- EMS research
- Public education
- Prevention
- Legislation and regulations
- System finance
- Human resources
- Medical direction
- Education systems
- Public access
- Communication systems
- Clinical care
- Information systems
- Evaluation

Reprinted from *Emergency Medical Services Agenda for the Future.* Washington, DC: US Department of Transportation, National Highway Traffic Safety Administration; August 1996.

BOX 23-2 EMS Agenda for the Future: Recommendations

Education Systems

- Ensure adequacy of EMS education programs
- Update education core content objectives frequently enough so that they reflect patient EMS healthcare needs
- Incorporate research, quality improvement, and management of learning objectives into higher-level EMS education
- Commission the development of national core contents to replace EMS program curricula
- Conduct EMS education with medical direction
- Seek accreditation for EMS educational programs
- Establish innovative and collaborative relationships between EMS education programs and academic institutions
- Acknowledge that EMS education is an academic achievement
- Develop bridging and transition programs
- Include EMS-related objectives in education for all healthcare professions

Reprinted from *Emergency Medical Services Agenda For The Future* (Washington, DC: US Department of Transportation, National Highway Traffic Safety Administration, August 1996).

of 1998 to discuss the EMS educational system and the scope of practice issues. Out of that task force, the *EMS Education Agenda for the Future: A Systems Approach* document was developed through the same extensive peer-reviewed process as was used for the original Agenda document. The *EMS Education Agenda* is a vision for the future of EMS education and a proposal on how to improve the structure of the system that will educate the next generation of EMS professionals. It builds on broad concepts from the 1996 *EMS Agenda* to outline steps to enhance the consistency, quality, and efficacy of EMS education, which will ultimately lead to increased competency among program graduates.

A task force representing the full range of professions involved in EMS education created the *Education Agenda*. The document proposed an education system with the following five integrated national EMS core components:

- Core content
- Scope of practice
- Education standards
- Education program accreditation
- Certification

The proposed system prescribes a high degree of structure, coordination, and interdependence among the five components. EMS, like many other allied health disciplines, will increasingly use a system that requires programs to be nationally accredited and that allows only graduates of these accredited programs to take national credentialing exams (Figure 23-1).

Both *Agenda* documents are important reading for anyone who wishes to attain credentials as an EMS instructor (Box 23-3). These documents may be obtained by contacting NHTSA, or by visiting the NHTSA Web site at http://www.nhtsa.dot.gov/people/injury/ems.

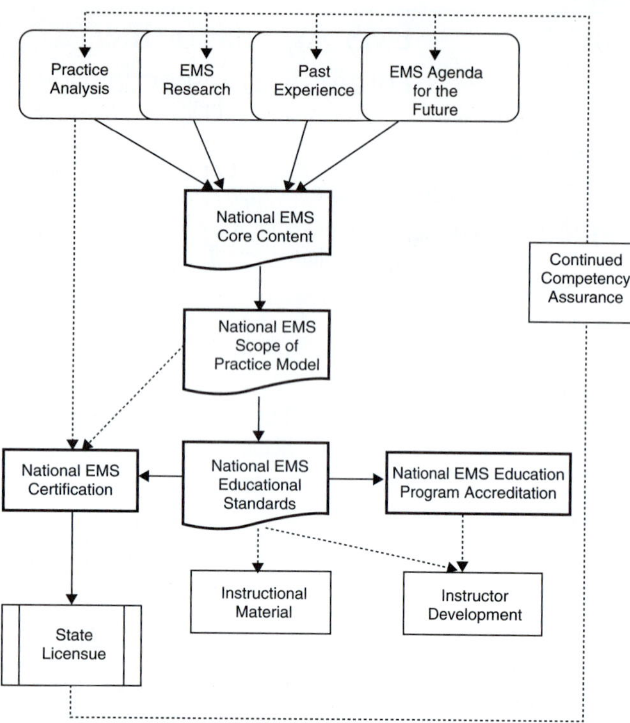

FIGURE 23-1 EMS education system components. (Reprinted from *Emergency Medical Services Education Agenda for the Future: A Systems Approach.* Washington, DC: US Department of Transportation, National Highway Traffic Safety Administration; January 1998:36.)

Accreditation

According to *The American Heritage Dictionary,* accreditation is "the act of accrediting or the state of being accredited, specifically, the granting of approval to an institution of learning by an official review board after the school has met specific requirements." In the United States, educational program accreditation is the most common way of judging the adequacy of an educational program or institution. In the context of education, accreditation is defined as a voluntary standard conferred by a nongovernmental organization. States, however, may require that educational institutions meet specific minimum regulations before beginning operations. This may include a mandate to become accredited. The states themselves do not accredit educational programs but rather approve the operation of institutions. Accreditation is by nature based on a structured self-appraisal that is overseen by professional peers—not by state regulators. In some states, institutions or programs may need state agency approval but may not be required to be accredited. The *EMS Agenda for the Future* advocates accreditation, and many states are actively moving in that direction.

The primary purpose of educational program accreditation is the protection afforded current and potential students when a program is evaluated according to specific standards and benchmarks. In addition, accreditation provides benefits for the program and the institution, for the healthcare community, and for society at large. Accreditation promotes the professionalism of emergency medical services as the profession itself identifies and achieves standards.

The program benefits from a comprehensive review based on the structured, self-study process mentioned previously, as well as a site visit and consultation with representatives of the accrediting body. These activities stimulate self-improvement, while assisting the program and its sponsoring institution with strategic planning, organizational development, and the allocation of resources.

Potential students can identify programs and institutions that have met established standards, a fact that likely provides reliable information, and are endowed with some assurance that their tuition will not be wasted. Although peer review does not guarantee quality, it is a reasonable indication that the educational program complies with commonly accepted practices. Accreditation also conveys a bonus that is important to the professionalization of EMS: credit for education is more easily transferable between academic institutions.

The healthcare community and EMS provider agencies benefit from the increased sophistication and flexibility that accredited programs offer. Likewise, the social good that flows from an accredited program is the assurance that a graduate is not only a "safe beginner" but also a provider who can quickly learn from experiences and adapt to an ever-changing clinical and operational environment.

Two types of accreditation can be provided: institutional and programmatic. Institutional accreditation addresses standards for the entire institution without making any judgment on specific programs of study within the institution (e.g., the Southern Association of Colleges and Schools [SACS] or the Western Association of Colleges and Schools [WACS]).

By contrast, programmatic accreditation, which may also be called *specialized accreditation,* pertains to a specific educational program, most typically one that is preparing students to practice for a particular occupation. These types of accrediting bodies apply standards for curriculum and profession-related specifics and may be associated with a professional organization. The only nationally recognized accreditation currently available for EMS education is provided through the Commission on Accreditation of Allied Health Education Programs (CAAHEP). CAAHEP has a special committee for EMS called the Committee on Accreditation of Emergency Medical Services Professions (CoAEMSP). It is one of 17 Committees on Accreditation of the Commission affiliated with CAAHEP. Before January 1, 2000, this committee was

BOX 23-3 EMS Education

The *Education Agenda* describes a future structure for our EMS education system and proposes a process by which this system will evolve. It is a vision that defines the EMS education system elements, describes their interrelationships, clarifies a decision-making process, establishes methods for input, and accommodates improved data and research. It defines a system which promotes national consistency and flexibility to allow for individual state variances, and facilitates rapid inclusion of innovative methods of patient care. The synergistic effects of the system are enormous; clearly, the whole is greater than the sum of its parts. The infrastructure laid out in this vision ensures a permanent, viable framework for national EMS education decision making and future planning. The shift toward this system will place new emphasis on educational quality and curriculum development, and on the performance of EMS instructors and educational facilities. However, instructor and program development are among the areas that receive the least attention in today's EMS educational system. To be successful in our implementation of the *Education Agenda,* we need to place a special focus on instructor and program development. This document was crafted with the expectation that quality EMS education will lead to superior EMS personnel, capable of providing the exceptional EMS care the public has come to expect and the EMS system was created to provide. The next steps in achieving this vision are to:

- Distribute this document to the appropriate stakeholders;
- Educate the stakeholders on the value of this vision;
- Seek stakeholder acknowledgment that the vision is shared;
- Begin development of the National EMS Core Content; and
- Establish a coordinating group consisting of representatives from major national EMS organizations charged with monitoring the implementation of the vision.

To guarantee the best EMS system in the future, we need to take action now. With this document, the EMS community is taking the first step, laying out a common goal that we can all work toward. This is a vision we can approach with confidence, knowing that it is the product of careful deliberation of our peers, technical experts, and leaders from across the range of EMS professions.

And while this vision reflects the best ideas from today's perspective, it is essential that as we follow this course we periodically assess our progress and ensure that our target continues to meet our collective needs. The basic concepts of system integration and instructional quality will stand the test of time, but we need flexibility in our means to these ends to allow for a changing environment.

Creating the vision was a challenging task, but the real work lies ahead. Implementing the vision will require commitment, determination, and persistence from EMS providers, educators, administrators, medical directors, and our public officials. But the rewards are compelling. We have the opportunity to achieve new levels of performance in our EMS systems and improve the quality of life of our patients and communities.

Reprinted from *Emergency Medical Services Education Agenda for the Future: A Systems Approach.* Washington, DC: US Department of Transportation, National Highway Traffic Safety Administration; January 1998:36.

called the Joint Review Committee on Accreditation of Education Programs for the EMT-Paramedic (JRCEMT-P). Other education programs accredited by CAAHEP include those for respiratory therapists, athletic trainers, medical assistants, medical illustrators, and other clinically related occupations.

At the time of this writing, the process of accreditation provided through the CoAEMSP is changing to include all levels of EMS education—not just paramedic education. EMT-Intermediate educational programs will soon have standards by which can they become accredited (Boxes 23-4 and 23-5).

Accredited paramedic programs also submit a program evaluation report, first with their initial self-study materials, then annually thereafter (Figure 23-2). This report is based on program outcomes and includes evaluation of program achievement toward their stated goal of graduating students who are competent in the three domains of learning: cognitive (knowledge), psychomotor (skills), and affective (behavior). These goals (which are sometimes called *benchmarks*) are evaluated through the use of internal and external tools such as graduate satisfaction surveys, employer satisfaction surveys, and credentialing exam success rates on both written and psychomotor skill tests. A report is created based on these and other measures that includes the analysis of data, a discussion of areas that need improvement, and the resulting plans for improvement. Each year, achievement of the objectives in each domain is revisited and continued attempts to improve the program are documented.

Accreditation also exists for EMS continuing education (CE) programs. The Continuing Education Coordinating Board of Emergency Medical Services (CECBEMS) accredits programs and institutions that offer EMS CE. CECBEMS accreditation is particularly useful because it makes it possible for students to earn CE at national or regional EMS conferences conducted outside the student's home state, or for students to

BOX 23-4 Standards for Accreditation

Standards for accreditation include the following:

1. Sponsorship
2. Program goals
3. Resources
   - Personnel
   - Program director
   - Medical director
   - Faculty
4. Curriculum
5. Resource assessment
6. Student and graduate evaluation/assessment
   - Student evaluation
   - Outcomes
7. Fair practices
   - Publications and disclosure
   - Lawful and nondiscriminatory practices
   - Safeguards
   - Student records
   - Substantive changes
   - Agreements

Source: www.CoAEMSP.org

BOX 23-5 Accreditation Process

- Self-study against established standards
- Written self-study document developed and sent to CoAEMSP
- Site visit to the program by site evaluators representing the accreditation body
- Written report provided to program by site evaluation team
- Program response and/or development of a plan for necessary improvements
- CoAEMSP review of program and recommendation to CAAHEP for accreditation
- Final decision of CAAHEP on accreditation

Source: www.CoAEMSP.org

obtain CE on the Internet. For more information on this type of accreditation, visit www.CECBMES.org.

National EMS Credentialing

The creation of a national scheme for EMS credentialing is another issue raised in the *Education Agenda* that has generated a good deal of discussion. For instance, there is considerable misunderstanding—and sometimes, broad disagreement—within the national EMS community regarding certification and licensure. This confusion has often begun in the legislative process of each state. Federal documents have provided some guidance on these issues but have not been followed by every state. According to the federal guidelines, a license is a document issued by a state government to a person who meets specific requirements established by state laws and regulations. Meeting those requirements grants the recipient the right to practice in a proscribed fashion within that state. Those who attempt to practice without license are subject to state sanction.

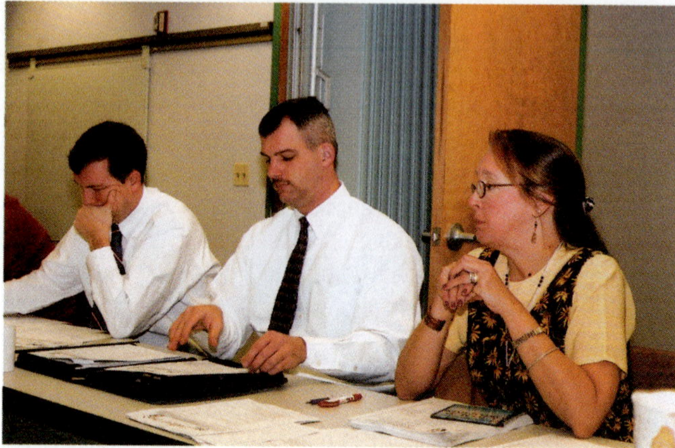

FIGURE 23-2 An accreditation site visit typically includes interviews with program officials, students, graduates, faculty, medical director, employers of graduates, and preceptors.

These same federal documents define certification as a document issued by a private agency based on a provider's meeting the prescribed standards of the agency, which are typically focused on entry level competency in a specialized field. The certificate is meant to convey the judgment that the individual who possesses it is competent and capable of performing the skill sets required for a particular occupation. Both licensure and certification carry specific legal responsibilities for the body that issues the credential.

The third credential used by EMS organizations is that of registration. A registry is simply a list of persons who have attained a defined professional status. In EMS, the National Registry of EMTs (NREMT, or "The Registry") is a listing of persons who have met the credentialing standards as determined by the NREMT Board of Directors, which has a long history of not only credentialing EMS providers but also supporting EMS since the establishment of the NREMT in 1970. Registration with the NREMT does not grant an individual the right to practice in any state. To work in a particular state, the EMT must possess a state-recognized or state-approved credential, in the form of either a license or certification, as defined within state law. The reciprocity that "The Registry" provides means that, in many cases, one needs only to present his or her NREMT card and pay a fee to the state EMS agency to receive a credential in that state.

The NREMT is also a recognized leader in providing valid and reliable EMS testing materials for states to use in their provider credentialing process. NREMT examinations and CE standards are based on an analysis of currently practicing EMS providers; examinations are authored by a multidisciplinary group of experts with input from various EMS-related organizations. These experts are also involved in the practice analysis used to develop and revise examinations for each level of provider identified in the National EMS Scope of Practice Model. Additionally, they are collecting information important to the professional development of EMS in their ongoing Longitudinal EMT Attributes and Demographics Study (LEADS). More information on this can be found at www.nremt.org.

Upon successful completion of the NREMT initial testing process, the applicant is granted a 2-year registration. At the time of this writing, nearly 40 state regulatory agencies currently use some form of the Registry's examinations in their credentialing process. This process may involve a single-level exam or the use of NREMT exams at all provider levels. In some states, CE and recertification or relicensure requirements are also managed through the biennial NREMT reregistration process.

STATE ADMINISTRATIVE ISSUES

As outlined previously, the governance of EMS is the responsibility of each state. Each state's laws or statutes and their attendant regulations or administrative rules contain specific directives regarding the education and training of EMS personnel. The location of each state's lead EMS agency varies, but it is typically found inside the Department of Public Health, the Department of Public Safety, or the Office of Emergency Management, or it is established as a separate state agency. The EMS agency is often organized into sections that usually include licensure and certification, training and education, trauma system development, data collection, disaster management, and ambulance service or other EMS responder authorization.

Each state should also have an EMS law or other enabling statute, which includes language delineating the following:

- Definitions
- Lead agency identification
- Establishment of oversight or regulatory councils or commissions
- Rule-making authority
- EMS responder types and program approval
- Education and training
- Certification and licensure renewal
- Disciplinary action
- EMS provider authority
- Prohibited acts

The lead agency is usually given the authority to develop, adopt, and periodically update rules and regulations that implement the relevant laws or statutes. The state legislature, however, is still responsible for ensuring that the intent of the statute is preserved. Time is generally allowed for input and feedback from all stakeholders who have an interest in the proposed changes in rules and regulations.

Each state has statutes unique to its jurisdiction; some are more prescriptive than others, and some delegate more responsibility to the state EMS agency or a local government office. In addition to the state EMS agency, frequently the Department of Education of each state has additional or similar laws, which regulate the establishment of educational institutions and the qualifications of instructors, including those who offer EMS education and training programs.

Regulations regarding EMS education are generally found within the administrative code chapter of each state, usually entitled, "EMS Provider Education, Training, and Certification." The EMS educator must be familiar with the state's rules and regulations regarding education and training and must be able to access the statutes when students request the information. It is also a good idea for the instructor to include copies of these documents, or instructions on how to access these documents, with the program orientation materials provided to students. In addition, many states require EMS instructors or course coordinators to have a particular kind of credential in that state so that they can give course lectures.

The information below is intended to be a guideline only. An instructor should contact the state EMS agency for information on and interpretation of a particular state's rules and regulations. A typical administrative rule or regulatory chapter outlining EMS education and training includes, but is not limited to, the following:

- Definitions of appropriate terms
- Enrollment requirements
- Certification standards
- Renewal of certification
- Fees
- Continuing education standards
- Endorsement/reciprocity
- Training program standards, application, inspection, and approval
    1. Approved curricula
    2. Clinical or field resources
    3. Facilities
    4. Staff
    5. Advisory committee
    6. Student records

7. Student selection
8. Financing and administration

- Complaints, investigations, and appeals

Also, some common characteristics are required within a state's educational program standards. The following are some examples:

1. Education programs typically must use, at a minimum, curricula approved by the state's lead agency. This may also include specialty curricula not available nationally. The curricula offered by NHTSA to train EMS personnel is not federally mandated; therefore, each state must decide what curriculum and possible enhancements or deletions must accompany EMS instruction
2. If clinical or field experience is obtained outside the structure of the educational program, then written agreements and/or state EMS agency approval must be obtained
3. Classroom, laboratory, and practice space, as well as a library with appropriate reference materials, must be adequate for student needs. Opportunities for the student to accomplish skill competencies in the field environment must be ensured
4. The educational program must have liability insurance and must offer liability insurance to students who are enrolled in the educational program
5. The educational program must have a physician medical director
6. Education program personnel, including program director, coordinator, and primary instructors, must be properly credentialed. This may involve state instructor or coordinator certification
7. Preceptors who supervise students in the hospital or field must be properly trained
8. An advisory council is essential for policy formation. An advisory group should include various stakeholders, including graduates and employers of graduates.
9. Individual student records must be maintained, including application, certifications currently held, transcripts of hours and performance, and documentation of clinical and field experiences (Figure 23-3)
10. The student selection process must be clearly outlined and followed
11. The educational program must supply information to each student at the beginning of each program, including the following:
    - Course objectives
    - Student handbook
    - Required hours or competencies
    - Minimum acceptable scores on testing
    - Attendance requirements
    - Disciplinary action that may be invoked
    - Grievance procedures
12. Practices that safeguard the health and well-being of students must be followed by each program

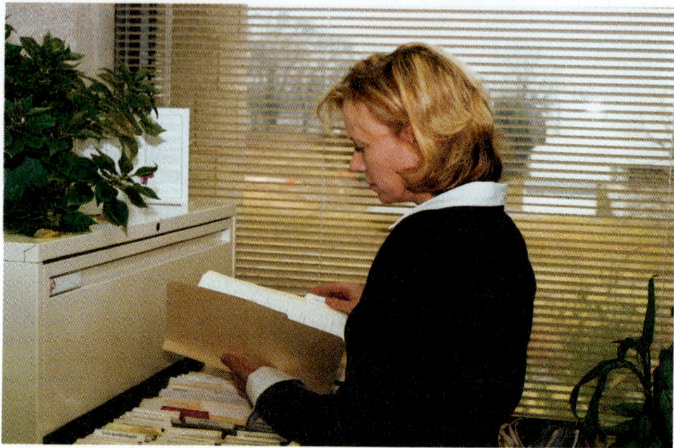

FIGURE 23-3 Maintenance of student records is important. A student's record should include his or her application, transcripts, documentation of achievement of objectives in all domains, and other relevant documentation.

LOCAL AND INSTITUTIONAL ISSUES

Admission Issues

Admission to an EMS program may be open to anyone with or without minimum criteria being in place. Some programs, particularly some at the paramedic level, require minimum reading, writing, and math assessment scores before admission, as recommended in the DOT EMT-paramedic NSC. This minimum requirement enables students to be admitted who have adequate basic learning skills; this enables students to concentrate on the paramedic material.

Some paramedic courses have a competitive admission process that gives higher standing for admission to those with high assessment scores, academic course credits, and EMS or other patient care experience. Regardless of the setting or type of admission process, clear criteria must be published and adhered to by the program. If a competitive admission process is used, prospective students should be told how to prepare academically and experientially to increase their chances of admission. In addition, the selection process should be fair and unbiased with objective and defendable criteria. Institutional policies and procedures should be closely followed and should be consistent with state laws and regulations.

Course Syllabus

The course syllabus is an important resource for guiding students and faculty and keeping them on the right educational path.[2] Educators should design clear, complete, updated documents that answer student's questions and prevent misunderstandings, complaints, and other problems.[3] Each student should receive his or her own copy of the syllabus at the first class meeting. Copies of these documents may also be available through electronic media and the Internet. Many programs and institutions of higher learning develop Web sites that archive these documents for quick access.

TEACHING TIP: A successful course begins with the first, crucial step of effective syllabus development.

The syllabus should contain certain course information and policies, including the following:

- Course title and description of course[4]
- Course objectives or learning outcomes
- Instructor(s) contact information and office hours
- Location of course meetings
- Days and hours the class meets
- Lab sessions and schedule
- Course calendar and/or schedule of topics
- Holidays or other dates when the class will not follow the established schedule
- Required texts and reading assignments
- Equipment or materials needed (e.g., stethoscope, penlight)
- Health and immunization requirements
- Grading scale
- Assignments and dates due
- Scheduled examination dates
- Attendance, tardiness, and class participation policies
- Explanation of final grade computation
- Statements/policies regarding academic dishonesty (e.g., cheating, plagiarism)
- Course drop dates and payment refund policy
- Policy on missed exams and late assignment submissions
- Grievance policy
- Instructional support services available
- Class rules, such as talking or eating in class
- Technology rules (e.g., beepers and cell phones off, no cell phones or PDAs on a student's person during exams)
- Classroom, lab, clinical, and field safety policies and procedures, including the emergent reporting and evaluation of body substance exposures
- Body substance isolation (BSI) methods and the proper use of personal protective equipment (PPE)

The syllabus is a contract between the instructor, who represents the institution, and the student. Consequently, the syllabus should be thoughtfully prepared, realistic, and changed as little as possible during the course. The student should sign a document acknowledging receipt of the syllabus, and that document should be retained in the student records.

Medical Director's Role in an EMS Program

The medical director is an essential component of an EMS educational program and can be a potent force for positive change in the classroom or in clinical and field settings (Figure 23-4). As has been mentioned, physician oversight is commonly required by the state EMS agency, and active participation of the medical director is required for the national accreditation of paramedic and EMT-Intermediate programs. As a practicing physician, the medical director can be a powerful advocate and therefore be instrumental in moving a program toward its organizational development goals; he or she can also be responsible for securing the financial and community support necessary to be successful. Too often, the medical director is not used to his or her full potential, and programs struggle to meet students' needs without the assistance of this important ally.

At a minimum, the medical director must do the following:

- Review and critique educational content and verify medical accuracy
- Review major examinations for accuracy and relevance
- Provide a measure of medical instruction, supervision, and evaluation of students, particularly in the clinical setting
- Monitor progress of students and the program

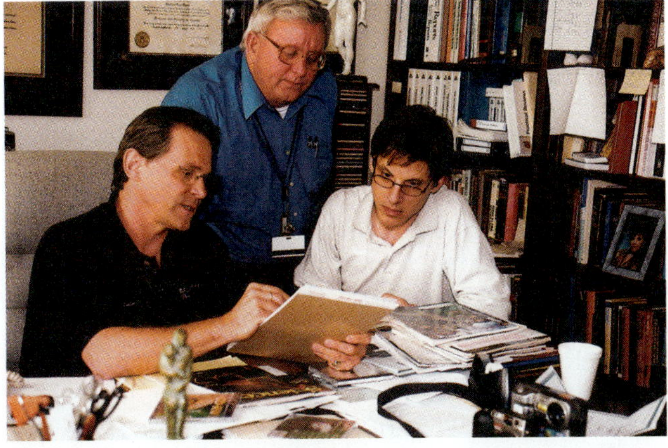

FIGURE 23-4 The medical director of an educational program should approve the medical accuracy of the course content and all examinations.

- Cooperate and collaborate with the program director
- Assume responsibility for the quality of the program and for delegated responsibilities
- Verify entry level competencies of students before graduation
- Understand EMS and have knowledge of the medical community
- Serve as an active advisory board member and facilitate interaction between the educational institution, the instructional staff, and community stakeholders[5]

For all these duties, and others that may arise during the course of the medical director's tenure, he or she may be considered for some degree of monetary compensation. Payment for serving as an EMS educational program medical director should be commensurate with the time and effort committed toward meeting the program's goals and objectives (Box 23-6).[5]

BOX 23-6 Position Paper

Medical Direction

Physician Medical Direction of Emergency Medical Services Education Programs

Approved by the ACEP Board of Directors January 1997

Reaffirmed October 2002 by the ACEP Board of Directors

As an adjunct to this policy statement, ACEP's Emergency Medical Services Committee developed a Policy Resource Education Paper (PREP) entitled, "Physician Medical Direction of EMS Education Programs."

The American College of Emergency Physicians (ACEP) and the National Association of EMS Physicians (NAEMSP) believe that changing technology, advances in research, and changing health care delivery systems require the active involvement of knowledgeable, identifiable, and responsible physician medical directors in the provision of emergency medical services (EMS) education programs, including initial and continuing education programs. The role of the physician medical director of an EMS education program is:

- To approve the medical and academic qualifications of the faculty, the accuracy of the medical content, and the accuracy and quality of medical instruction given by the faculty; to routinely review student performance and progress and attest that the students have achieved the desired level of competence prior to graduation; and
- To have a significant role in faculty selection and curriculum development, authority over presentation of medical content, and authority to assure that faculty teach established medical practices.

The physician medical director's qualifications should include:

- Knowledge of current EMS scope of practice and legislation relating to education programs
- Training and experience in emergency care delivery and medical direction of EMS systems
- Appropriate credentials attesting to experience in coordinating and teaching related education programs

Reprinted with permission from the American College of Emergency Physicians (ACEP) and the National Association of EMS Physicians (NAEMSP). *Physician Medical Direction of Emergency Medical Services Education Programs.*

Academic Dishonesty

Academic dishonesty is defined as a breach of the standards of academic integrity and typically includes cheating, plagiarism, collusion, falsifying academic records, and any act designed to give unfair advantage to the student. In many programs, the cost of academic dishonesty can be suspension or permanent expulsion from the institution. A failing grade may also be a consequence, along with a disciplinary record that may affect the student's future employment or educational opportunities.[7] A dishonest or incompetent student who becomes a dishonest or incompetent EMS practitioner produces unconscionable consequences.

Academic integrity and honesty are essential for all allied health providers who care for patients, and even more critical for EMS personnel. Of all allied health providers, EMS personnel, especially paramedics, most often care for patients who require the most urgent and invasive therapy available. Their independent knowledge and skills affect patient mortality and morbidity, and educators must be sure that these practitioners possess the knowledge, skills, and behaviors required to perform the job.

Although instructors may believe that cheating does not occur in the classes they teach, academic dishonesty should be a concern for every instructor in every educational setting. Those who would like to dismiss the concern should consider the following research by Donald McCabe from the Center of Academic Integrity:

- More than 75% of students on most campuses admit to some cheating. A 1999 survey of more than 2000 students on 21 campuses in the United States revealed that approximately one third of students admitted to serious cheating on tests. In addition, half the students admitted to at least one instance of serious cheating on written assignments (see http://www.academicintegrity.org/cai_research.asp)
- A 2000-2001 study of approximately 4500 students at 25 high schools revealed that 74% of respondents admitted to one or more instances of serious cheating[8]

Educators can and should take steps to minimize the likelihood of cheating in the classroom and in other settings. An understanding of how students may cheat helps instructors deter dishonest activities. The document, "Southwestern Allied Health Sciences School, Academic Dishonesty Recommendations, a Guide for Faculty," describes ways in which students may cheat and details how instructors can prevent various types of academic dishonesty (Box 23-7).

Institutional policies vary as to what an instructor should do when he or she suspects that academic dishonesty is occurring or has occurred. All instructors should be familiar with policies on confronting a student and taking up an exam. In general, when academic dishonesty is suspected, nothing should be done to prejudice the student's rights. Calling in a witness to the event is important.

Instructor Evaluation

The instructor plays a central role in the educational process. Therefore, the performance of the instructor, in any learning activity, is critical and must be considered when course and overall program performance are evaluated. Thus, every educational activity must provide a means by which instructor performance is evaluated.

Purpose of instructor evaluation

For a proper instructor evaluation to occur, it is imperative that the purpose of the evaluation be clearly defined and stated. Instructor evaluations fall into two broad but overlapping categories: evaluations done to evaluate and rate the performance of the instructor, and instructor evaluations obtained for the purpose of improving the instructional experience. It may seem that both approaches ultimately accomplish the same objective, that is, to improve the learning experience, and they ultimately do, but for different reasons.

Instructor performance evaluations

Almost all educational programs require some sort of official evaluation of instructor performance conducted on a regular basis. In institutions of higher education, such evaluations serve a number of purposes, such as forming the basis for contract renewal, pay increase, tenure review, accountability, or union contract requirements. Most evaluations follow an approved and standardized format and are conducted by a program director, chair, or dean.

In the case of EMS education, instructor evaluation is required by accrediting bodies and often by state regulatory agencies. This is especially true for educational programs that result in professional certification.

When conducting a performance evaluation, the assessor should do the following:

- Use a standardized form that has been institutionally or agency approved
- Provide a means for the instructor to acknowledge that the evaluation has occurred, most often by

BOX 23-7 Southwestern Allied Health Sciences School, Academic Dishonesty Recommendations—A Guide for Faculty

The Responsibility of the Faculty

Confronting academic dishonesty is the shared responsibility of faculty and students, although faculty members are called upon to play a leadership role. An attitude of intolerance by faculty can play an important role in its prevention. In keeping with a "no tolerance" policy, faculty members should add the following statement to their examination papers to be signed by all students: "I have neither given nor received assistance on this exam (paper, project, presentation, etc.)." Or, faculty may choose to have students hand-write the statement and sign it.

Ways in Which Students May Commit Scholastic Dishonesty

During examinations:

- Signaling to another student with coughs, hand signals, or other body language
- Concealing notes on hands, caps, or shoes, or in pockets
- Writing in blue books prior to an examination
- Writing information on boards or desks, or keeping notes on the floor
- Obtaining copies of a test in advance, without permission (e.g., during an earlier exam period offered by the faculty member)
- Passing examination information from an earlier class to a later class that day or week
- Leaving information in the restroom
- Exchanging exams after they have been distributed so that neighbors have identical test forms
- Changing a graded paper and requesting that it be regraded
- Failing to turn in a test and later suggesting that the faculty member has lost it
- Stealing another student's graded test paper and writing one's own name on it
- Recording two answers—one on the test form, one on the answer sheet

Continued

BOX 23-7 Southwestern Allied Health Sciences School, Academic Dishonesty Recommendations—A Guide for Faculty—cont'd

- Marking an answer sheet to enable another student to see the answer
- Transmitting answers for an exam to a student in a testing area via a pager
- Encircling two adjacent answers and claiming to have had the correct answer
- Stealing an exam for someone in another section or for placement in a test file
- Using a programmable calculator to store test information

On a paper, lab, or other type of assignment:

- Destroying or removing library materials to gain an academic advantage
- Obtaining reports or assignments from Web sites
- Fabricating data for lab assignments
- Failing to contribute as an equal partner in group assignments

General Tips for Combating Scholastic Dishonesty

1. Incorporate professional ethics content into program curricula and reemphasize on a regular basis
2. At the beginning of the program, use the UT System's standard scholastic dishonesty language from the Guidelines for Students and orient students to the information. Emphasis should be placed on the fact that scholastic dishonesty will not be tolerated

   Standard language: "Any student who commits an act of scholastic dishonesty is subject to discipline. Scholastic dishonesty includes but is not limited to cheating, plagiarism, collusion, the submission for credit of any work or materials that are attributable in whole or in part to another person, taking an examination for another person, any act designed to give unfair advantage to a student or the attempt to commit such acts" (Regents Rules Section III, 3.2)
3. At the beginning of each course, review scholastic dishonesty guidelines in course syllabi and reiterate the importance of honesty
4. Make a clear distinction, in front of the class, between group assignments and expectations of sole effort

Tips for Combating Scholastic Dishonesty During Examinations

1. Separate students and/or assign seats. Move a student who appears to be copying from another student to another seat
2. Distribute different test forms (or rearrange the order of test items) and inform students of that practice, particularly for large classes. Change tests each semester
3. Require that proctors remain in the testing room, and occasionally walk around the room throughout the testing period
4. Enforce silence during the testing period
5. Do not return exams for students to keep or to write down exam items
6. Check desks and the surrounding area for unauthorized materials, including textbooks and papers
7. Issue a blank piece of paper for students to use to cover their answer sheets
8. Require students to remove caps, hats, and sunglasses during the testing period
9. Use caution in allowing students to use programmable calculators
10. Provide clear directions concerning rules to follow for the examination period (e.g., whether the student can go to the restroom, whether the student can access anything from his or her backpack)
11. Collect pagers and cell phones

Tips for Combating Scholastic Dishonesty on Papers/Assignments

1. Provide clear directions on each paper/assignment concerning allowable collaboration or absolute independence
2. Do not use take-home exams
3. Assign paper subjects or assignments in such a way that the student is unlikely to be able to purchase assignments from a "paper mill" or find a relevant paper on the Internet
4. Be attentive to higher vocabulary or more journalistic than academic writing style and other clues that may flag a paper as inconsistent with the knowledge and style of the student writing it
5. Share with your colleagues Web sites offering papers for students
6. Have students write the following statement on each independent assignment: "I have neither given or received aid on this assignment."
7. Search the Internet by topics assigned so as to be familiar with offerings on the Net

Tips for Combating Scholastic Dishonesty on Clinical Assignments/Experiences

1. Thoroughly orient preceptors to student objectives and expectations
2. Have clinical faculty/preceptors sign off student assignments in clinical settings, including papers or logs
3. Have faculty present in the clinical area

Reprinted from University of Texas Southwestern Medical Center, Southwestern Allied Health Sciences.

signing the form. This acknowledges that the evaluation has taken place, but not that the instructor necessarily agrees with or accepts the findings of the evaluation

- Provide a time for consultation with the instructor after the evaluation has been completed, to discuss the findings and to identify strengths and weaknesses
- Provide the instructor with a copy of the evaluation
- Provide a means by which the instructor can refute evaluation findings in a formal manner. This is especially important when the evaluation has a direct effect on continued employment and promotion
- Consider using videotape during the evaluation as a means of recording instructor performance[10]

It is important to note that some institutions use student evaluations of the instructor for performance evaluation. This approach would seem reasonable given that the instructor's role is to assist students in meeting course objectives. However, such evaluations must be taken in the context of the course material, the instructional process, and the standards established by the instructor. The question to be constantly asked is whether the student evaluations reflect a true measure of the instructor's performance, or the personal feelings and whims of the students. A "hard" instructor may receive low marks because of the high standards he or she has established for the class, even though he or she is doing an effective job of teaching. Likewise, the nature, motivation, and ability of the students must be considered in any performance evaluation. Often, instructors teach entry level EMS courses to personnel who have other interests but are required to complete EMS training as part of their job training. Such students may express their frustration or lack of motivation through the instructor evaluation process.

Regardless of the purpose or nature of the performance evaluation, the institution or agency should have in place a support system for assisting instructional personnel. This applies not only to inadequate or marginal instructors, but to "good" instructors as well. A faculty development center or teaching laboratory can provide help in evaluating an instructor's classroom performance and in providing strategies for improvement.

Like any evaluation, the performance evaluation is merely a snapshot in time of the instructor's performance. Everyone has good and bad days, and some topics and subjects are taught better than others. To provide a more complete picture of an instructor's performance and teaching, a more comprehensive tool, such as a teaching portfolio, is needed. The teaching portfolio provides an opportunity for the instructor to present his or her "teaching life" in a complete and organized manner. A teaching portfolio should contain at least the following items:

- List of all courses taught over a particular time
- Syllabi of all past and present courses
- Past evaluations—both performance and student based
- Examples of innovative or creative teaching approaches or strategies developed by the instructor
- Examples of visual aids and teaching materials developed by the instructor
- Instruction-related continuing and advanced education completed by the instructor
- A statement of the instructor's teaching philosophy and what he or she expects to accomplish through teaching
- The instructor's future plans related to instruction and teaching

More information on teaching portfolios can be obtained through the Center for Teaching and Learning (CETaL) at the University of Texas at El Paso (see http://www.utep.edu/cetal/).[11]

Instructor course evaluation

The second type of instructor evaluation is conducted for the purpose of improving course delivery by the instructor. This evaluation usually occurs at the end of the course and is often completed by course participants. End-of-course instructor evaluations are often mandated by institutions and accreditation bodies. Feedback to the instructor is provided so that he or she may recognize strengths and areas for improvement or change. Some institutions use a two-part evaluation consisting of a standardized form that may be machine-readable and a second form that contains open-ended questions. The open-ended form is designed exclusively for feedback given directly to the instructor; the machine-readable form is used to rank instructors on an institution-wide basis and may be used as a performance evaluation.

The common practice of gathering course evaluations from participants at the end of the course has positive and negative aspects. Positive aspects include the following:

- Convenience—Participants are in class and have scheduled time to complete the evaluation
- Response rates are high because the participants are in class
- Students have the entire course perspective on which to base their evaluation
- Evaluations given after final participant course evaluation and results are anonymous, so students have no fear of retaliation by the instructor

However, some disadvantage to this approach should be considered, including the following:

- Participants may feel "forced" to complete an evaluation
- If the evaluation is the last thing to be completed before the student leaves, especially with 1-day

seminars, the participant may rush through the evaluation and not give it much thought

- Any positive feedback given to the instructor about the course is lost because the course has already been completed
- The participant may be "motivated" or "pumped-up" about the course, especially if it will result in a new certification with the expectation of being able to perform at a new level. This may cause the participant to have a positive bias toward the instructor and the course
- The participant may focus unduly on a recent negative or positive event in the course instead of on the whole course experience

Given the limitations of the traditional end-of-course evaluation, some instructors and institutions wait for a time after the course has been completed to send participants an evaluation. The main advantage to this approach is that students have had time to reflect on, and maybe even use, the knowledge and skills taught in the course. This gives them a better perspective on the true usefulness of the course in relation to their work and lives. The downside is that return rates may be poor in that participants can self-select to respond. In addition, responses may be slanted toward those participants who feel strongly, either positively or negatively, about some aspect of the course.[12]

If evaluation of the instructor is to be truly useful for course improvement, consideration should be given to conducting the evaluation during the course. This allows the instructor to receive feedback and make changes to improve student outcomes. A good time to give such evaluations is at midterm or after a major evaluation activity in the course. Conducting such evaluations also lets students know that the instructor values their input and is willing to make changes in their best interest. Instructor evaluation also sends the signal to students that the evaluation is not punitive and that they should provide constructive feedback. Depending on the course length, the instructor may provide multiple opportunities for student evaluation. Because such midcourse evaluations are often not "official," the instructor can tailor the evaluation to obtain the most feedback from students. If the sponsoring agency or institution requires an end-of-course evaluation, that too can be done as needed.

Course Evaluation

The process of course evaluation can be very extensive, involving a number of different evaluative dimensions. However, for the purposes of this book, a simple approach designed to help the individual instructor evaluate a course will be presented. It is important to recognize that individual course evaluation is just part of a larger scheme of evaluation that includes both instructor and program evaluation.

Evaluation of a course of instruction can be divided into two major approaches: formative and summative evaluations. Formative evaluation involves an ongoing evaluation designed to assess course effectiveness while the course is in progress. Ideally, formative evaluations will provide feedback on all aspects of the course, including instructional effectiveness and student performance. The formative evaluation can serve as verification that the stated goals and objectives are being attained, or as identification that they are not being met, so corrections can be made. A summative evaluation is a retrospective review of the course after it has been completed. Ideally, formative and summative evaluations should complement each other and provide a total evaluative picture of the course.

Another set of terms often associated with course and program evaluation is *outputs and outcomes.* Outputs are the statistical results of the course; they include measures such as number of students completing the course, student contact hours, tuition generated, and so forth. Outcomes are nebulous and difficult to measure directly. An outcome is designed to measure the impact of a course on a group or area. For instance, if a service conducts a training course on geriatric mental emergencies for its paramedics, the outcome that one would expect to see would be an improvement in the quality of care provided to geriatric patients with mental conditions and, ultimately, a decrease in negative outcomes as a result of these conditions. Although outcomes are important, they are often not used or required for evaluation of an individual course because they cannot be directly measured in most cases and effects take time to occur.

Paramount to performing any type of evaluation is deciding on the measures to be used in the evaluation. These should be decided during the course development process and not as an afterthought once the course has begun. Possible measures or sources of measurement include the following:

- *Course objectives.* This is the "gold standard" for evaluation because this measures whether or not the participant met each of the objective requirements for the course
- *Student completion rates.* The number of students successfully completing the course provides some indication as to the effectiveness of the course, provided a uniform standard for determining successful completion is applied
- *Comparison with other courses.* This will work only if the courses are identical, such as with a comparison of two EMT-B courses that are conducted to the same national standard
- *Certification/licensure rates.* If a course prepares the student for some level of certification or licensure, attainment of that certification level is a good measure of course success

- *Job placement and continued employment.* Are students who have completed a course able to obtain jobs and function effectively in that job?
- *Standardized testing.* The use of standardized tests or other evaluations given to students at the end of a course that compare them according to an established norm
- *Student satisfaction evaluations.* How did the student feel about the course and what was its value to them? Such surveys can be given at the conclusion of the course and followed up some time later, perhaps after the provider has been employed in the field for a specified time

Most of the evaluative strategies listed earlier provide a summative evaluation of the course in that they occur after the course has been completed. However, the conscientious instructor will want to make sure that the course is accomplishing its objectives while it is ongoing. If a problem is noted, it can be corrected to ensure a positive learning experience. Gagne and Briggs, in their book, *Principles of Instructional Design* (1979), list the following as examples of data that can be collected during a formative evaluation[13]:

From the observer:

- In what respects are (are not) the materials and media employed in the manner intended by the designer?
- In what respects does (does not) the teacher carry out the procedures and make the decisions intended?
- In what respect do (do not) the students follow the general procedures specified?

From the teacher:

- What practical difficulties are encountered in conducting the lessons?
- How would you estimate the degree of interest or absorption of students in the lesson?
- What difficulties were encountered in carrying out the intended teaching procedures?

From the student:

- How likely are you to choose to do the things you learned in this lesson?
- How likely are you to recommend this lesson to a friend?
- What are the results of a test of performance based on the lesson's objectives?

How the instructor goes about obtaining these data will depend on a number of factors, including course length, course type, number of students, and available time. Some possible approaches to evaluation include the following:

- Giving course evaluation questionnaire to students periodically
- Taking time out from class to discuss with students how the course is going
- Using standardized measures such as giving the same test to all sections of a course, or comparing results of previous course measures with those of the current course
- Using an outside observer of a course lesson as a resource
- Having a "neutral third party" visit with students alone and discuss the course(s)
- Asking students to list the pros and cons of the course anonymously

Regardless of the input received by the instructor through either a formative or a summative evaluation, the important thing is that the instructor must be prepared to render some judgment as to the course's worth. Boyle lists the following as program characteristics that should be considered when one is making a judgment about an educational course or program: quality, suitability, effectiveness, efficiency, and importance.[14] By using a combination of formative and summative evaluations, the instructor will be better able to evaluate a program in the many dimensions required to provide an effective learning experience.

SUMMARY

EMS educational program administration involves many facets. The program director must remain current on many issues, including national standards and curricula, national accreditation, national and state credentialing, and state standards and requirements for course oversight and administration. Local and institutional requirements must also be met so the integrity of the program can be maintained and the institution and its employees protected. Attention to administrative matters may become tedious at times, but it is essential for safeguarding the reputation of the program and its faculty and for raising the professional standards of EMS. Beyond the legal and ethical considerations, doing so will save the instructor and course coordinator many headaches in the long run and will enhance the quality of the program.

REFERENCES

1. US Department of Transportation. *Emergency Medical Services Agenda for the Future.* Washington DC: National Highway Traffic Safety Administration; August 1996.
2. Royse D. *Teaching Tips for College and University Instructors, A Practical Guide.* Boston: Allyn and Bacon; 2001.
3. Helms LR, Weiler K. Suing programs of nursing education. *Nursing Outlook.* 1991;39:158-161.
4. McCabe D, Drinan. *Toward a Culture of Academic Integrity. Chronicle of Higher Education.* October 15, 1999.
5. NAEMSE. Domain 3 from summer 2003.
6. NAEMSE. Domain 3 from summer 2003.
7. University of Texas Southwestern. *Medical Center Handbook of Operating Procedures.* University of Texas Southwestern; January 1998.
8. McCabe DL. CAI research. The Center for Academic Integrity, Duke University. Available at: http://www.academicintegrity.org/cai_research.asp

9. McCabe DL. CAI research. The Center for Academic Integrity, Duke University. Available at: http://www.academicintegrity.org/cai_research.asp
10. Steingold FS. *The Employer's Legal Handbook.* 3rd ed. Berkley, Calif: NOLO; 2000.
11. Center for Teaching and Learning (CETaL) at the University of Texas at El Paso. Available at: http://www.utep.edu/cetal/
12. Kerlinger FN. *Foundations of Behavior Research.* 2nd ed. New York: Holt, Rinehart, and Winston; 1973.
13. Gagne RM, Briggs LJ. *Principles of Instructional Design.* 2nd ed. New York: Holt, Rinehart, and Winston; 1979.
14. Boyle PG. *Planning Better Programs: The Adult Education Association Professional Development Series.* New York: McGraw-Hill.

Resources for the EMS Educator

Agency/Organization	Description	Contact Information
Professional Organizations		
AED Instructor Foundation	Instructor support and training materials for AED programs	Front & Main Streets Suite 911 Upland, PA 10915 610-872-7447 www.aedif.org
American Academy of Pediatrics	The mission of the American Academy of Pediatrics is to attain optimal physical, mental, and social health and well-being for all infants, children, adolescents, and young adults	National Headquarters 141 Northwest Point Boulevard Elk Grove Village, IL 60007 847-434-4000 www.aap.org
American Ambulance Association	Information on employability of EMTs, ambulance operations standards, and legislation regarding ambulance operations	1255 23rd Street NW Washington, DC 20037 202-452-8888 www.the-aaa.org
American College of Emergency Physicians	Position papers and current information on clinical topics regarding emergency and prehospital medicine	P.O. Box 61991 Dallas, TX 75261 214-550-0911 www.acep.org
American College of Osteopathic Emergency Physicians	Supports quality emergency medical care, promotes interests of osteopathic emergency physicians, supports development and implementation of osteopathic emergency medicine education, and advances the philosophy and practice of osteopathic medicine through a system of quality and cost-effective health care in a distinct, unified profession	142 East Ontario Street, Ste. 1250 Chicago, IL 60611 312-587-3709/800-521-3709 www.acoep.org
American College of Surgeons	Dedicated to improving the care of the surgical patient and to safeguarding standards of care in an optimal and ethical practice environment	633 North Saint Clair Street Chicago, IL 60611 312-302-5000 www.facs.org
American Heart Association	Current cardiac care standards and educational programs	7272 Greenville Avenue Dallas, TX 75231 www.heart.org

Agency/Organization	Description	Contact Information
American Public Health Association	Promotes the scientific and professional foundation of public health practice and policy, advocates the conditions for a healthy global society, emphasizes prevention, and enhances the ability of members to promote and protect environmental and community health	800 I Street NW Washington DC 20001 202-777-2742 www.apha.org
American Red Cross	The mission of the American Red Cross Disaster Services is to ensure nationwide disaster planning, preparedness, community disaster education, mitigation, and response that will provide the American people with quality services delivered in a uniform, consistent, and responsive manner	National Headquarters 2025 E Street, NW Washington, DC 20006 202-303-4498 www.redcross.org
Association of Standardized Patient Educators	Group devoted to simulated patient encounters	1 Crested Butte Dr Huntington, WV 25705 304-733-4562 www.aspeducators.org
The Brain Trauma Foundation	To improve the outcome of patients with traumatic brain injury (TBI) nationwide	523 East 72nd St 8th Floor New York, NY 10021 212-772-0608 www.braintrauma.org/
Citizen CPR Foundation	Community education and service programs	P.O. Box 15945-314 Lenexa, KS 66285 913-495-9816 www.citizencpr.org
Emergency Medical Services for Children	Clearinghouse for EMS-C products and publications	111 Michigan Avenue, NW Washington, DC 20010 202-884-4927 www.ems-c.org
Emergency Nurses Association	Legislative, clinical, and educational updates on emergency medical issues involving the nursing profession	915 Lee Street Des Plaines, IL 60816 www.ena.org
International Association of Fire Chiefs—Emergency Medical Services Program	Serves as the foremost advocate and spokesperson for the interests of fire-based EMS before the media, other EMS industry organizations, federal and state regulatory agencies, and the Congress. The EMS program communicates EMS news and developments on a national scale to IAFC membership. In addition, the EMS program serves as a liaison to the IAFC EMS Section, ensuring that the expertise of the section is reflected in EMS-related policies and initiatives of the IAFC	4025 Fair Ridge Drive, Ste. 300 Fairfax, VA 22033 703-273-0911 www.ichiefs.org/departments.ems
International Association of Fire Fighters	A valuable and comprehensive source of information and comments on issues concerning fire fighters, fire fighting, emergency medical services, and the fire service	1750 New York Ave, NW Washington, DC 20006 202-737-8484 www.iaff.org
International Fire Service Training Association	Educational materials specific to EMS in the fire service	930 North Willis Street Stillwater, OK 74078 www.iftsa.org

Agency/Organization	Description	Contact Information
National Association of EMS Educators	Professional development and educational support for EMS educators	Foster Plaza 6 681 Andersen Drive Pittsburgh, PA 15220 412-429-9550 www.naemse.org
National Association of EMT's	Professional development and support for career and volunteer EMTs and paramedics	408 Monroe Street Clinton, MS 39056 800-34-NAEMT www.naemt.org
National Association of EMS Physicians	Leadership in clinical, educational, and legislative issues in medicine	P.O. Box 15945-281 Lenexa, KS 66285 800-228-3677 www.naemsp.org
National Flight Paramedics Association	The largest independent paramedic association in the country. Our focus is the professional paramedic and our purpose is to serve as advocates for the profession on a national basis	383 F Street Salt Lake City, UT 84103 800-381-6372 www.flightparamedic.org
The National Council of State EMS Training Coordinators	Promotes the training of EMS personnel based on sound educational principles	201 Park Washington Court Falls Church, VA 22046-4513 703-538-1794 http://www.ncsemstc.org/
National Collegiate EMS Foundation	Support for EMS on college campuses	P.O. Box 113 Delmar, NY 12054-0113 208-728-7342 www.ncemsf.org
Prehospital Care Research Forum	Promotes, educates, and disseminates clinical and educational research for prehospital care	11303 W. Washington Blvd Suite 200 Los Angeles, CA 90066 310-572-2060 www.pcrf.mednet.ucla.edu
Society for Technology in Anesthesia	A diverse group of educators focused on using technology in medical education. The group sponsors the annual international meeting on medical stimulation	PMB 300, 223 N. Guadalupe Santa Fe, NM 87501 505-983-4923 www.anestech.org
Tactical EMS Association	Specialized training and equipment for tactical EMS	P.O. Box 504 Farmington, Michigan 48332-0504 248-476-9077 www.tems.org
US Medical Licensing Examination	This site has a wealth of information on clinical skills, examinations, and assessments, including links to research	3750 Market Street Philadelphia, PA 19104-3190 215-590-9700 www.usmle.org
Resources for Certification, Licensure, and Accreditation		
Commission on Accreditation of Allied Health Education Programs	Major accreditor of health science programs; parent organization to CoAEMSP	35 East Wacker Drive Suite 1970 Chicago, IL 60601 312-553-9355 www.caahep.org

Agency/Organization	Description	Contact Information
Committee on Accreditation of EMS Professions	Accrediting body for EMS educational programs	1248 Harwood Road Bedford, TX 76021 817-283-9403 www.coaemsp.org
Continuing Education Coordinating Board for EMS	Establishes guidelines and approves credit for continuing education programs	5111 Mill Run Road Dallas, TX 75244 972-387-2862 www.cecbems.com
National Association of State EMS Directors	Professional organization for state directors of EMS, liaisons to public health departments, administrators and developers of prehospital care policies	111 Park Place Falls Church, VA 22046 703-538-1799 www.nasemsd.org
National Council of State EMS Training Coordinators	Organization responsible for development of training standards and programs for prehospital care providers	201 Park Washington Court Falls Church, VA 22046-4513 703-538-1794 www.ncsemstc.org
National Registry of EMTs	Agency responsible for national testing standard and registration of EMTs and paramedics	6610 Busch Blvd PO Box 29233 Columbus, OH 43229 614-888-4484 www.nremt.org
Textbook Companies		
Brady Publishers	Publisher of EMS educational materials	One Lake Street Upper Saddle River, NJ 07458 800-638-0220 www.bradybooks.com
Channing L. Bete Company, Inc.	Offers an array of nationally acclaimed products and programs that focus on areas such as smoking prevention and cessation, substance abuse and violence prevention, and school success	One Community Place South Deerfield, MA 01373 413-665-7611 www.channing-bete.com
Delmar Learning	Delivers lifelong learning products and services to customers from age 16 to 60. Delmar Learning offers learning solutions for all points along a customer's career, from introductory course work to professional certification and continuing education	Thomson Learning—Customer Service 10650 Toebben Drive Independence, KY 41051 800-354-9706 www.delmarlearning.com
Jones and Bartlett Publishers	Publishers of EMS educational materials, including AAOS EMT, GEMS, and PEPP	40 Tall Pine Drive Sudbury, MA 01776 800-832-0034 www.EMSzone.com
Mosby Publishers	Publishers of educational materials for EMS	Elsevier Publisher Mosby Books 625 Walnut St. Philadelphia, PA 19106 800-523-1649 www.mosby.com www.uselseveierhealth.com

Agency/Organization	Description	Contact Information
Worldpoint ECC, Inc.	Publishers of American Heart Association educational materials	151 S. Pfingsten Road Suite E Deerfield, IL 60015 800-322-8350 www.worldpoint-ecc.com
Periodicals		
Annals of Emergency Medicine	Peer-reviewed journal of the American College of Emergency Physicians	National Headquarters 1125 Executive Circle Irving, TX 75038-2522 800-798-1822 www.acep.org
EMS Magazine	Periodical that includes clinical, legislative, and professional information for prehospital personnel	Summer Communications 7626 Densmore Avenue Van Nuys, CA 91406 800-224-4EMS www.emsmagazine.com
EMS Insider	Professional journal for EMS and ambulance service administrators	JEMS Communications 525 B Street Suite 1900 San Diego, CA 92101 800-266-5367 www.jems.com
EMS Village	The leading Internet application destination for individuals, services, and businesses that are members of the emergency and prehospital care community. Helps EMS professionals to improve individual and organizational performance	168 Twinbrook Terrace Monroe, CT 06468 800-503-7032 www.emsvillage.com
Journal of Emergency Medical Services	Periodical that includes clinical, legislative, and professional development information for prehospital personnel	JEMS Communications 525 B Street Suite 1900 San Diego, CA 92101 800-266-5367 www.jems.com
MERGINET	A virtual reading room where you can come to get the latest EMS news and information. Warehouses all kinds of information about EMS clinical care, administration and management, operations, professional development, products, technology, and trade associations	860-826-3708 www.merginet.com
Prehospital Emergency Care	Peer-reviewed journal of the National Association of EMS Physicians	210 South 13th Street Philadelphia, PA 19107 412-578-3245 www.elsevierhealth.com
Teaching Resources		
Agency for Healthcare Research and Quality	Evidence-based information on healthcare outcomes	540 Gaither Road Rockville, MD 20850 301-427-1364 www.ahcpr.gov

Agency/Organization	Description	Contact Information
American Medical Identifications, Inc.	Serves the medical community and the public at large by offering quality medical identification products that, in a medical emergency, allow medics or other medical personnel to administer aid in a more prompt and efficacious manner than might otherwise be possible	4001 N. Shepherd, Suite 100 Houston, TX 77018 800-363-5985 www.americanmedical-id.com
American Safety & Health Institute	Designed to deliver cost-effective instructional programs in the areas of first aid, CPR, workplace safety/disaster preparedness, child and babysitting safety, driving safety, aquatic training, and rescue and pet first aid, among others. ASHI successfully targets all areas of safety and health, helping to educate the lay public and emergency service professionals alike	4148 Louis Avenue Holiday, FL 34691 800-682-5067 www.ashinstitute.com
Boundtree Medical	Distributors of medical supplies and training equipment	Corporate Offices 6106 Bausch Road Galloway, OH 43119 800-533-0523 www.boundtree.com
CE Solutions	Online continuing education	888-447-1993 www.ems-ce.com
EmCert	A company dedicated to bringing you quality medical education through the Internet. The advisory board includes physicians who are board certified in anesthesiology, cardiology, emergency medicine, neurology, and trauma; EMS professionals; and registered nurses	P.O. Box 7510, Beaumont, TX 77726 1-877-EMS-HERO (1-877-367-4376) www.emcert.com
EMed Professional	Timely news articles on EMS in the United States	800-522-1018 www.emedprofessional.com
EMS Network	Search engine for EMS topics, research, and education	www.emsnetwork.org
ERIC database	Clearinghouse for educational research materials	1131 Shriver Lab Building 075 University of Maryland College Park, MD 20742 www.eric.ed.gov
FARMEDIC Training Inc.	To design, develop, implement, and evaluate training programs for emergency providers and agricultural workers to reduce mortality, injury, and property loss resulting from agricultural emergencies	Cornell University Ag Health & Safety Program 777 Warren Road Ithaca, NY 14850 607-255-5492 www.farmedic.com
Ferno	Is the leader in emergency response equipment and solutions, including cots, backboards, stair chairs, and a full range of emergency response tools	70 Weil Way Wilmington, OH 45177 800-733-3766 www.ferno.com
FISDAP	Your gateway into our unique paramedic student field internship and hospital clinical tracking cyber-software	2136 Ford Parkway #168 Saint Paul, MN 55116 651-690-9241 www.fisdap.com

Agency/Organization	Description	Contact Information
Gaumard Scientific Company	Your direct source for health care education needs	14700 SW 136 Street Miami, FL 33196 305-666-8548 www.gaumard.com
Healthcare Providers Service Organization	Providers of professional liability insurance for students and instructors	159 East County Line Road Hatboro, PA 19040 800-982-9491 www.hpso.com
Healthstream	Online continuing education	209 10th Avenue South Suite 450 Nashville, TN 37203 615-301-3100 www.healthstream.com
Human Anatomy Online	Comprehensive guide to human anatomy	1528 E. Missouri, Suite 100 Phoenix, AZ 85014 888-214-1415 602-230-0333 www.innerbody.com/htm/body.html
Image Perspectives	Moulage and simulation training and supplies	2650 Damon Road Carson City, NV 89701 775-882-6257 www.moulage.net
Laerdal	Manufacturers of medical training equipment, manikins	167 Meyers Corners Road Wappingers Falls, NY 12590 877-523-7325 www.laerdal.com
MD Choice CyberPatient Simulator	Online human patient simulation activities	908-203-5200 www.mdchoice.com/cyberpt/cyber.asp
Med-Eng Systems, Inc.	The world leader in the research, design, and manufacture of personal protective systems for explosive ordnance disposal (EOD, including chem/bio blast protection), Demining, crowd management, and body temperature control	2400 St. Laurent Blvd Ottawa, ON. K1G 6C4 Canada 613-739-9646 www.med-eng.com
Medical Devices International	A 25-year-old company committed to manufacturing only the highest-quality products. The market-leading CPR Microshield has become the most recognizable CPR barrier in the United States	3849 Swanson Court Gurnee, IL 60031 800-323-9035 www.cprmicroshield.com
Medic First Aid International, Inc.	A worldwide leader in CPR, first aid, and emergency care training programs for business, industry, and the general public	500 S. Danebo Ave. Eugene, Oregon 97402 541-344-7099 800-800-7099 www.medicfirstaid.com
Medtronic Physio-Control	Manufacturers of medical training equipment, cardiac monitors	11811 Willows Road NE P.O. Box 97006 Redmond, WA 98073 800-442-1142 www.physiocontrol.com

Agency/Organization	Description	Contact Information
Moore Medical Corp.	An Internet-enabled multichannel marketer and distributor of medical, surgical, and pharmaceutical products	P.O. Box 1500 New Britain, CT 06050 800-234-1464 www.2mooremedical.com
Nasco	Markets Life/form© training manikins and simulators that are ideal for EMT, ACLS, paramedic, and nursing training at every level	901 Janesville Avenue Ft. Atkinson, WI 53538 920-563-2446 www.enasco.com
National Association of EMS Educators Trading Post	The Web was seen as a perfect tool for this exchange of ideas and goods. The Trading Post is our first attempt at a "Swap Meet" of sorts. Only NAEMSE members can obtain (download) and contribute (upload) digitized educational resources	Foster Plaza 6 681 Andersen Drive Pittsburgh, PA 15220 www.naemse.org/members/trading_post.asp
Northern California Training Institute	The premier leader in paramedic education in California, and the largest institution of its type in the Western United States, providing education to more than 2500 students annually	333 Sunrise Ave, Suite 500 Roseville, CA 95661 916-960-6284 www.ncti-online.com_
PEPID, LLC	Help your students save time, reduce errors, and prepare for any emergency situation: tap into PEPID:EMS, the leader in PDA medical resources	8001 Lincoln Ave, Suite 725 Skokie, IL 60077 847-329-7744 www.pepid.com
Philips Medical Systems	Delivers one of the world's most robust portfolios of medical systems for faster and more accurate diagnosis and treatment	3000 Minuteman Road-MS 0395 Andover, MA 01810 978-659-2863 www.medical.philips.com/cms
Pulse Emergency Medical Update (Fire & Emergency Training Network)	Develops and delivers the training that empowers emergency personnel to react safely, swiftly, and capably. Quality training, education, and information that are delivered directly to your department	4101 International Parkway Carrollton, TX 75007 800-845-2443 www.pwpl.com/fire/pulse.asp
The RALE Repository	Respiratory sounds for training	208-3111 Portage Avenue Winnipeg, MB, R3K 0W4 Canada 204-885-4936 www.rale.ca
RxList Top 200	Search engine for drugs and pharmaceuticals	500 3rd Street, Suite 530 San Francisco, CA 94107 www.rxlist.com/top200.htm
Simulaids	Manufacturers of medical training equipment	P.O. Box 807 Woodstock, NY 12498 800-431-4310 www.simulaids.com
Zoll Medical	Manufacturers of medical training equipment, cardiac monitors	Worldwide Headquarters 269 Mill Road Chelmsboro, MA 01824 800-348-9011 www.zoll.com

Agency/Organization	Description	Contact Information
Federal EMS Resources		
Americans with Disabilities Act of 1992 (ADA)	Specific legislation prevents discrimination against mentally or physically challenged individuals	US Department of Justice 950 Pennsylvania Avenue, NW Civil Rights Division Disability Rights Section—NYAV Washington DC 20530 800-514-0301 http://www.ada.gov/
Center for Disease Control and Prevention	Protecting the health and safety of people—at home and abroad, providing credible information to enhance health decisions, and promoting health through strong partnerships	1600 Clifton Rd. Atlanta, GA 30333 404-639-3311 www.cdc.gov
The Federal Emergency Management Agency (FEMA)	Its mission is to lead America to prepare for, prevent, and respond to and recover from disasters	500 C Street, SW Washington DC 20472 202-566-1600 http://www.fema.gov
Maternal Child Health Bureau of the Health Resources and Services Administration (HRSA)	Information about Emergency Medical Services for Children (EMSC)	US Department of Health and Human Services Parklawn Building 5600 Fishers Lane Rockville, Maryland 20857 http://www.hrsa.gov
National Highway Traffic Safety Administration	Funding and distribution of national standard curricula and guidelines for EMT, paramedic, and EMS instructors	10 regional offices throughout the United States www.nhtsa.dot.gov
National Institutes of Health	Health information, current health events, grant and funding opportunities	9000 Rockville Pike Bethesda, MD 20892 301-496-4000 www.nih.gov
National Trauma Data Bank	Site operated by ACS; serves as a repository of trauma data	633 N. St. Clair 26th Floor Chicago, IL 60611 800-435-3590 www.facs.org/trauma/ntdb.html
Occupational Health and Safety Act (OSHA) of 1970	Regulates employment environments and practices to ensure health and safety of the nation's workforce	200 Constitution Avenue, NW Washington DC 20210 800-321-6742 http://www.osha.gov/
US Department of Health and Human Services	Community and family health initiatives, educational materials, and funding opportunities	200 Independence Avenue SW Washington, DC 20201 202-619-0257 www.hhs.gov
US National Library of Medicine	National library for medical research, documents, and books; MEDLINE search engine host	800 Rockville Pike Bethesda, MD 20894 301-496-6308 www.nlm.nih.gov

APPENDIX B

Correlation to Guidelines Matrix

This matrix cross-references the chapters of this book with the corresponding topic coverage in the modules of the "Guidelines for Educating EMS Educators" document.

Text Chapters	Guidelines for Educating EMS Educators Modules
1. Attributes of Effective Educators	1, 2, 5, 14, 15, 23
2. EMS Educator Roles	1, 2, 3
3. Principles of Adult Learning	7, 15
4. Learning Styles	7
5. Diversity	21
6. The Learning Environment	6, 11, 14, 19, 22
7. Domains of Learning	8, 16, 17, 18
8. Goals and Objectives	9
9. Lesson Plans	10
10. Legal Issues for the Educator	3, 4, 5, 19, 20
11. Audiovisual Basics	11, 22
12. Introduction to Teaching Strategies	11, 13, 14
13. Teaching in All Domains	16, 17, 18
14. Tools for Individual Learning	11, 16
15. Tools for Small Group Learning	11, 13
16. Tools for Large Group Learning	11, 13
17. Tools for Distance Learning	11
18. Tools for Field and Clinical Learning	17, 18
19. Principles of Evaluation of Student Performance	12, 14
20. Using Written Evaluation Tools	12
21. Other Evaluation Tools	12
22. Remediation	20
23. Administrative Issues	1, 3, 4, 22

APPENDIX C

Study and Test-Taking Skills for EMT Students

STUDY AND TEST-TAKING SKILLS FOR EMT STUDENTS*

Before the Test

1. If you have a history of not doing well on written examinations, you may suffer from a reading or learning disability. Professionals at the counseling center of a college or university can help you determine if this is the case. If you have a diagnosed learning disability, they can help you identify strategies to help compensate for it. Also, in some cases, certifying agencies will allow reasonable accommodations, such as increased time to take a test, if you have a documented learning disability.
2. Keep up with the course material. Try to schedule time to study every day. As part of your schedule allow some time each week to review all course content presented up to that point.
3. Try to identify and learn the major concepts before you learn the details. Understanding the major concepts gives you a structure to associate the details with.
4. Do NOT simply memorize the material. Take the time to understand why patients with specific problems present with specific signs and symptoms or why you manage particular problems in a specific way. If you understand the material and try to make it meaningful to yourself, you'll be able to remember and apply it more effectively and efficiently.
5. Schedule time for both personal and group study. When you study alone, you have a chance to go over material you are unsure of. When you study in a group, you can learn from your partners and help others.
6. Do NOT study and review with the goal of passing the test. Study and review to prepare yourself to be the best EMT you possibly can be. If you remain focused on this goal, you also will be able to pass the tests.
7. Get plenty of rest. Do not pull an "all nighter" just before a test.
8. Do NOT cram. Cramming tends to clutter your mind and lead to confusion. Also, material you study during a "cram" session will not be stored in your long-term memory where you can use it later. Study regularly and learn the material in small steps.
9. On the day of the test, dress comfortably. Wear layered clothing so you can add or remove clothing if the testing room is too hot or too cold.
10. Eat a low-fat, complex carbohydrate meal before coming to a test. Avoid over-eating or eating foods that may be hard to digest.
11. Avoid too much caffeine, which can affect your attention and concentration. Do NOT drink alcohol before a test. While you should NOT self-medicate, there are a number of medications your doctor can prescribe if you suffer from severe test anxiety that hampers your performance.
12. Try to arrive at the test site early. Running late will raise your anxiety. Also, by arriving early, you may have an opportunity to choose a seat in an area that is as free from distractions as possible. Avoid last-minute reviewing or quizzing with others. They can confuse you.
13. Use the restroom immediately before you go to the testing room. You don't want to be distracted or have to stop during the test if at all possible.
14. Try to relax. Sitting up straight, closing your eyes, and taking 5 slow, deep breaths are a simple, non-disruptive way of relaxing yourself.

During the Test

1. Read all the directions carefully before starting the test.
2. Read every question completely before attempting to answer it. Important background information may be contained in the sentences leading up to the actual question.
3. After reading the entire question, try to answer it without looking at the choices. Then look at the choices to see if your answer is the same as, or close to, one of the choices.
4. Read ALL of the choices. Even if the first choice seems to be the correct answer, read the other choices so you do not overlook a better choice.
5. Read carefully. Give all the words in the question and answer choices equal attention. A missed or misread word can mean the difference between a correct answer and an incorrect answer.
6. Look for key words or phrases in the question such as "first," "most important," "next," or "least."
7. Skip questions you don't know the answer to and come back to them later. If you answer all questions you know the answer to first, you will be reviewing the course material and forming associations that may help you answer questions whose answer you don't immediately remember. Also, a question further on in the test may contain information that will help you answer a question you are having difficulty with.
8. Be sure the number on the answer sheet corresponds to the number of the question you are answering. Check periodically to ensure the question number and answer number correspond.
9. Do NOT change an answer to a question unless you realize you marked the wrong spot on the answer sheet or misread the question. Your first choice will almost always be correct.

---

*From Nagell K, Coker N: *EMT-Basic review: A case-based approach.* St. Louis, 2005, Mosby.

10. If you are having difficulty with a question, read the question using each of the answer choices given. Reading the question and each answer choice together in their entirety allows you to focus on choices that make sense logically and grammatically.
11. Remember the fundamentals. In most cases, confirming scene safety, ensuring an open airway, ensuring adequate oxygenation and ventilation, and correcting life-threatening problems take precedence. Look for answers that deal with these aspects of patient management.
12. If you do not immediately know the correct answer, eliminate any choice you are sure is incorrect before you make a guess.
13. Be wary of answers that contain words or information you have never heard of before, even if they seem to be plausible choices. If it wasn't mentioned in lecture or in your textbook, it's probably NOT correct.
14. Base your answers on the material presented in lecture or in your textbook. Do NOT rely on personal experience or the experiences of EMS personnel you may know.
15. Know how the test will be scored. If no penalty is applied for guessing, answer EVERY question. However, to discourage guessing, some tests are scored with a system that applies a penalty for each incorrect response. For example, a correct response is worth 1 point, an unanswered question is worth 0 points, and an incorrect response is worth –0.25 points. On this type of test it is better to leave questions unanswered unless you are very sure of the correct response.
16. Use all of the allotted time. You are being tested on your knowledge, NOT on the speed with which you can take a test.
17. Use any time remaining near the end of the exam to be sure you marked the correct spots on your answer sheet. But do NOT change an answer unless you know you marked the answer sheet incorrectly or you discover you misread an question. Your first choice will almost always be correct.

Choosing the "Best" Answer for a Question

Multiple choice test items usually consist of a "stem" (a question or incomplete statement) followed by 3 to 5 "responses." One of these responses, the "keyed response" is the correct answer. The other responses are called "distractors" because they are designed to distract you from selecting the keyed response as your answer. Distractors are designed to seem right without being the best answer to the question. The following tips may help you eliminate distractors and identify the best response to a question.

1. The best response to a question may not be the perfect response. It is just the best choice among those presented for the question.
2. If the responses to a question consist of a series of steps in a procedure, the correct answer will be the series that is most complete and in the correct order.
3. If two or more responses seem to be correct, be sure all of them relate directly to the question. A common strategy used by test writers to develop distractors is to include statements that are correct but that are not related to the question. For example, a question related to management of airway and breathing might include a true statement about management of circulation as a distractor. Although the statement might be true, it doest not relate to the question, so it is not the best choice.
4. If two or more responses seem correct, look for one that is more specific. For example, a medical-legal question might present a scenario in which you knowingly write information in a patient care report that is not true and that damages the patient's reputation. You might then be asked what you could be sued for and presented with choices that include "slander," "libel," "defamation of character," and "an intentional tort." The best choice is libel. Although both slander and libel are legally classified as defamation of character, which in turn is an intentional tort, libel is the most specific response to this question.
5. If three responses seem correct, look for one that includes the other two. For example, you might be asked what kinds of ingestions administration of activated charcoal is inappropriate for. The answers might include "aspirin," "alkalis," "acids," and "corrosive substances." Aspirin clearly is NOT a correct response. Alkalis and acids both appear to be correct. However, the choice "corrosives" includes both acids and alkalis. Therefore, it is the best response.

Glossary

360-Degree evaluation: Evaluation by superiors, subordinates, and peers. Used in the educational setting to refer to evaluation of a student by other students.

Adobe Acrobat Reader: A software program for creating and viewing Portable Document Files. The file can be distributed electronically and enables the document to be viewed exactly as the author intended.

affective domain: Describes learning in terms of feelings/emotions, attitudes, and values.

alternate form reliability: Form equivalence.

analytic learner: Logical thinker who tends to process information logically, sequentially, and in small parts, building toward the whole.

anecdotal records: An evaluation instrument used in the clinical setting on which the examiner can make free-form notes regarding a student's performance when the observation is not clearly covered by other records.

Angoff method: A system used to determine the cut score, consisting of an expert panel that predicts the difficulty level of examination items.

assumption of risk: Doctrine indicating that a person who is participating in an activity and is known to have an inherent risk is barred from recovering damages, because that person willingly assumed the risks involved.

asynchronous learning: Learning that is done independently and without direct contact with the teacher.

attribution: The cause or reason a student fails an evaluation.

audiovisual: Of or relating to both hearing and sight; items and equipment used to transit messages for hearing and/or sight.

auditory learner: A person who uses predominantly the sense of hearing to learn.

behavioral anchor: A description of observable behaviors linked to specific ratings in an evaluation.

"bias cueing" Clues within the wording of a limited response exam item that lead the student to the correct response, without knowledge of the subject. Examples include plural/singular agreement and/or grammatical clues.

bias: Unjustified negative feeling(s).

blackboard: A hard, smooth, usually dark surface used especially in the classroom for writing or drawing on with chalk.

blueprint: A test plan describing the percentage of test questions allotted to each content area and the level of thinking required for successful completion.

breach of contract: Failure to comply with contractual terms into which an individual or party has entered.

camera: A device that consists of a lightproof chamber with an aperture fitted with a lens and a shutter through which the image of an object is projected onto a surface for recording (as on film) or for translation into electrical impulses (as for television broadcast).

CD-ROM (compact disk read-only memory): A computer disk that can hold many times the data of a floppy disk.

chat room: An Internet site where the user logs in to communicate with other Internet users, usually in real time. Many LMSs offer this feature.

cognitive domain: Describes learning that takes place through the process of thinking—it deals with facts and knowledge.

collaborative learning: An instructional method in which a small group of students work together toward a common goal.

computer: A programmable device that can store, retrieve, and process data.

conceptual map: An outline of the course that identifies how all sections fit together to make the whole.

content validity: The degree to which the content of an examination is an accurate, representative sample of the wider body of knowledge that the examination purports to assess.

contributory negligence: Plaintiff's behavior or action fell below the acceptable standard that should have been met for self-protection and is a contributing cause to the injury.

covered entity: Healthcare providers who transmit patients' protected health information, insurance providers, and other medical facilities (as defined in HIPAA).

criterion validity: The degree to which an examination can accurately predict performance of a specific aspect of performance that is typically much more difficult to directly assess. Also known as *predictive validity*.

criterion variable: Refers to an aspect of predictive validity; the criterion variable is the measurement that is being predicted through variation of the predictor variable. In research terms, this would be referred to as the *dependent variable*. The criterion variable is indirectly assessed through examination of the predictor variable.

criterion-referenced grading: Grading strategies that assign grades according to a student's performance relative to an objective standard, such as mastery of the course objectives.

critical incident form: An evaluation instrument used in the clinical setting that provides a list of characteristics with space on which the examiner can make comments regarding observations that apply to a given characteristic. Distinguished from observation logs in that observation logs typically have clear linkage to course objectives, while critical incident forms do not.

cultural competency: Degree to which one is aware of and knowledgeable about the cultures in his/her social setting; this is not an *all or nothing* condition, it is instead a continuum from very little to very much.

cultural disconnects: Occasions on which one's action or lack thereof displays ignorance about a particular culture (usually resulting in an uncomfortable situation).

culture: General term describing a group with commonalities, including social customs, religious practices, and language.

curriculum-based evaluation: An evaluation based on the objectives of an educational program.

cut score: The minimum passing grade for an examination.

declarative material: Component of the lesson plan that contains the "meat," or content, of the lesson. This material should provide guidance for the instructor and should address the depth and breadth of content as described by the verbs used in the lesson objectives.

defamation: False statement that damage a person's reputation.

defendant: The party against whom charges are brought by a plaintiff.

didactic: The instructional theory, the lesson content.

difficulty index: The percentage of students who correctly answer an examination item.

digital: Relating to an audio recording method in which sound waves are represented digitally (as on magnetic tape) so that in the recording, wow and flutter are eliminated and background noise is reduced.

distracter: Incorrect potential student responses offered with multiple-choice items.

diversity: Degree of difference within an identified population, including physical, psychological, ideologic, and sociologic characteristics.

DLP projector (digital light projector): High-end projector most commonly used for very large-screen and large-room applications; has extremely high light output (up to 15,000 lumens) and high scan output.

document sharing: A feature that allows a group of users to view and write on the same document by enabling a control button.

domain: A category of learning. *See* Affective domain, Cognitive domain, and Psychomotor domain.

DVD (digital videodisk): Type of CD-ROM that holds a minimum of 4.7 gigabytes.

easel: A frame for supporting something (such as a flip chart).

elements: Components of the strands of a learning style inventory.

E-mail: Electronic mail.

enabling objectives: One of several strategies for describing goals and objectives. With this strategy, the enabling objective, upon successful completion, "enables" the goal to be met.

***et seq.*:** And following.

ethnic minority: All non-White (or Euro-American) racial groups within the context of the US population.

ethnocentrism: A worldview that focuses on a particular ethnicity or race (usually that of the person).

face validity: A "commonsense" assessment of validity performed by one or two people who review the item and assess appropriateness. Not scientific.

flip chart/posterboard: Paper pad supported on an easel.

form equivalence: The ability of different forms of evaluation to produce consistent results. It is used to test reliability. Also known as *alternate form reliability*.

formative evaluation: An evaluation conducted primarily to provide the feedback needed to modify learning and instructional strategies.

fraud: Same as misrepresentation.

global learner: Learner who thinks in terms of the big picture and needs to see the whole before the parts.

global performance rating: A performance evaluation tool that provides a characteristic linked to a rating scale. Typically used in the clinical and internship settings.

goal: Overarching statement of intended learning that states the expected outcome but does not generally provide the measurement criteria.

Health Occupations Basic Entrance Test (HOBET): A diagnostic test used to assess an applicant's academic and social skill preparation for health-related education.

high-fidelity simulations: Simulations that provide very realistic portrayals of patients and emergency scenes. Usually refers to simulations that allow the student to actually perform invasive skills on a realistic manikin.

high-speed Internet connection: Internet connection that enables fast downloading of files or programs.

high-stakes evaluation: An evaluation with major impact on student grade or passing of the educational program.

***in loco parentis*:** In place of the parents.

independent learner: A learner who prefers to learn alone as opposed to working in a group.

infra-: Below.

instructional design: The model that determines how instruction will be delivered, the sequence of delivery, and how the objectives for learning will be achieved. Instructional design includes the instructor's choice of teaching methods to ensure that each of the domains of learning is used in the lesson. It may involve video clips, print, or computer conferencing.

instructor-centered learning: The instructor is in control of the learning process.

intelligences: Basic components of the multiple intelligences concept.

Internet: A transglobal computer network that allows persons and institutions to exchange information via telephone wires, cable, and satellite links.

interrater reliability: The ability to produce consistent results with different people grading the examination.

item discrimination: The degree to which a question distinguishes between students who know the material well and those who do not know the material well.

Java script: Computer programming language for creating scripts that add functions to Web pages. It contains a large number of tasks that enable key tasks to be carried out at one time, thus speeding up programming times.

JPEG (joint pictures expert group): Digital picture format.

key: The correct potential student response offered with multiple-choice items.

key informants: Persons identified as influential members of a community who can provide insights about that group.

kinesthetic learner: A person who learns best with his or her body, as when movement and physical activity are incorporated as part of the learning experience.

lavaliere microphone: A small microphone that is clipped onto clothing to allow a speaker to move around while presenting.

LCD projector (liquid crystal display): Used to project presentations from a computer, DVD, VCR, or digital HDTV signal; forms images by shining (or transmitting) light through one or three LCD panels, which are built into the projector; produces bright, high-resolution images.

Learning Management System: A program that provides a range of functions required to deliver instructional material and to manage administrative matters associated with educational courses.

learning style: The sensory and contextual preference used by a learner to receive and process information.

learning style inventory: A test designed to assess one's learning style.

lectern microphone: A microphone attached directly to a lectern on a flexible metal gooseneck for adjusting.

libel: Written or printed defamation.

Likert scale: A numeric rating used to quantify otherwise qualitative aspects of statement.

litigation: Lawsuit.

low-stakes evaluation: An evaluation with minor (or no) impact on grade.

lumen: A unit of luminous flux equal to the light emitted in a unit solid angle by a uniform point source of one candle intensity.

message board: A feature on a Web site that allows visitors to post a message, which is then seen by other visitors who in turn can post a contribution.

microphone: An instrument through which sound waves are caused to generate or modulate an electric current, usually for the purpose of transmitting or recording sound.

misrepresentation: False statements.

moulage: Simulation of injuries by the use of makeup.

multiracial: An ethnic identity increasingly used to acknowledge a diverse racial/ethnic background.

Myers-Briggs Type Indicator: A test designed to determine a person's personality type.

negligence: The failure to exercise the standard of care that a reasonably prudent person would have exercised in a similar situation.

norm-referenced grading (normative): Grading strategies that assign grades according to a student's performance relative to the performance of other students. Commonly known as "grading on the curve."

objective: Subcomponent that follows a goal. The objective articulates the intended audience, expected behavior, measurement tool or criteria, and any conditions imposed upon the performance of the behavior.

observation log: An evaluation instrument used in the clinical setting that lists objectives with space for the examiner to make comments as to observations that apply to a given objective.

outcome: A measurement of the impact of a course on a group or area, based on changes in results.

output: The statistical measures of course results, including number of students completing the course.

overhead projector: Audiovisual equipment designed to project and magnify an image from a transparent sheet and acetate.

pedagogy: Principles, practice, or profession of teaching.

performance agreement: A process of evaluation used during several stages of instruction. It is used to confirm the strengths of the interrelationships between components. Examples include goals compared with objectives, instructional content compared with goals and objectives, and the material delivered to students compared with expected material described in the lesson plan. Performance agreement evaluations can take many forms and should be performed in both directions (i.e., goals should be compared with objectives, then objectives should be compared with goals). This process should identify areas of weakness or non-agreement, which can then be addressed.

performance checklist: A list of component steps of a skills, used as an evaluation instrument for psychomotor skills in practical examinations and in the applied care setting.

PHI: Protected health information as defined in HIPAA.

pixel: Any of the small discrete elements that together constitute an image.

plaintiff: The party bringing a complaint against the defendant.

portfolio project: Project that provides a collection of the student's work, usually in a variety of formats for evaluation.

practice analysis: A formal assessment of the skills and competencies needed to perform a role or skill, conducted by survey or observation of actual performance of the task by providers in context.

preceptor: An instructor who teaches and evaluates performance in the applied care setting.

predictive validity: *See* criterion validity.

predictor variable: Refers to an aspect of predictive validity; the predictor variable is the measurement that is being directly assessed, along with analysis made of the impact on the criterion variable. In research terms, this would be referred to as the *independent variable*.

***prima facie*:** Evidence that is strong enough in favor of the plaintiff that a defendant may be required to respond to charges.

primary instructor: A person who possesses the appropriate academic and/or allied health credentials, an understanding of the principles and theories of education, and the required teaching experience necessary to provide quality instruction to students.

proctor: An instructor who supervises a written examination.

proctored exams: Exams supervised by a person who has been delegated the responsibility by the educational organization.

programmed patient: An actor trained to simulate a patient's reactions during a situational assessment.

projector screen: Surface on which images are displayed.

psychometrician: A specialist in the measurement of knowledge gathered from written examinations.

psychomotor domain: Describes learning that takes place through the attainment of skills and bodily, or kinesthetic, movements.

qualitative: A qualitative measure describes the expected standard or character. Qualitative measures speak to dimensions of quality that cannot easily be scored. For example, a student may be required to perform skills with a pleasant demeanor and to demonstrate professionalism and customer service. Such affective traits are difficult to quantify, but lack of these traits can be observed.

quantitative: A quantitative measure provides a numeric score that may be used to conduct an evaluation. For example, a skills check-off sheet will include points that are awarded to the student as the student performs the step.

QuickTime: A multimedia program; it allows sound and video to be embedded in Web pages. It also supports videoconferencing.

RealPlayer: A multimedia player and browser plug-in.

regression analysis: A mathematical test of the strength of the relationship between two variables.

release of risk: An agreement in which a person relinquishes claim, duty, or obligation against another part.

reliability: The trait of an examination that is able to produce consistent results with minimal impact of measurement error.

remediation: The process of analysis and identification of deficits (or problems) and the creation of a plan for retraining and/or improving performance.

resolution: The amount of detail the projector can capture.

risk control: Method of risk management conducted by alleviating potential liability in the classroom by eliminating or reducing the risk of harm.

risk management: Process of preventing, or at least minimizing, physical or material harm or loss to a school, program, instructor, or student.

risk transfer: Method of risk management conducted by transferring liability to another party, such as with waivers, releases, and insurance.

rubric: An evaluation instrument that converts a vaguely worded characteristic to a list of observable behaviors that can be scored.

schema: A mental plan used by a person to organize and respond to a stimulus.

secondary instructor: A person who possesses the appropriate academic and/or allied health credentials and an understanding of the principles and theories of education, and who may have *limited* teaching experience.

self-direction: In adulthood, a process in which the learner assumes primary control of what he or she desires to learn.

senses: The five physical senses of sight, hearing, touch, taste, and smell.

situational assessment: Type of practical examination that tests practical skills in context; useful for evaluating high levels of psychomotor domain.

skill evaluation: Type of practical examination that tests rote practical skills without context; useful for evaluating mid levels of the psychomotor domain.

slander: Spoken or oral defamation.

slide projector: Equipment designed to project the image of a slide onto a viewing screen.

social learner: A learner who prefers to learn in a group or in the company of other people.

split-half test: A test of internal consistency of an examination completed by comparing different items within that examination that test the same content. It is a method of testing reliability.

standardized patient: An actor trained to simulate a patient's reactions during a situational assessment.

statute: A law.

stem: The first part of a limited response examination item.

stereotype: A generalization of a particular group, commonly accenting characteristics that are unflattering and/or unfounded.

stimuli: The five dimensions of a learning inventory.

student-centered learning: The onus for learning lies with the student; the student controls the learning process; the student decides how, when, and what is to be learned.

summative evaluation: An evaluation conducted primarily to verify mastery of the content of an educational program by the student.

supra-: Above.

SXGA (super-extended graphics adapter): The display resolution of a computer.

synchronous learning: Students and instructor come together at a specific Web site to discuss course material at a scheduled time.

task analysis: A detailed list of component steps necessary for performance of a skill. Used to construct performance checklists.

teleconference equipment: Two-way voice communication between several people using telephones.

teleconferencing: The holding of a conference among people remote from one another by means of telecommunication devices (such as telephones or computer terminals).

terminal objectives: One of several ways of describing goals and objectives. In this strategy, another level is placed between a goal and an objective. This level is called a *terminal objective*. Objectives that are related are grouped together under a terminal objective. Several related terminal objectives are then grouped together under a goal.

tort: A wrong or injury.

transcultural: Reaching across the boundaries from one culture into another.

U.S.C.: US Code.

validity: The ability of an examination to actually measure what it purports to measure.

VCR: Videocassette recorder.

videoconferencing: The holding of a conference among people at remote locations by means of transmitted audio and video signals.

virtual classroom: The Internet classroom.

visual learner: A learner who predominantly uses the sense of sight to learn.

whiteboarding: A feature of videoconferencing systems that allows the placement of documents on an on-screen shared space or "whiteboard"; participants can edit and mark up the document just as on a physical whiteboard.

whiteboard utility: A feature of some Learning Management Systems. It allows one or more users to draw on the screen while others on the network watch. It can be used for instruction in the same way that a blackboard is used in a classroom.

XGA (extended graphics adapter): Display resolution of a computer.

Index

Note: Page numbers followed by f indicate figures; t, tables; b, boxes.